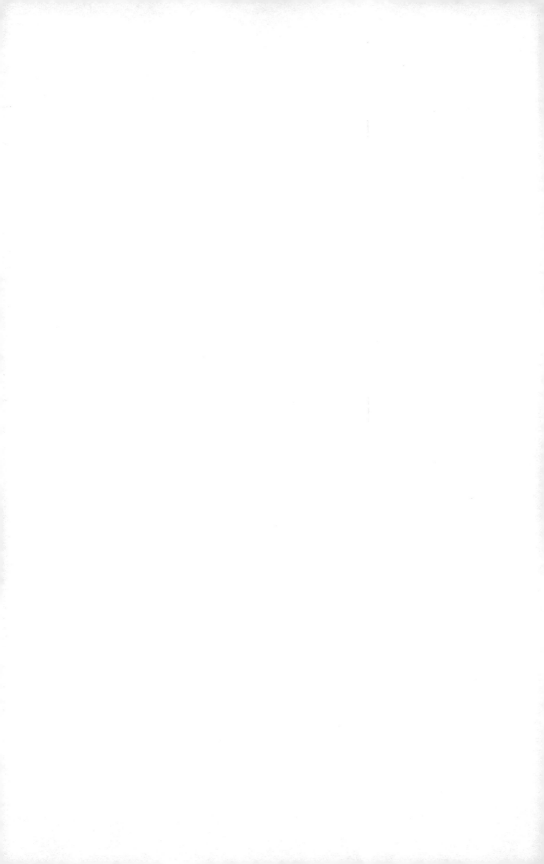

Women, Weight, and Hormones

Women, Weight, and Hormones

A WEIGHT-LOSS PLAN FOR WOMEN OVER 35

Elizabeth Lee Vliet, M.D.

M. Evans and Company, Inc.
New York

Your Hormone Power Plan and *Your Hormone Power Life Plan* are registered trademarks of Elizabeth Lee Vliet, M.D.

M. Evans and Company, Inc.
216 East 49th Street
New York, New York 10017

Library of Congress Cataloging-in-Publication Data

Women, weight, and hormones : a weight-loss plan for women over 35 / Elizabeth Lee Vliet
    p. cm.
    Includes index.
ISBN 0-87131-932-2
    1. Middle aged women—Health and hygiene. 2. Hormones. 3. Weight loss.
  I. Vliet, Elizabeth Lee, 1946–
RA778 .W746 2001
613'.04244—dc21   2001023420

Printed in the United States of America

9 8 7 6 5 4 3 2 1

This book is dedicated to

⋄ *The courage and persistence of my women patients—and their partners—who have struggled with inexplicable weight gain and often felt devalued about their observations, yet continued to pursue answers to their health questions. I hope you find validation in the connections and current international research I have presented in this book.*

⋄ *My husband, Gordon Cheesman Vliet, who has worked hard with me to see that this book was completed, and who has shared the "health" journey of trying to keep up heavy work demands and yet maintain healthy meals and exercise. You've been a terrific encourager and exercise buddy!*

⋄ *My mother and her mother, who always understood the critical role of sound nutrition and a healthy lifestyle and who taught me the basics so well.*

⋄ *Our Creator, who has provided insight, guidance, and strength to bring these words to those who need them, and to continue my life's work in women's health.*

Contents

Acknowledgments

My deepest thanks and appreciation to all who have made this book possible—from the dedicated researchers and clinicians worldwide who have led the way in providing the science to show how women's bodies function differently from men's, and clarified our understandings of these hormone connections in metabolism, weight gain, and weight loss, to those on my team at *HER Place* who have put in the additional time and hard work to see that our patient needs are met while I took the time and energy to focus on getting the book written. I am grateful to all of you!

My deepest admiration and thanks to Gordon Vliet and Kathy Kresnik, incredible supporters and encouragers, who labored long hours, "above and beyond," working with me to bring this book to fruition while keeping the offices running. You both have been "the wind beneath my wings"—I couldn't have done it without you and all your efforts!

My thanks to my clinical colleagues, James Talmadge Boyd, M.D., F.A.C.O.G., and Carolyn Margraf, M.S., R.N., C.S., who have provided caring and capable patient care at *HER Place* and helped me to focus on my writing to broaden our work beyond our office walls. Your support for me, your dedication to these crucial areas of women's health in serving our patients, and your strong faith have been an inspiration to all of us.

Special thanks to Brandi McCoy, a young woman who has truly blossomed in her role as medical assistant and organizer of the Texas office. Your dedication, quick mind, and commitment to support my work in women's health and to be a caring presence for our patients have been invaluable. Even when you have felt overloaded, you have always been cheerful and willing to go the extra mile to help others.

My appreciation to Glenda Silsbee and the rest of my loyal office staff in both Tucson and Texas, who continue to work hard to keep our clinical offices responsive to the needs of our patients during all my writing responsibilities.

Thanks also to Tom Wadkins, computer whiz par excellence, who has always willingly been available to solve my technical challenges and glitches.

To Linda Snyder, "mother hen of the books," my appreciation for all the ways you take care of business matters and relieve pressure on me. You're the best! And my appreciation to my business advisors, David Cohen, Tony Rickert, and his A-1 assistant, Debbie White—you guide me through the complexities of running this organization—I couldn't get the writing done without your guidance on the business side.

Thanks to Dr. Virginia Armstrong, Donna Gilson, and Victoria Hahn: friends, colleagues, and "readers" who reviewed the early stages of the manuscript and meal plans and gave me important guidance and feedback to make this book even better.

My appreciation for the skills and insights of PJ Dempsey, Kate Kelly, and Sandra Noelle Smith, the editors who guided my writing and helped hone and refine this book to make it helpful to readers, yet keep the scientific grounding that women need to make informed decisions.

Thanks to my publisher, George C. de Kay, who saw the need for a weight book written specifically for women, based in research on women rather than men. I am grateful he has been committed to seeing that my work and message reached a broader audience of women who have been misled too long with other "diet" books.

And I also thank you, the women who have honored me by sharing your experiences and have allowed me to help guide you on the journey to health. We are students and teachers of one another in this "marvelous and maddening hormone journey" through our lives as women. Your insights and observations have taught me much that goes beyond the textbooks of medicine. This book becomes part of your legacy, too, as I pass on your words so that they can touch and help others.

Introduction

"Middle Spread and Mental Pause" is my humorous view of my midlife body, I told an audience of women recently. They laughed, and I laughed, but inside, many of us are crying silently about what is happening to our bodies. In my office we have a sign on the scales: *"Don't be alarmed. This scale measures IQ."* But it does little to alter the seemingly inexorable "upward mobility" of the numbers for us midlife women.

Midlife, women, and weight gain. It feels inevitable.

Maybe you have struggled with weight all your life as I have, or maybe you just noticed it becoming a problem when you hit your thirties or forties. Either way, it's a trauma for those of us dealing with being overweight in a culture that idolizes young, *thin,* and unwrinkled women. "Pound-creep" and "scale-inflation" make you wonder, "Where did my waist go? Why doesn't last year's belt fit anymore?" Or you avoid belts altogether and try the elastic waist skirts and untucked tunic tops. Then you cut back on food . . . you cut back some more . . . and back . . . and back some more until you feel like you couldn't possibly eat any less and still survive, and that "#@*!*#" scale *still* won't budge a single notch. Finally, you erupt: "What on Earth is going on? What do I have to *do* to lose weight?"

Weight loss is difficult. I know. I have been there. As you'll read in chapter 1, I've been *fat.* I have been fat and unfit. Interestingly enough, I have also been fat and fit. And I have been, with a lot of hard work, trim and fit. Yet even when I reached a size 8 and 20 percent body fat, I still felt fat because I didn't look like the models in the magazines! It seems like we women can never feel satisfied with our weight and how we look.

Now, at midlife and through menopause, I am there with you, in a constant struggle to keep off excess body fat. *What have I learned as a physician and as a woman on this journey of dealing with weight and hormones? What do we as midlife women have to do to lose weight and keep it off? That's what this book is all about.*

I have read just about all the diet books written recently (and trust me, picking up and putting down diet books is not sufficient exercise to lose weight). Despite the vast number of books that have been written about losing weight, something crucial for women is missing from every one: I have not found a single diet book that accurately describes how women's hormones regulate weight from puberty to menopause and beyond. Even books written by physicians that purport to talk medically about women's weight don't provide correct information about estrogen, progesterone, and testosterone and their effects on weight gain. So far, not one that I have seen really gives us answers fully tailored to our bodies.

Nor do any tell the truth about hormone therapy and weight gain. What really causes you to gain weight when you start hormone replacement therapy (HRT)? What causes you to gain weight at midlife if you don't start HRT? What kinds of foods make the problem worse for women and why? What changes do women need to make to avoid getting fatter during perimenopause and menopause? So many questions. So few accurate and complete answers. The remarkable advances in our scientific understanding of women's body metabolism, women's hormone balance, and women's unique patterns of weight gain at important "hormonal shift" milestones in our lives have not been *reliably* addressed by any of the diet book authors I have read. No wonder women tell me they feel confused and bewildered.

Just like you, I have struggled with these issues for most of my life. I have also been working with the brain/mind-body effects of women's hormones for over twenty years as an active practicing physician, seeing women daily for medical evaluations. To help find the answers, I have become a hormone specialist, a "hormone detective" of sorts, trying to figure out how all these complexities intertwine and affect one another. I continue to be fascinated by the myriad ways that our unique women's hormones interact with each other and play a crucial role in the function of each and every cell and organ in our bodies . . . far beyond just their reproductive effects. I often refer in my talks and seminars to "Those Marvelous and Maddening Hormones!" They certainly are both. So how do we learn to capture more of the "marvelous" part and less of the "maddening" part about our wonderful hormones, especially where our body weight is concerned? Read on.

I am excited to be able to share these ideas with you, because I know firsthand the very real and frustrating struggle you must be going through daily, trying to figure all this out and make some sense of all the conflicting claims out there. My book isn't a typical diet book in the sense of a "deprivation regimen" or a "crash diet." (If you want a short-term, quick-fix kind of diet book, you may need to buy someone else's.) I have in this book some exciting advances in our research to share with you that will help you eat more successfully. I will help you better understand your unique body hormone balance and how this can work for or against you in your efforts to maintain a healthy body weight and recapture your energy and zest. I will teach you what I have learned over the years of working with thousands of women (and myself) about hormones, hormone balance, weight gain and loss, which types of hormones women need to help them lose weight in a healthy way, and which types of hormones (and hormone therapy) to avoid if you are gaining weight.

After you finish reading this book, you'll understand how your hormones have affected your eating patterns and weight control, and you'll be well prepared to talk knowledgeably to a medical professional who can help you achieve the right hormone balance for you. And don't worry, I won't leave you on your own without meal plans and lots of suggestions regarding exercise routines—important elements in fighting "midlife middle spread."

HOW TO USE THIS BOOK

Part One and Part Two of *Women, Weight, and Hormones* provide all you need to know about your weight control issues and hormones. Part One is primarily devoted to helping you understand your unique health risks and why weight loss is so difficult at this time of life. By understanding better why it's so necessary, yet challenging, to lose weight, you'll find it's much easier to figure out how to go about losing what you want to. (*Hint:* Men created most diets, and most diets are tested on men.)

Part Two explains your hormones. Which ones are important when it comes to weight loss? How do they function, and how does the loss of some hormones at critical times of our lives affect how our bodies work? By understanding what constitutes "optimal functioning," you'll be able to decide how best to help your body function better as you go through these changes.

Part Three of the book is your "Action Plan." From suggestions on hormone supplementation to specific recommendations on meal planning, vitamin and mineral supplements, exercise, and mental attitude, you'll find what you need to know to conquer midlife scale inflation.

I wish you well. Let's go!

Part One

When and Why Women Gain Weight

A Self-Test: Is This Book for You?

1. Do you now, or did you, have PMS?
2. Do you have, or did you have, premenstrual food cravings?
3. Have you gained more than 5 pounds since age 18?
4. Have you gained more than 5 pounds since the birth of a child?
5. Have you gained more than 5 pounds since a tubal ligation?
6. Have you gained more than 5 pounds since a hysterectomy?
7. Have you gained more than 5 pounds during perimenopause?
8. Have you gained more than 5 pounds since starting birth control pills or hormone therapy?
9. Do you exercise more than 3 times a week and still have difficulty losing weight?
10. Have you changed to a low-fat diet and still have difficulty losing weight?

11. Have you changed to a vegetarian or high-soy diet and still have difficulty losing weight?
12. Do you frequently have out-of-control sweet cravings?
13. Has you appetite become *ravenous* as you have gotten older?
14. Do you feel like you could *kill* for chocolate at certain times of the month?
15. Are you putting on fat around your waist?
16. Is your waist circumference more than 33 inches?
17. Are you considering hormone therapy (or birth control pills) and worried about weight gain?
18. Is your energy flagging to the point that your "get-up-and-go" got up and went?
19. Do you get uncontrollably sleepy after you eat?
20. Do you suffer from noticeable mood or "blood sugar" swings?

If you answered yes to three or more of the above questions, this book is a must read for you! I'll explain all of these, and more. Read on.

Chapter 1

MY STORY

I started looking like a little balloon in the third grade. I hated being fat. I hated being teased. I hated not being able to climb trees easily like my friends. And then, to make it worse, I had to get glasses. Four-eyes and fat. You can imagine what the other kids did with that. My parents couldn't quite figure out why I suddenly started gaining weight, since everyone else in the family was slender. My mother didn't allow much in the way of junk food, and the family meals were a healthy combination of fresh vegetables from the garden, meats or fish or chicken, and fruits.

We were also active children. I was not a couch potato (or computer-potato as we call it today), and we weren't allowed to spend hours in front of the TV instead of being outside playing. So why on earth was I getting so fat? I didn't put it all together at the time, but of all my cousins, it was only my two *female* cousins who got fat at about the age of third grade. None of the boys did. Hmmm . . . mmm. Could there be something hormonal here in this picture? Stay tuned. It took me years to put the pieces of the puzzle together in a way that made some sense about this pattern in my family tree, and what can affect women in general to make us fatter.

Then in adolescence, puberty arrived, and with a healthy diet and more exercise I slimmed down, though taunts from childhood and the fear of being fat lingered in my soul. Overall, high school was a time of lots of activity, a healthy body, and a desirable body weight. Then college came, along with the "freshman fifteen"—you know, those pounds that suddenly appear as soon as you hit dorm life? My friends and I quickly discovered that if we started smoking cigarettes, we could be cool and lose weight all at the same time. I did that for a few years until I realized smoking was dumb and dangerous, and I quit. But overall, with the physical activity of walking around campus, appetite-suppression through smoking, lots of dancing on the weekends, and the ubiquitous "quick fix" diets, I kept the weight under control in college and was generally pleased with how I looked and felt. (The young can get away with "dumb" health decisions, but eventually, age and body changes dictate that smarter decisions are necessary.)

After college, my twenties were filled with working full time, graduate school, a busy social life, parties, eating out, and enjoying my new hobby of gourmet cooking, and the pounds seemed to stick to my body like flies to glue. I wasn't exercising at all then, and I was taking *birth control pills*, which I didn't realize were adding to my struggles. I was on a high progestin pill that made me hungrier than ever and made my blood sugar swings worse. Another fifteen pounds added. A friend said, "Why don't you run after work?" I said to myself, "What do you mean, go out and run after work. Are you nuts? I don't have the energy to put one foot in front of the other, much less *exercise*." Little did I know then what I know now: Exercise revs up your energy and helps *fight* fatigue!

During this time, I tried every diet in the book, from Atkins to Zen and everything in between. Like many of you, I would lose a few pounds, hit that plateau, get frustrated, and go back to what I normally ate; the pounds would come flying back with a vengeance. Each time I went on a crash diet, I lost more muscle, and when the weight came back later, it was all fat. Then my metabolism was even slower than before, so it was harder to lose the next time. What a vicious cycle. Recognize this pattern? I had no way to evaluate the fad diets I tried or to understand my body chemistry and hormone balance so I could figure out the best approach for *my* body.

Then at age 28 I started medical school. Talk about *stress*. Living away from my husband in order to attend school, I felt lonely and overwhelmed with the work load of a three-year, year-round curriculum. Chocolate became my consolation and solace, and I gained thirty pounds the first year—all-night studying, turning pages with one hand and emptying chocolate-chip-cookie boxes with the other.

I finally came to my senses and realized I couldn't continue this crazy pattern. A classmate encouraged me to start jogging with her. Of course, she was thin, fit, and ran three-plus miles a day! That seemed pretty overwhelming to the "cookie monster" me, barely able to walk a mile, much less *run* one. Finally, Colleen's coaxing won out. I started by walking the mile lap around the neighborhood, and then slowly jogged the last block. Each week, I added one more block for the jogging part, until finally, after ten weeks, I had built up to being able to jog the entire mile. I was thrilled with my success and accomplishment! I kept up the jogging through my medical school years, and also ate much more reasonably. As a result, the excess pounds slowly dropped away, and I felt *tons* better. I had more energy, I slept well, and I had more stamina and concentration for studying. I noticed very quickly that when you are pulling all those pounds along on the jog, the cookies and ice cream don't seem nearly as desirable. Plus, I got my brain cleared and my body refreshed with movement instead of becoming lethargic from overeating. My present to myself on my thirtieth birthday was to *run* five miles, something I had not been able to do even at eighteen, much less twenty or twenty-five. It made me proud.

My postresidency years were marked by a new job, the stress of leaving friends and family, moving across the country, noticing more of those premenstrual chocolate cravings (and giving in to them), and getting out of the exercise habit and into the Häagen-Dazs habit. The pounds piled back on. I pretended I didn't notice, but after awhile, I couldn't hide the body changes anymore. I got together with a friend who was also out of shape and overfat and we went back to exercising. This time instead of jogging, I went to aerobic dance classes that were terrific fun, even though I felt awkward being there at my size. Progress was slower, since I was older now, though I hadn't fully made that connection at the time.

This time I again began to lose weight through exercise and healthy eating, going down to a size 8–10 and 22 percent body fat. I was understanding the mind-body connections better now, and I felt so much better about myself being fit than fat. I wasn't a size 4 or even a 6, but I sure did feel good. I decided those Madison Avenue types weren't going to make me feel less of a woman because I was bigger than a 6. I took perverse delight in surprising the "perfect body" exercise instructors with my level of fitness and stamina in the classes.

A few years went by, I sustained these postive changes, and I felt great. Then something seemed to go awry. The PMS was getting worse, the chocolate cravings were back in force, my energy was down, I wasn't sleeping as well. My clothes didn't fit the same; all the waists seemed to be shrinking at the same time. Now the low-fat diet just wasn't working, even though I was scrupulous about cutting out the fat and focusing on the complex carbs, healthy pasta, bread without any butter or margarine. These previously successful approaches suddenly weren't working . . . which meant more weight gain, less energy, sluggishness, and I didn't feel like exercising. My formerly boundless energy seemed to have gotten up and gone. I felt like I was dragging though my days. I was getting older though I hadn't really paid attention to that. Though I was "only" in my mid-thirties, no one—including me, who had developed a special program for helping women with PMS—had thought to check my own PMS. Along with heart palpitations, I spent night after night waking up looking at the clock and wondering when I would fall asleep and *stay* asleep. I went to my doctors, who felt I must just be "stressed" from a busy medical practice and needed to take more time off. Does any of this sound familiar?

Then I had two different surgeries for herniated disks in my neck. I was out of work for months, couldn't exercise as intensively as I had been, and those "@#*!#%" pounds piled on *again*. Before I could finish the full rehabilitation from my neck surgeries, I found I needed a hysterectomy, bringing on a sudden menopause many years before I thought I would face that milestone. What a shock.

While I struggled to find the right hormone balance, I gained even more weight. The middle body fat problem escalated, and hypothyroidism, insulin resistance, and glucose intolerance resulted. I went through it all, in part made worse by a low-fat, high-carb meal plan. Boy, after the hysterectomy, that approach *really* didn't work! (I'll share more about why as you take the journey with me through the pages of this book.)

After a lifetime of searching, and reading and trying every diet there is, I have several conclusions to report—some of which you have probably already figured out on your own:

⬦ Weight loss is difficult. Period.
⬦ There is no "magic pill" after all.

⋄ Men lose weight easier than women, at all ages through-out life (decidedly unfair!).

⋄ Diets that work like "magic" for men, don't work for women, or if they do, you have to work at it three times as hard and four times as long as a man to lose half the weight he did!

⋄ Deep inside, you and I both know that "diets" don't work in the long run. (Haven't you always regained the weight you lost?)

⋄ We get fatter as we get older (women blame this on "hor-mones"; men blame this on "beer").

⋄ Women think—and tell me every day in my office— "Hormone therapy at menopause causes weight gain—I don't want to take hormones." What I will show you in this book is that this "conclusion" is wrong. Hormone *imbalance* causes weight gain.

Maintaining a healthy body takes work. Many times, I get tired of "working" at it, just like you probably do. I think I have always wanted to find a "cure" or miracle diet that would take the weight off easily, perma-nently, and without a lot of bother or fuss or effort. Have I found a "magic pill"? No.

Have I finally found some clues that will help you put the "weight prob-lem" in better perspective for you as a woman? Yes.

Have I found some ways to deal with "midlife middle management" with greater success? Yes.

Have I found some ways to help you "take hormones" and *not* gain more fat? Yes.

Is there some good news to follow my earlier statement that *weight loss is difficult?* Yes.

It has taken me twenty years of detective work; study; and searching the international medical literature on hormones, weight, nutrition, and exer-cise to come to the understandings that I will be sharing in this book.

Finally, I feel better equipped to put all these life lessons together into a rational plan that will help you, and me, keep the pounds off as we head into the second half of our lives. And that's why I decided I had to write this book. I want to help women like me, who struggle every day with unwanted weight and can't seem to find a way out of the maze of conflicting infor-mation and meal plans.

There *are* answers to help you in your struggles. You need this book, just as I needed all of this information to help *me*. There's a lot to share with you on all this, and I hope you will find the journey through this book to be both exciting and encouraging. There is *hope* for keeping your weight down without letting diets rule your life and destroy your energy. Come with me on the journey and find out the *real* story behind the "hormones-and-weight hoopla."

Chapter 2

HEALTH RISKS OF WEIGHT GAIN:

WOMEN ARE HIT HARDER

Most of you already know the long litany of health risks that obesity presents: high blood pressure, early heart attacks, strokes, and diabetes to mention only a few. *But did you know that there are several conditions, worse in women or unique to women, that are even more serious in women who are also obese?* The unique ways that obesity hits women haven't been adequately addressed in our current health care system, and you need to be aware of some special vulnerabilities that you have as a woman who is in midlife and overweight—or heading that way.

The scientific evidence is overwhelming and consistent: Women, *but not men*, show a sharp increase in obesity between the ages of forty-five and fifty-four as demonstrated in a recent Swedish study. We women intuitively knew this all along. Ask any woman who has lived to see "over forty" and watched her waistline disappear! Now, you can have the satisfaction of knowing that your "inner knowing" has been validated by scientific study. Earlier studies from the 1960s clearly demonstrated that women over thirty-five have decreasing lean body mass (i.e., loss of muscle and bone) and increasing percent body fat, particularly in the abdominal area. Even studies from Asian countries, with high soy intake and lower overall rates of obesity, have shown that as women get older and become menopausal, they begin storing excess fat in the middle of the body (central or android, "malelike" fat pattern) instead of around the lower tummy, hips, and thighs (the premenopausal female or gynecoid fat pattern).

Women around the world have given this midlife "middle" fat a variety of funny names ("meno-pot," "Buddha belly," and others), but the end result isn't funny at all. Today, in the United States, 53 percent of women between the ages of forty and forty-nine are overweight or obese. That number jumps to 65 percent in women fifty to fifty-nine years old, with almost 40 percent of this group obese (body mass index over 30). With all of us baby boomers now over forty, the overweight problem is an epidemic. Why is this important to *you?* This "middle spread" of menopause makes you have a much higher risk of serious medical problems and even early death: high blood pressure, diabetes, cancers of breast and uterus, high cholesterol, high triglycerides, sleep apnea, arthritis, gallstones, and other problems.

If you are already overweight, you have additional concerns to consider when deciding about birth control or hormonal replacement options that may be appropriate for perimenopausal and menopausal problems. The synthetic progestins found in birth control pills and HRT products, some more so than others, have appetite-stimulating and mood/energy-depressing properties, along with the potential for negative effects on lipids and glucose control. And these effects can also occur with natural progesterone. (More about these specifics in chapter 13.) However, before you swear off the pill or HRT, you should know that the increase in fat around the middle of the body is even more true for menopausal women *not* taking hormones than for women who do take hormones at menopause. *Taking* hormones doesn't make you fat; *losing* the right ones does. Higher levels of the wrong hormones at menopause, and in the years afterward, make you fat. I'll go into more detail on this in upcoming chapters and outline *Your Hormone Power Plan* to help you overcome these problems.

OBESITY HITS WOMEN HARDER

The following disorders and illnesses create greater health problems for women who are overweight than for men. What's more, an underlying illness such as any one of the following may simply make it much harder for women to lose unwanted weight.

Diabetes and its complications are worse in women, and obesity leads to an increased risk of becoming diabetic.

Heart disease, increased by obesity, tends to lead to earlier deaths in women than in men and often goes unrecognized because doctors still don't think women are at high risk.

Hypothyroidism (low thyroid) is already eight to ten times more common in women; being obese intensifies the complications of hypothyroidism as well as making it even harder for women to lose weight even with treatment of the thyroid problem.

Breast cancer, endometrial cancer—Four- to sevenfold increased risk in women who are obese.

Depression, already three times more common in women, increases even more with obesity in women, more so than is seen in obese men. The reasons for this are still being explored and are, in part, related to the very hormone changes I am addressing in this book.

Trauma to self-esteem—obese women face more stigma, isolation, and discrimination than do men who are obese. Women are seen as slovenly, lazy, lacking in motivation. Obese men are often seen as "powerful," and don't have the same negative labels applied.

© 2001 Elizabeth Lee Vliet, M.D.

DIABETES

Obesity leads to a much higher likelihood of insulin resistance and the development of diabetes, a condition of high blood sugar that leads to serious health problems. If not treated and controlled, the high blood sugar levels in diabetes cause damage to the arteries throughout the body, leading to high blood pressure, kidney damage, nerve damage, vision loss, cognitive loss and memory damage, as well as early heart attacks and death in both men and women.

However, diabetes is a much greater problem for women than for men for two reasons: more women *get* diabetes, and women tend to have more severe and more frequent complications than men. Women of African-American, Native American, and Hispanic descent are at even greater risk than Caucasian women, with diabetes striking 30 to 40 percent of women in these groups. High levels of blood glucose sustained over long periods of time are thought to cause decreased bone-building processes, meaning an increase in bone loss and osteoporosis in women with Type 1 diabetes. Type 2 diabetes is the form caused by excess body fat, and this type of diabetes is far more common in women.

Oral contraceptives and hormone therapy regimens require careful selection and monitoring in women with diabetes to reduce side effects such as depression, weight gain, impaired glucose control, and yeast infections that are already more prevalent due to the diabetes.

HEART DISEASE

Obesity is one of the most significant risk factors for heart disease. Women are more likely than men to be misdiagnosed early, and more women die with their first heart attack. Heart disease poses some unique risks for women who are also moving into the perimenopausal years when estradiol (the form of estrogen that prevails prior to menopause) declines. In my earlier book, *Screaming to Be Heard,* I explained how many different ways our premenopausal estradiol acts to reduce our risk of vascular disease leading to heart attacks and stroke.

Obese women have a triple whammy in this regard as they move into menopause:

- ◇ They are losing the protective effects of the estradiol at the same time they have higher levels of the "unhealthy" estrone (more about this in Part Two).
- ◇ They have higher levels of the androgens made in fat tissue that promote dangerous "middle-body" fat storage.
- ◇ They have a greater incidence of significant insulin resistance than do men, and this is another risk factor for all types of cardiovascular disease and diabetes.

Diabetes then increases the risk of heart disease, so it is a vicious cycle. As you've just read, overweight women are at greater risk of diabetes. It's a very serious picture, and doctors don't really explain this gender difference in risk very well. Patients are usually told, "You're overweight, so eat less and exercise more." It isn't that simple for women!

HYPOTHYROIDISM (LOW THYROID)

Hypothyroidism is another disorder far more common in women than men. It leads to significant weight gain in the early phases of the illness, long before the thyroid stimulating hormone (TSH) has elevated to a point that most doctors would say requires medication. The weight gain, high cortisol and cholesterol, as well as changes in glucose-insulin regulation that are caused by hypothyroidism, can end up leading to increased risk of diabetes later if not recognized and treated aggressively in the early stages.

Sadly, even though all medical textbooks describe weight gain as a complication of hypothyroidism, most doctors don't take complaints of "weight gain" very seriously and don't consider doing a detailed thyroid evaluation early on. Most doctors believe that thyroid problems cause only a small fraction of obesity problems, and will tell you that it "can't be your thyroid" if your TSH is normal. Just remember, your body's "normal" may be different from numbers we have arbitrarily decided are "normal" on a laboratory range. Women may have a "normal" TSH but still have markedly elevated thyroid antibodies that can lead to impaired thyroid function.

BREAST CANCER

Obesity is a significant risk factor for breast cancer, with obese women having almost a four- to sevenfold increased risk of developing it. Excess body fat contributes to higher levels of estrone and a male hormone called dehydroandrostenedione (DHEA) circulating in the blood. It is not known for certain which of these hormones is the culprit in the increased risk of breast cancer in women. Two factors imply that it is estrone: First, 80 percent of breast cancers arise in women after menopause, when estrone is the primary estrogen present in the body (produced in the fat tissue and the adrenal glands) and there is very little 17-beta estradiol (the premenopausal "good" estrogen) remaining. Second, the location of the fat on the body is important—there is about a sixfold increase in risk of breast cancer in women who have excess upper-body fat (i.e., from the belly button to the shoulders) compared to women whose fat is distributed more around the hips, buttocks, and thighs. For example, a 1991 summary of nutrition and breast cancer risk in Japan revealed that Japanese breast cancer patients differed from the control group because they had an increase in abdominal body fat. Upper-body fat distribution is associated with lower levels of estradiol and higher levels of estrone, androgens, and cortisol.

DEPRESSION

About three times more women than men will have at least one episode of depression in their lifetime. On average, there are about 11 million women in the United States affected in a given year. This gender difference is found at all ages after puberty. In addition, more depressed women gain instead of lose weight with their depressive episode. Depressed men tend to lose weight. More women than men suffer from Seasonal Affective Disorder (SAD or "winter depression"), dysthymia, and cyclothymia. All of these "atypical depressions" are more associated with weight gain than with weight loss.

Biological and psychological changes can partially explain the gender differences in depression. Elevated cortisol, decreased serotonin, and sleep disruption, which can result from depressive illness, make it more likely that someone will gain weight. In addition, there are a host of psychological factors. If you're depressed, you feel lousy about yourself; you feel you'll never look like the magazine ads say women should look; you feel hopeless, so it doesn't make a difference if you lose weight; you're discouraged about ever getting better; you're tired all the time . . . as well as many more negative thoughts that contribute to overeating as a way of trying to feel better.

Depression also tends to zap energy so that you don't feel like doing all the work that's needed to have healthy, balanced meals (making grocery lists, buying the food, preparing it, cooking it, and cleaning up), so you just eat whatever is handy that makes you feel better—usually "comfort" foods such as sweets and prepared foods that are high in sugar, salt, and fat.

And if our energy level is zapped from our diet, as well as depression and discouragement, then it's not surprising that we don't get out and exercise! So you become more of a couch potato, less and less active, all the while snacking on carbohydrates hoping you'll have a serotonin boost and feel better. No wonder the pounds creep on. You know this pattern, because if you are overweight and have been depressed, you have probably gotten caught in this vicious cycle, just as I have in years past.

Add to all this the fact that more than three times as many women than men are obese, a number that rises as women get older, and obesity itself increases the likelihood of a depressive episode. Women end up being hit especially hard when the two are combined.

CONDITIONS MORE COMMON IN WOMEN THAT ARE AGGRAVATED BY WEIGHT GAIN

In addition, the following conditions are more common in women and made worse by obesity:

Alcoholism complications are worse in women. We have lower tolerance for alcohol, and that is made worse by obesity, which increases the risk of "fatty liver" damage. Women who drink alcohol heavily also have a greater tendency than men to become obese and to develop insulin resistance and diabetes from the effects of alcohol. This is especially true with the metabolic changes of menopause that slow down metabolism, decrease estradiol, and make the empty calories from alcohol even more of a factor in weight gain.

Gallstones, already more common in women, increase more with obesity and further increase in menopause when loss of estradiol causes decreased gallbladder emptying.

Gastro Esophageal Reflux Disease (GERD) is increased by obesity and is more common in women during perimenopause, menopause, the progesterone-dominant luteal phase of the menstrual cycle, and the last trimester of pregnancy because progesterone slows down muscles that control stomach emptying.

Sleep Apnea, or episodes of stopping breathing during sleep, is a serious disorder more common in women than men. The likelihood of your developing it increases as you gain weight, and also increases with the menopausal loss of estradiol that causes more fragmented sleep. Sleep apnea affects many metabolic pathways in the body, leading to further weight gain, early heart attacks, loss of sexual function, and increased likelihood of depression.

WOMEN ALSO HAVE OTHER HEALTH ISSUES THAT AFFECT WEIGHT GAIN

While the above information should convince you of the importance of addressing being overweight, I have a little more bad news: Women have unique health issues that make it more challenging—but not impossible—to prevent weight gain and to effectively take off excess weight. Here's a sampling of what all women have to contend with.

Menopause

Menopause causes a number of metabolic changes. If you are obese (more than 20 percent above desired body weight) before you hit menopause, your problems are compounded when the menopausal endocrine changes occur. You would have had to have had your head in the sand for the last twenty years to avoid hearing about osteoporosis as a consequence of menopause and loss of estrogen. But have you heard much about the ways that a decrease in 17-beta estradiol, your most active premenopausal estrogen, causes your metabolism to change in unwanted ways? I'll bet you haven't.

I will talk in future chapters about the many metabolic effects that occur when women experience the hormone shifts of perimenopause and menopause. But there are other body changes happening around "the change" that cause midlife obese women to have special risks: the further shift to increased central-body fat stores (i.e., "middle spread"), less responsiveness to insulin (increases fat storage), higher blood pressure, more risk of heart attack and stroke, increased cortisol that in turn increases fat storage around the middle, increased bad cholesterol, increased triglycerides, and a host of others that will be described as you read further.

All of these changes make women store fat more efficiently and store more of their fat around the waist, again contributing to the risk of diabetes. So the "middle spread" weight gain is like throwing gasoline on a fire! This is why it's often called "toxic" weight gain.

Polycystic Ovary Syndrome (PCOS)

Obese women are more likely to suffer from PCOS, a woefully under-diagnosed, profoundly serious disorder that affects many body systems and causes complex metabolic damage. The main focus by gynecologists has been that PCOS causes infertility, so women who aren't trying to get pregnant rarely get diagnosed in the earlier stages of the disease.

PCOS is such a devastating metabolic disorder that it is imperative to screen women early for the presence of this disease in order to reduce later development of diabetes and premature heart attacks. The metabolic syndrome caused by PCOS triggers marked weight gain, insulin resistance, upper-body fat, excess facial and body hair, acne, and infertility.

Since many women don't even know they have PCOS, they end up becoming morbidly obese before anyone even thinks about the fact that this severe weight gain may have been caused by PCOS. In my medical practice, we rarely see our PCOS patients describe "binge" behavior in their food consumption, even though most of these women are seriously obese as a result of PCOS. Since women with PCOS often do not ovulate normally and do not have the typical cyclic rise and fall in progesterone that tends to trigger the cravings for increased food and sweets in particular, it fits that they don't have the same intense "food cravings" that I hear from women with PMS or who tend to binge and/or purge.

Figure 2.1
WOMEN'S MIDLIFE BODY SHAPE CHANGES

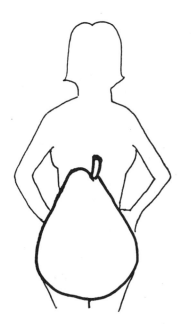 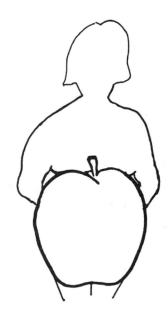

PEAR-SHAPED BODY
Characteristic of women prior to menopause, when estradiol (E2) is greater than estrone (E1); normal female level of androgens.

APPLE-SHAPED BODY
Characteristic of women after menopause (if *not* on hormone Rx); E1 greater than E2. Associated with higher level of androgens (DHEA, testosterone, etc.) and higher risk of heart disease, hypertension, insulin resistance and diabetes. Also seen in PCOS due to higher androgens.

© 1995, revised 2001 by Elizabeth Lee Vliet, M.D.

Binge Eating Disorder (BED)

This syndrome affects twice as many women as men and is found in about 10 to 20 percent of obese people. I have frequently found that my women patients with BED are more likely to engage in their binges in the two weeks of the menstrual cycle (luteal phase) when progesterone levels are high, leading me to conclude that the ratio of estradiol to progesterone is a major factor with this disorder.

People with BED consume excessively large amounts of food, usually high calorie and high fat, in relatively short periods of time, several times a week. They typically describe feeling "out of control" with their eating at the time of a binge. For women, this often occurs seven to ten days before menses.

In spite of these observations from many clinicians who work with women who have eating disorders, the menstrual cycle hormone fluctuations are rarely taken into account either for evaluation or for treatment.

◇   ◇   ◇

Does all this make you think seriously about how important it is to work on a healthy weight-loss plan? I hope so. Your life and health are too important not to! The years of perimenopause and menopause are a time to get control, restore your hormone power balance, and recapture your energy and zest for the years ahead. We now have the opportunity to go through menopause and live an average of thirty to forty years beyond menopause. That was not the case for our great-grandmothers and their ancestors. Let's make these added years great ones!

You've now seen the negative aspects of not paying attention to weight gain. Resolve now to make the most of your additional years. Don't focus on just whether you have symptoms of menopause or not. If you are having difficulty with middle-spread weight gain, whether you have hot flashes or not, this book is critical to your long-term health. This book is all about recapturing the power of healthy hormone balance so you can turn it into *Your Hormone Power Life Plan* for healthy, permanent loss of excess fat.

Chapter 3

ARE YOUR HORMONES MAKING YOU FAT?

METABOLISM BASICS

For women, our distinctive ovarian hormones play especially important roles in total metabolism and, therefore, weight gain and loss. As we travel together on the journey through my book, you'll see how changing hormone levels at midlife affect your weight and where body fat gets stored on your body, and why the eating habits you got away with when you were younger are now getting you into trouble with excess body fat. It isn't only the actual levels of these hormones that's critical, it is also the *ratio* of the various ovarian hormones that will determine how much and where we gain body fat. As you will see, you have to look at all of these hormones in an integrated approach if you are going to understand how you gain weight, and how to lose it.

The foods we eat provide the metabolic fuels that keep us alive and help us grow and function normally each day. When we eat, digestion breaks food down into smaller, simpler molecules that can be absorbed into the bloodstream and carried throughout the body to be taken up by the trillions of cells that make up our organs and tissues. Once in the cells, these simple molecules are combined with oxygen and "burned" to provide energy to run the cells. This process of burning food to make energy is called *metabolism*. What are some of these simple molecules or building blocks? They include simple sugars from carbohydrates, amino acids from proteins, fatty acids and ketones from fats. Together with the vitamins and minerals needed to make the chemical reactions and metabolic enzymes work, these simple molecules provide fuel for the chemical reactions that keep us humming along, able to function each day.

The female hormonal ebb and flow, which occurs in a cyclical manner, has widespread effects on the brain-body processes, as well as on our weight. When you understand the specific effects and roles of each of the primary female hormones, you can see how beautifully orchestrated the female endocrine system is for its role in bringing new life into being and for keeping the species alive. These hormonal actions make sense from an evolutionary standpoint for the tasks that they govern in the body. The problem today is that in our culture, food is no longer scarce. For most people, food is overly available. We don't eat as much fiber in fruits, whole grains, and vegetables; we have too much sugar, caffeine, and alcohol easily at hand. We are not getting pregnant as often, we are living longer, and we are trying to do multiple tasks every day, which causes a marked increase in overall stress levels. Consequently, some of the natural survival roles for our hormonal metabolic effects are now working against us. With our current lifestyles and diet, these former "survival functions" now cause unwanted physical-psychological "symptoms" that make us both feel lousy and gain weight faster. This is one of many reasons that we see so many more women today struggling with their weight as they get older. Before we explore the way our hormones may be contributing to our weight problems, let's first understand what a hormone is, what our hormones do, and introduce you to your hormone cast of characters.

WHAT IS A HORMONE?

I think of hormones as "chemical communicators" or "connectors" that carry messages to and from all organs of the body and serve to connect one organ's function with another organ's function to keep the body balanced and functioning optimally. Hormones are very potent molecules, and it usually takes minuscule amounts, sometimes as little as a billionth of a gram (nanogram), to exert their effects on cells of the target organs.

Without our hormones to keep the connections and messages flowing smoothly and our organs functioning in a balanced and an integrated manner, we would die. It's that simple. The secretion and interaction of hormones throughout our bodies every day is a highly complex and ongoing process. Each hormone provides a specific set of directions or messages to the target cells to enable the cells to perform certain functions. The cells of the body are like manufacturing plants, making the many chemicals the body needs to function. Hormones have a variety of functions, some similar to those of assembly-line supervisors directing the manufacturing processes, and some similar to those of team facilitators acting as catalysts for chemical processes to occur in the cell.

The interactions of the hormones and our cells is quite complex. To simplify it, I have often used the visual analogy of a "key in a lock" to describe the way hormones bind at their specific receptor sites all through the brain and body to trigger their action on the target cells. The receptor sites may be located on cell surfaces or inside cells at the nucleus, our cellular "command central." Each hormone, or other chemical messenger, is a specific molecular "key," and each has a "lock" (receptor site) into which it fits (see figure 3.1). As also with keys, similar keys may fit in a lock but will not be able to turn it. Some keys fit partially and turn the lock slightly. This model is too simplistic based on our current knowledge of the complexities of the hormone-receptor interaction, but at least it helps you to get the idea that it is important for a proper fit between the hormone and its receptor in order to have optimal function. If you use this visual picture when you read about the many types of medications available to restore or mimic hormone effect, it will help you understand the differences in how women respond to various types of hormone products and the phytoestrogens in foods.

In the figures that follow, you can see some of the major hormones, where they are produced, and what they do. With such an array of hormone messengers, something has to coordinate their action in the body, especially for metabolism and optimal use of food, which is so crucial to our survival. The brain is the organ that directs this complex interplay of our hormones and their target organs.

You can think of the brain as a "master conductor" of a hormone "orchestra." In its role as conductor, the brain directs and coordinates the actions of all these various players (hormones) to produce the "symphony" of our body rhythms and functions. Then the "music" generated by the action of the various hormones is "heard" by the brain in a feedback loop that allows the brain conductor to direct the next responses. It is a two-way process: the brain directs the output of hormones, and the hormones in turn affect the brain's responses.

Figure 3.1
HORMONES AND RECEPTORS:
A LOOK AT HOW THEY WORK

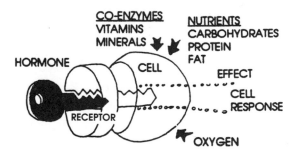

Each hormone has its own receptor site "lock" at target cells throughout the body. The body's own hormone molecular "key" fits into its receptor to trigger hormone effects. Molecules with different shapes may also occupy the "lock" for that hormone, but *may or may not* trigger the hormonal action in the way your body's molecules do. These different shaped molecules (e.g., equilin, genistein, SERMS) may actually block the body's own hormones from working properly, or may make it work differently.

© 1995, revised 2001 by Elizabeth Lee Vliet, M.D.

Figure 3.2
THE ENDOCRINE SYSTEM:
A LOOK AT KEY HORMONES AND WHAT THEY DO

I. STEROIDS

Hormone	Primary Actions
◇ Cortisol	many metabolic actions, especially to *store* more body fat; produced in higher amounts under stress and may suppress normal immune function due to anti-inflammatory actions
◇ Aldosterone	regulates fluid balance by stimulating kidneys to retain sodium and water and excrete potassium; contributes to excess *water* weight gain when progesterone levels are high in second half of menstrual cycle and stimulate more aldosterone secretion
◇ Androgens (DHEA, others)	enhances sex drive, produces male features in women (e.g., facial hair, male body shape), stimulates appetite, contributes to middle-body and waistline fat gain when levels too high

◇ Estrogens (three)
  ◇ Estradiol
  ◇ Estrone
  ◇ Estriol
	female secondary sex characteristics; key role in menstruation, pregnancy, over 400 other crucial functions throughout the body and brain, including increased metabolic rate, improved insulin sensitivity and carbohydrate tolerance, role in body temperature regulation

◇ Progesterone	helps maintain pregnancy; many metabolic effects, including increased appetite, increased fat storage, and reduced sensitivity to insulin; high levels give sedative, analgesic effects at brain, may produce depressed mood
◇ Testosterone	produces male secondary sex patterns, triggers sex drive and arousal in both males and females, many metabolic effects (bone and muscle growth, increased metabolic rate, etc.)

Figure 3.2 (continued)
THE ENDOCRINE SYSTEM:
A LOOK AT KEY HORMONES AND WHAT THEY DO

II. AMINES

Hormone	Primary Actions

◇ Thyroid hormones
  ◇ Thyroxine (T4)
  ◇ Triiodothyronine (T3)
	stimulate body metabolism by increasing cell energy release, heart rate, heat production, and brain activity; helps maintain normal regulation of metabolic pathways, normal growth and function of nervous and musculoskeletal systems

◇ "Adrenaline" hormones
  ◇ Norepinephrine (NE)
  ◇ Epinephrine
	"fight or flight" (stress) hormones, prepare body for emergencies by increasing heart rate; act on brain to lift mood (or, in excess, cause anxiety), increase alertness; dilate arteries to key organs to provide more oxygen, glucose, and nutrients

III. PEPTIDES AND PROTEINS

Hormone	Primary Actions
◇ Insulin	*lowers* blood sugar (moves glucose into cells to be used for fuel in muscle or stored in fat cells), stimulates fat storage and protein synthesis
◇ Glucagon	*raises* blood glucose (glycogen breakdown and glucose release from liver, gluconeogenesis)
◇ Somatostatin	mild effect to raise blood glucose
◇ Parathyroid (PTH)	major role: increase blood calcium levels by stimulating bone breakdown, calcium release
◇ Calcitonin	involved in regulating blood calcium levels by inhibiting bone breakdown, calcium release
◇ Thymosin (thymus gland)	major role in development of immune system

© 1995, revised 2001 by Elizabeth Lee Vliet, M.D.

III. PEPTIDES AND PROTEINS (continued)

Hormone	Primary Actions
◇ Adrenocorticotropin (ACTH)	stimulates part of the adrenal gland to make cortisol
◇ Follicle Stimulating Hormone (FSH)	stimulates ovaries, activates and promotes follicle growth to produce estrogen
◇ Lutenizing Hormone (LH)	triggers ovulation, formation of the corpus luteum, secretion of progesterone, estrogen
◇ Growth Hormone (GH)	oversees entire process of normal body growth, stimulates formation of more muscle and less body fat, declines during menopause with loss of estradiol; improved with estrogen therapy
◇ Thyroid Stimulating Hormone (TSH)	stimulates the thyroid gland to release T3, T4; TSH will be *high* in low, or *hypo*thyroid conditions, and *low* in *hyper*thyroid conditions
◇ Prolactin	stimulates breast enlargement during pregnancy and regulates milk production after delivery, increases appetite and body fat to support nursing; often elevated in PCOS
◇ Anti-Diuretic Hormone (ADH)	prevents dehydration by stimulating kidneys to increase reabsorption and retain water
◇ Oxytocin	stimulates uterine contractions during labor, helps trigger milk release after delivery
◇ Melatonin (pineal gland)	regulation of sleep cycles, body rhythms; promotes fat storage by increasing appetite, especially for carbohydrate foods (e.g., to prepare for winter hibernation); plays a role in winter depression (SAD) syndromes that are characterized by low energy, weight gain, daytime sleepiness, depressed mood

© 1995, revised 2001 by Elizabeth Lee Vliet, M.D.

BRAIN-BODY HORMONAL COMMUNICATION PATHWAYS

The brain and body are interconnected by an incredible array of chemical and electrical circuits, each one interacting with and affecting others. The brain has a multitude of ways to direct the orchestra of the body to respond to what it (the brain) perceives, from inside the body physically, from inside the mind's thoughts and feelings, and from outside the body. In women's bodies, the entire process is even more complex, with the menstrual cycle rhythm of changes causing the brain-body systems to continuously adapt to the changing hormonal environment. Unlike the male body, which maintains a fairly steady production (*tonic* pattern) of testosterone all month, the female body has a *cyclic* pattern of ovarian hormone rise and fall.

The major underlying influence of these crucial female hormonal rhythms has rarely been fully appreciated for the diverse effects on all parts of the female body, not just reproduction. Figure 3.3 shows these monthly hormonal changes; these stimuli (stressors) of all kinds require the body processes to change and adapt. Hormonal change is another one of those stimuli that triggers the body systems to constantly change and adapt. When the body systems are overstressed, a variety of things may occur: We call these changes *symptoms* if they feel unpleasant to us, or we call them *phenomena* if they are just normal and don't bother us. These changes themselves may then become additional "stressors" on the body and contribute to more overload and possible illness. The interconnections and the ways in which hormonal production may in turn be altered by stress on the body are often overlooked when women seek medical care. Keep in mind that Mother Nature's protective plan is to prevent pregnancy when animals or humans are stressed or sick. It shouldn't be a surprise that prolonged stress can suppress the ovaries and cause decreases in hormone production. The two-way nature of these pathways is a critical connection throughout all facets of women's health, and is so often overlooked in dealing with weight management.

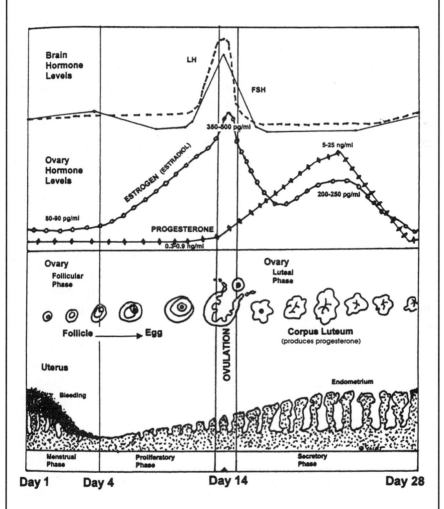

Figure 3.3
THE MENSTRUAL CYCLE HORMONE RHYTHM

© 1995, revised 2001 by Elizabeth Lee Vliet, M.D.

YOUR MONTHLY HORMONE RHYTHMS

It takes all of the hormones in proper balance, each carrying out its own tasks yet working together, to produce a normal menstrual cycle. It really is an amazing interplay. When our hormone balance goes awry, we develop problems with weight gain and other symptoms. If estradiol is falling and progesterone, testosterone, and DHEA are still in the mid- to high-normal range, we start gaining fat around our middles. In the *less common* situation of high estradiol relative to progesterone, we will gain fat around our hips and lower tummy rather than around the waist and upper body.

The ratio of the ovarian hormones is crucial to determining how and where we gain fat. When any hormone system is out of balance, it may trigger weight gain. So we have to look at all of them as an integrated whole. Whether we are experiencing a decline in hormone production with natural or surgical menopause or due to another cause, and whether we lose optimal hormone function at the expected age of menopause or at an earlier-than-normal time, the end result is a similar pattern of middle spread. With all the many unwanted effects of hormone decline, gaining weight certainly ranks high on the list of women's concerns and drastically affects our self-esteem as well as our overall health. So let's now meet the key players and unmask those that are really culprits in our hormonal "middle spread."

MIDLIFE HORMONES AND THEIR EFFECT ON YOUR WEIGHT

In Part Two of this book, you'll learn in more detail about hormones and what they do for you, but here I'd like to briefly introduce those that particularly have to do with metabolism and weight regulation.

Estrogen

Our bodies have three types of estrogen: estradiol, estrone, and estriol. As you'll read, these estrogens are *not* interchangeable, and you will want to understand the difference because of estrogen's major effect on women in midlife.

17-beta estradiol (E2) is the predominant human estrogen produced by the ovaries; it is also the one we lose completely at menopause. Estradiol contributes to improved insulin response, enhanced energy and mood, as well as clarity of thinking, sharper memory, ability to concentrate, normal blood pressure, optimal bone density, better quality of sleep, a better sex drive, and a healthy, active metabolic rate.

Declining estradiol during midlife also contributes to a decrease in serotonin production. Loss of optimal serotonin, in turn, causes depression, increased irritability, increased anxiety, increased pain sensitivity, eating disorders, increased obsessive-compulsive thinking, and increased disruption of normal sleep rhythms. Each of these effects can make your metabolism more sluggish, so the cumulative result of losing your optimal estradiol is that it is now harder for you to lose excess fat.

Estrone (E1) is made in the ovary and fat tissue of our bodies before and after menopause. When estradiol declines at menopause or after hysterectomy or tubal ligation, the balance shifts toward more estrone. Higher estrone levels are associated with a slower metabolism and, you guessed it, more gain in body fat. Estrone does not prevent the unwanted postmenopausal changes in skin, bone, hair, heart and blood vessels, brain, and other organs. High estrone is also associated with higher risk of breast and uterine (endometrial) cancers.

Estriol (E3), the weakest of the human estrogens, is produced by the *placenta* during pregnancy and is not normally present in measurable amounts in nonpregnant women. It is often promoted as a "safe" estrogen because it is weak, but what you don't hear is that it doesn't have the same benefits for the body as estradiol (E2) does. Since estriol does not replace the metabolic functions of the estradiol you lose at menopause, it is not helpful in maintaining the premenopausal estrogen balance necessary to keep your metabolism more active. If you take enough estriol to relieve symptoms, it also stimulates the uterus and breasts.

Progesterone

Progesterone is the hormone responsible for preparing the body to sustain a pregnancy, so it makes you want to eat more for you and the baby. Progesterone is high the second half of your cycle and contributes to the food cravings you notice during this time of the month. They aren't imaginary! Other changes—water retention and breast enlargement—are also part of this pregnancy-promoting effect of progesterone.

Progesterone also slows the movement of food through the gastrointestinal tract, which then permits a woman's body to absorb more nutrients from what she eats. During times of famine, this would have been particularly helpful to women trying to sustain a pregnancy. (This is also why you feel bloated during this phase of your menstrual cycle.) Due to its specific effects on the brain, progesterone may be calming and sedating, but for a lot of women this also leads to a decreased activity level, increasing the potential for weight gain.

Testosterone

Yes, women have testosterone (in minuscule amounts compared to men), and yes, it declines with age. Women lose more than half of their normal testosterone production with menopause, but it can start declining at a much younger age. Testosterone not only promotes a healthy sex drive, but it also has a crucial effect for healthy weight management. Testosterone is an *anabolic* hormone, which means it helps *build* muscle and lean body mass *and* it uses fat for fuel, which in turn helps decrease your excess body fat.

I talk more about all this in Part Two, where you will see that estradiol, along with testosterone, has many effects that help us maintain a healthy body balance of more muscle and less fat tissue. Since women lose up to 95 percent of their estradiol, and over 50 percent of their testosterone, when the ovaries no longer function optimally, it's no wonder women are struggling with weight problems at midlife. This is a dramatic loss of muscle-building, lean-mass-sustaining, metabolism-stimulating hormones!

DHEA

DHEA is another "male" hormone primarily produced in the adrenal gland, but also made by our ovaries before menopause. DHEA has been promoted as a hormone that helps weight loss, but these results were actually found only in men. More recent studies of DHEA typically show that *women gain* weight taking it, and women also experience a host of other negative effects such as hair loss, facial hair, acne, marked sweet cravings, restless sleep, and irritability. DHEA supplements are sold over the counter, but since most of these doses are too high for women, negative side effects are common.

Thyroid Hormones

T3 and T4 are the two primary thyroid hormones produced by the thyroid gland. These are your major metabolic regulators, along with the ovary hormones, since they govern energy use and production in every cell and tissue in the body. All of our metabolic pathways depend upon normal thyroid function for the chemical reactions to take place at the cellular level. When thyroid function is too low, especially when our ovary hormones are also out of balance, women will gain body fat very easily, even when cutting back to very low calorie levels. Sometimes, even in conditions of *excess* thyroid hormone production, women will gain weight in the early phase due to the appetite-stimulating effects of overactive thyroid hormones.

Cortisol

Cortisol is known as our *stress* hormone, and it rises in response to immediate stressors as well as longer lasting ones. Short-term or acute stress also triggers a rapid release of adrenaline, known as the "fight or flight" stress response. Interestingly though, both short-term and ongoing persistent stress responses promote middle-body weight gain and storage of fat in the abdomen instead of promoting fat breakdown. Why? After acute stress you often feel really hungry as a result of the adrenaline outpouring; this can lead to food cravings, especially for sweets, that make you eat more than normal to compensate. Chronic stress, on the other hand, leaves you feeling fatigued, with low energy levels and general loss of your zip, and craving the classic "comfort foods" like carbs and sweets.

Insulin and Glucagon

Insulin and glucagon have important effects that regulate our blood glucose ("sugar") and govern the amount of body fat and muscle, among other functions. They are called counterregulatory hormones because they have opposite effects on blood sugar (glucose). Insulin lowers glucose levels by moving glucose from the blood into muscle cells, where it can be burned for immediate energy, or moving glucose into fat cells, where it is used to store more body fat. The speed and amount of insulin release is triggered by the type of food we eat, when we eat it, and what other foods are eaten at the same time. Glucagon has the opposite effect. When the brain senses falling blood sugar, glucagon stimulates the liver to send the glucose out of storage, into the bloodstream to be delivered to the cells for fuel. Insulin release is affected by the ovary hormones and vice versa. Too much insulin being produced, or insensitivity to insulin action, called *insulin resistance,* makes us store more fat around the middle of our bodies. This abnormal insulin response pattern is seen in PCOS and when our estradiol levels decline.

Prolactin

Prolactin is a hormone produced by the pituitary that may cause significant excess weight gain if it is abnormally elevated. I will not be discussing prolactin later in the book, so I present highlights here, since prolactin should be checked if you have any of the body changes or symptoms described below. You are probably familiar with prolactin as the hormone that regulates the release of milk during nursing. In nonpregnant women and in men, prolactin is normally less than about 15 to 20 ng/ml, but in the third trimester of pregnancy, prolactin levels rise to almost 300 ng/ml. Then it slowly decreases in the first few months after delivery, even if a mother continues nursing.

When prolactin is higher than about 15 to 20 ng/ml, it typically causes menstrual cycles to become irregular and suppresses estradiol levels. If prolactin elevations continue for a prolonged time, you may lose menstrual periods (*amenorrhea*) and notice a milky discharge from the breast (*galactorrhea*). These are the obvious findings when prolactin is higher than normal, but there are some less obvious problems that are common, but less often recognized by many physicians: *weight gain, breast enlargement, headaches, and depression.*

Elevated prolactin likely triggers significant weight gain by mechanisms—similar to the increase in appetite seen in nursing mothers—that stimulate increased food intake to support the caloric needs of mother and baby. The problem is, if you are not nursing, then you don't need to be eating for *two,* so the extra calories just get stored as more body fat. Prolactin may also trigger gain in body fat by suppressing ovarian production of estradiol and testosterone—both of which keep our metabolism revved up, help to maintain normal insulin-glucose regulation, and boost muscle mass and bone growth. In fact, women with high prolactin not only gain body fat, they also lose muscle and bone. Early bone loss leading to premature osteoporosis is one of the complications of untreated high prolactin levels.

Prolactin levels increase as women get older and go through menopause, so this is another factor in the midlife increase in body fat. High prolactin may also be caused by other things: stress; strenuous exercise training; hypothyroidism; nipple stimulation; and a number of common medications such as SSRIs (Prozac, Paxil, Zoloft, Celexa, Luvox), tricyclic antidepressants (Pamelor, amitriptyline, etc.), H2-blockers (Tagamet, Pepcid, etc.), and neuroleptic medicines (Navane, Haldol, Mellaril, etc.). Prolactin-secreting tumors of the pituitary are a potentially serious cause of elevated prolactin because they may cause problems with loss of vision due to optic nerve pressure, even though the tumor itself is usually benign. If you suspect high prolactin, there is a simple blood test your physician can order for you. For most accurate results, the test should be done between 7:00 and 8:00 A.M.

Leptin

Leptin is a recently discovered protein produced in fat cells and it has major roles in regulating the amount of our body fat and where it is deposited in the body. I will not be discussing this hormone elsewhere in the book, so here are the highlights. It is another hormone that goes awry around midlife and menopause, thereby adding to our middle spread. *Leptin* comes from the Greek word *leptos,* meaning "thin." Although it is made in fat cells, Leptin actually circulates in the bloodstream and helps to signal the brain about the body's amount of fat mass. Leptin appears to play a role in maintaining healthy glucose balance by its effects at brain centers.

Leptin has also been found to play a role in reproductive function. Fertility is impaired in both anorexia and extreme obesity; both conditions have been found to have abnormal leptin levels along with impaired leptin regulation. Researchers think that leptin is one of the crucial regulators to help *decrease* food intake and *increase* the body's energy use, which in turn uses fat for fuel, decreasing our body fat.

One of leptin's major actions appears to be inhibiting synthesis and release of another chemical in the hypothalamus, called Neuropeptide Y (NPY). NPY has the opposite effect of leptin, making us eat more, decreasing our energy expenditures, and increasing insulin and cortisol. In addition, leptin acts via effects on several other brain chemicals to carry out its role in helping to regulate changes in the body's needs for food, such as with pregnancy and nursing. Leptin also affects both thyroid and adrenal hormones, which we know are involved in regulating food intake, metabolic rate, and amount of body fat stores.

All of us have observed the obvious male-female differences in the amount and placement of body fat, both in humans and animals. Because of these differences, researchers believe that estrogen, testosterone, and progesterone also play a role in regulating leptin. Studies have looked at the variation of leptin levels during the menstrual cycle, during pregnancy, and during in vitro fertilization. At menopause, women show increases in body fat amount as well as the "apple" distribution of fat. They also show abnormal changes in leptin levels and function of the leptin system. One emerging theory is that as women reach midlife, we become more resistant to the normal effects of leptin, and this is another factor in our gaining excess weight. *Leptin resistance* is also thought to explain why we find *high* leptin levels along with obesity and insulin resistance in PCOS.

In summary, when leptin is present in normal amounts and the body is responding to it properly, we have a *reduction* in body-fat mass and leaner bodies. If leptin production is too low, or the target cells are *resistant* to the circulating leptin, we have more abdominal fat, along with higher rates of Type 2 diabetes. The interactions are quite complex and we don't yet have clear answers about how all these pieces of the puzzle fit together. Current research suggests that estrogen replacement at menopause helps improve leptin sensitivity, so this is another reason to review carefully the points I describe in chapter 13 on restoring ovarian hormone balance.

THE REST OF THE STORY . . .

While these are not all of the hormones involved in weight loss or gain, they are some of the most important metabolic players that affect us as women, particularly at midlife. I will tell you more about these hormones, and all that they do for us, in Part Two. In Part Three, you will learn ways of re-balancing these critical metabolism regulators to help you lose excess fat and regain your energy. There are many good options available to replen-ish what we are losing. Unfortunately, the headlines and sensational news stories related to hormones are often based on inaccurate interpretation of scientific studies and, as a result, scare women away from the very answers that can help them the most. If we truly understand how our bodies work, the role our hormones play in weight regulation, the healthy options avail-able, and a sensible fat-loss approach with realistic goals—we might actual-ly achieve a healthy weight and personal satisfaction in midlife and beyond. We have a long way to go because of the misinformation out there about what your hormones do, so this book is the start of your journey.

HORMONAL "HEAVYWEIGHTS": PMS, PCOS, FMS, CFS, AND DEPRESSION

Up until this point in the chapter we've been discussing natural decline and imbalance in your hormones, which can lead to weight gain. There are several specific conditions, however, that also contribute to hormonal imbalance and weight gain. Here are a few of those, and I think this illus-trates why you must consult a physician for a thorough evaluation before you undertake a weight-loss plan.

Premenstrual syndrome (PMS), polycystic ovary syndrome (PCOS), fibromyalgia syndrome (FMS), chronic fatigue syndrome (CFS), and sev-eral types of depression are all predominately female disorders that have profound hormone triggers and increase in both frequency and severity as women get older. All of these syndromes have another important dimension in common: They are *all* major culprits in women's midlife weight gain.

First, a few definitions: Generally, *premenopausal* refers to a woman who has healthy optimal hormone levels and is still menstruating regularly; *peri-menopausal* refers to a woman who has begun to have declining estradiol and/or progesterone levels that result in erratic, inconsistent periods with changing flow patterns (may be heavy one month, lighter and shorter the next); *PMS* refers to the cluster of physical and emotional changes occurring between ovulation and menses, which then clears for a symptom-free interval each month. PMS may occur in both pre- and perimenopause, since women are still having their natural ovary cycles. *Menopause* technically is defined as cessation of menses and loss of the ovary cycles and, on average, occurs at about age fifty. Natural menopause is not considered to have occurred until there has been no menstrual period for a full year. Surgical menopause is the removal of the uterus and ending of menstruation, even if the ovaies are not removed. *Postmenopause* refers to the years after the complete cessation of menses. These terms may be used very differently in various articles and books, and even by health professionals, so keep that in mind as you read other information.

PERIMENOPAUSE AND WEIGHT GAIN

The *climacteric* refers to the years of hormone decline from our full reproductive hormone levels toward the lower, nonfertile levels of menopause. It encompasses all the pre- and perimenopausal years. Some women make this transition without difficulty or gaining weight. But about 80 to 85 percent of us do experience weight gain around the waist, along with mild to moderate symptoms like insomnia, loss of sex drive, memory loss, low energy, worsening PMS, irritability, mood swings (lability), tearfulness, allergies, and palpitations. Early effects of estradiol decline usually manifest as restless sleep, fatigue, and middle-body weight gain, often long before we have a hot flash! During this time when our body is subtly changing, we may also notice some irregular menstrual cycles with changes in the flow (lighter or heavier). There are many ways that our normal estradiol levels help us maintain a healthy metabolic rate, as you will see in chapter 5. While we may also be experiencing many midlife stresses and changes—balancing home, career, children, aging parents, community roles—it is also true that declining estradiol and changing hormone balance increase our susceptibility to situational stressors and increase release of stress hormones that promote fat storage. The loss of estradiol, coupled with the rise in cortisol, leads to increasing health risks for illnesses like diabetes, heart disease, high blood pressure, and bone loss. We end up with a vicious cycle: The physical hormone changes and psychological stressors act together and then turn around to further decrease our ovarian function. Loss of ovarian hormones added to the increase in stress hormones then makes us gain more weight. Round and round we go, and our middles spread even more. This cycle is even more pronounced if you aren't exercising regularly because you feel too "stressed" and tired!

"Well," you may be asking, "how do I know if I am perimenopausal or if this is just PMS?" We generally use the term *PMS* if your symptoms are cyclic, related clearly to your menstrual cycle, and your FSH and LH are still low (premenopausal levels), and you still have regular menstrual periods. "Perimenopausal" usually refers to *erratic* menstrual periods, rising FSH and LH, and is often considered to be the four years before menopause and four years after menopause. But, keep in mind, "perimenopause" and the decline in estradiol, testosterone, and progesterone may actually occur for a full ten to twelve years before your periods completely stop (menopause). The real answer will be found in actually checking your hormone levels, as I explain in chapter 11. Ultimately, it doesn't really matter what name we give it; the end result is that our bodies are changing in some undesirable ways! I think that we will come to understand that the patterns of worsening PMS and worsening middle spread in the mid-thirties are just different sides of the same coin: the beginning of ovarian decline with loss of the metabolically active 17-beta estradiol and, sometimes, lower-than-optimal testosterone. I think the weight gain is another manifestation of our midlife endocrine changes.

Other factors contributing to the rising incidence of weight gain and obesity in midlife women include:

⋄ Postponing pregnancy and having fewer pregnancies than women did years ago leads to more years of ovulatory cycles, which depletes our follicles (egg supply) sooner, and triggers earlier decline in optimal estradiol production.

⋄ Increased conversion of androgens in fat tissue to estrone (E1). This shifts the estrone-to-estradiol (E2) ratio, as well as the estrogen-to-progesterone ratio, leading to more fat storage. Androgen conversion to estrone does not replace the estradiol produced in the ovary, so even though there is more "estrogen," it isn't the type that gives optimal effects at key brain-body estrogen receptors.

◇ The fact that the typical American diet is "super-sized" in portions and high in fat, salt, refined sugars, refined carbohydrates, alcohol, soft drinks, and caffeinated beverages—all of which have been shown to significantly aggravate weight gain.

◇ Our tendency to have a deficit of magnesium in our diets, which adversely affects metabolism, appetite, and glucose regulation. Magnesium has an important role as cofactor in the synthesis of many appetite and mood-elevating chemical messengers.

◇ Deficient calcium intake for many American women has now been found to be associated with difficulty losing weight.

◇ Inadequate intake of vitamin B6 (pyridoxine), a vitamin cofactor for our bodies to make the mood- and weight-regulating neurotransmitters and one involved in the liver metabolism of estrogen, testosterone, and progesterone.

◇ Sedentary lifestyles and chronic dieting—both slow down our metabolism and lead to more gain in body fat over time.

POLYCYSTIC OVARY SYNDROME AND SYNDROME X—SERIOUS TRIGGERS OF WEIGHT GAIN

PCOS is an overlooked serious metabolic endocrine condition affecting about 6 percent of premenopausal women, including teenagers. The metabolic derangements in PCOS cause very serious, marked weight gain that is often quite rapid. Patients of mine have reported gaining over fifty pounds in six months in spite of careful dieting and regular exercise. They tell me it often feels like they are gaining weight if they just look at food. PCOS is a devastating disorder. It hits women in many serious ways, including causing high blood pressure, high androgen levels, insulin resistance, glucose intolerance, and marked increase in risk of early heart attacks and diabetes mellitus, as well as apple-shaped bodies (this is especially upsetting to teenagers). For women aged forty to forty-nine years old who have PCOS, there is a *fourfold* increase in risk of heart attacks compared to women this age without PCOS. PCOS also causes major mood symptoms that often get mistaken for bipolar illness and lead to overuse of psychotropic medications, some of which then make the PCOS worse.

Syndrome X, another mysterious metabolic-endocrine disorder common in women, is seen in premenopausal women and also known to be associated with a particularly high risk of having an early heart attack. Syndrome X is characterized by obesity, insulin resistance, high blood pressure, and high cholesterol. Both PCOS and Syndrome X, are often overlooked because gynecologists have been taught that you can have PCOS only if you have stopped menstruating (called amenorrhea) or have problems with infertility. Waistline weight gain, excess facial hair, and irregular menstrual periods were seen as "minor" or "cosmetic" problems that didn't need further evaluation. Unfortunately, even today, many physicians don't realize that PCOS has life-threatening consequences for the rest of a woman's life, possibly causing early death from a heart attack long before menopause. Don't let your concerns be dismissed with "Just lose weight" if you think you may have PCOS or Syndrome X.

CHRONIC FATIGUE AND WEIGHT

CFS is characterized by extreme tiredness, low energy, and a number of other symptoms, which I wrote about in my earlier book, *Screaming to Be Heard.* Seventy percent of patients with CFS are women. A large percentage of these women are also struggling with middle-body weight gain. I think it is crucial to look at what hormonal changes could be playing a role. If you recall that the hormone changes of midlife (declining estradiol, increasing levels of the male hormones, decreasing thyroid function, increasing insulin with insulin resistance, etc.) cause a great deal of weight gain and changes in blood sugar that provides our "energy," it is not surprising that fatigue is more common in this group of women as well. Since we know that the ovarian hormones have metabolic effects on every organ system in the body, we must check these hormone levels, as I outline in chapter 11, when we are evaluating fatigue problems in women.

CFS, as a syndrome of severe unrelenting fatigue, may have many causes and contributing factors. Loss of ovarian hormone levels may be only a part of the picture. But milder forms of fatigue and loss of "vitality" or "zest" are described by a large number of women experiencing major ovarian hormone changes: adolescents with PCOS, postpartum women with low ovary hormones as a result of suppression by nursing, or women with infertility and lower-than-optimal hormone levels, perimenopausal and menopausal women with naturally declining ovary hormone levels. Along with the fatigue, many of these women are also gaining excess body fat. Estradiol and testosterone in particular have significant activating or stimulating effects on energy level as well as our metabolism. Losing your optimal levels of these key metabolic hormones makes you feel more tired, slows down your metabolism, and contributes to weight gain that in turn makes you more tired, even if you don't have full-blown CFS.

FIBROMYALGIA AND WEIGHT

Fibromyalgia is a chronic pain syndrome characterized by diffuse muscle pain, multiple tender points throughout the body, weakness, sleep disturbance, and fatigue. More than 80 percent of sufferers are women, and most of these are in the midlife years. In *Screaming to Be Heard,* I wrote extensively about fibromyalgia and effects of estradiol loss in triggering and aggravating this syndrome; you may want to refer to that book for more information on these hormone-pain connections. So how does the chronic muscle pain of fibromyalgia contribute to your gaining weight, or becoming fatter?

One way is that this syndrome saps your energy and ability to exercise. In addition, when your muscles are stiff and sore, you don't feel like exercising. Lack of exercise added to the effects of low estradiol and testosterone, makes you lose more muscle mass with age, which shifts your body composition toward more fat tissue. Even if you have actually lost pounds, or haven't changed in dress size, the inactivity of fibromyalgia causes you to gradually and insidiously lose muscle and become fatter as time goes on. Fibromyalgia may also make you fatter because persistent pain itself is a trigger for increased cortisol output. Higher cortisol causes us to store more fat and break down muscle. Excess cortisol also makes you more insulin resistant, and means that you have more blood-sugar swings as your glucose-insulin pathways become unbalanced, as I describe in more detail in chapter 9.

DEPRESSION, MOOD CHANGES, AND WEIGHT GAIN

Nearly everyone has occasional times of down moods or bouts of sadness and discouragement that may last for a while. Women, more so than men, gain weight when they are depressed. How do we begin to sort out when these mood changes and "out-of-control" appetites mean hormonal problems or when they may indicate a major depression? One important clue is whether the low moods come only during the seven to ten days before your period, or whether they are there most all the time. Hormonal decline typically causes the mood changes to occur either during the premenstrual week (likely due to estradiol and progesterone being out of balance) or a day or two before bleeding begins, and the first few days of bleeding (likely due to the low estradiol at this time). Tearfulness, crying spells, fragmented sleep, anxiety attacks, palpitations, and irritability typically are intensified for these few days.

There is an additional mechanism by which perimenopausal women may experience anxiety attacks, depressive mood changes, and weight gain: When estradiol levels fall, this triggers hot flashes or night sweats that wake you up frequently. This may occur at night for several years prior to the beginning of skipped periods in perimenopause. When you aren't sleeping well night after night, coupled with a lot of stress and poor eating habits, you can expect to feel depressed, lethargic, and irritable! Plus, you can't remember things, you can't concentrate, and you just don't feel *well.* Then the stress of not sleeping, added to your daily woes, leads to increased cortisol and insulin, causing more fat storage. When these mood changes are happening as a result of low estradiol, women often respond better to hormone balancing than to antidepressants, antianxiety medications, or sleeping pills. Take a look at chapter 13 to see all the options you have to help you feel better.

STRESS: VICIOUS CYCLE EFFECTS ON HORMONES AND WEIGHT

We think of stress as just things that happen outside us in our lives. But *stress* refers to changes that may also occur in our internal body chemistry even when our life is going along well. Our brain is designed to take note of all these changes and stimuli, whether they come from inside our body or from outside in our daily life. The brain is a *physical* organ, as well as the psychological organ of "mind" that expresses our personality, psyche, and behavior. Many times what are labeled "psychological" symptoms may in fact be caused by biochemical changes in our body's physiological balance. Whether we are having external stressors or whether we have internal physiological changes that require the body to change and adapt, our body is the "final common pathway" through which these changes act and operate. An example is the "anxiety" feeling that comes when estradiol falls sharply with menstruation or when your blood sugar falls rapidly after you eat candy. This anxious feeling is the same response that occurs when you are also worried about something in your life. How do you tell the difference, since the symptom and feeling state is the same? This is where having lab tests can be very helpful to sort out the various causes, as I describe in chapter 11.

How does stress make you fat? This happens primarily through the extra release of various stress hormones, such as cortisol, that make our body store more fat in preparation for that "emergency." More cortisol release, or abnormal daily rhythms of cortisol production, causes more insulin resistance and more fat storage around our middles. Prolonged stress also disrupts the body's balance, or homeostasis, leading to symptoms from "adrenaline" overactivity, such as headaches, high blood pressure, panic attacks, colitis, irritable bowel, muscle tension, fatigue, and many others. Prolonged stress also causes illnesses due to adverse effects on the immune system. You may experience problems related to overactivity of the immune system such as asthma and allergies, or you could have problems related to an underactive immune system such as frequent infections, poor wound healing, or cancers. Sometimes, the immune system runs amuck and attacks your own body, leading to autoimmune disorders such as lupus or thyroiditis. All of these are manifestations of the combined effects of stress-induced biochemical changes on the body pathways, occurring over time.

For women, chronic stress packs another punch by decreasing ovarian hormone production, and it alters thyroid function as well. Since estradiol helps regulate the action of important chemical messengers that regulate mood, eating behavior, appetite, memory, and sleep (norepinephrine, serotonin, dopamine, and acetylcholine), the loss of estradiol then makes it harder for us to cope with psychosocial stressors when we used to be able to cope just fine. Once again, the role of stress is a two-way street: Life

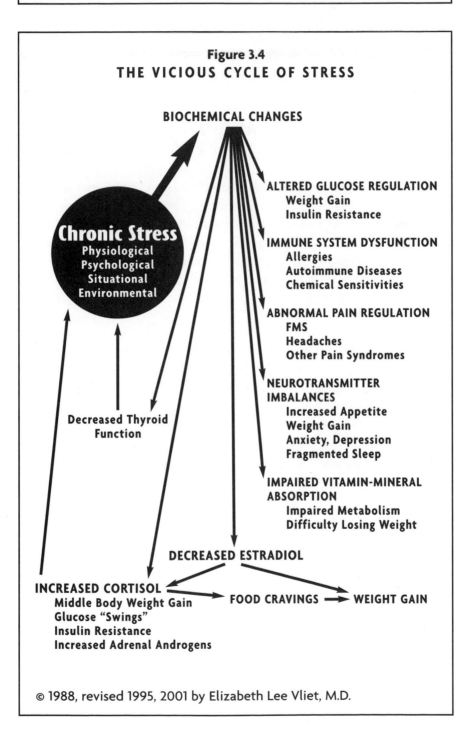

Figure 3.4
THE VICIOUS CYCLE OF STRESS

© 1988, revised 1995, 2001 by Elizabeth Lee Vliet, M.D.

stress suppresses the ovaries, which decreases estradiol production, which disrupts sleep, and so on. Getting older also decreases estradiol, which alters brain chemistry, which affects our ability to cope with stress, and we are stuck in another one of those vicious cycles, as I show in chapter 9.

HOW ARE ALL OF THESE PHENOMENA RELATED?

I have diagrammed these connections in figure 3.4 to show how I see these various stress and hormone factors coming together to cause some of the weight gain problems we see in women with the hormone changes I have been discussing. I see it much like a vicious cycle, with one event affecting another until it all snowballs on us. Think about these various pieces of the puzzle as they relate to your life, and your lifestyle habits, and see if it helps you identify some healthy ways to "break the cycle."

HORMONE IMBALANCE CAN BE A CULPRIT . . . HORMONE BALANCE AN ANSWER

PMS. PCOS. Postpartum depression. Premature menopause. Perimenopause. Weight gain. Depression. Fatigue. All have important implications for your health. All share common connections in occurring when you have lower-than-optimal levels of estradiol, with an imbalance of other important hormones, such as an excess of cortisol and/or your androgens.

Contrary to the popular myths and incorrect information about hormones perpetuated in a number of books and articles, it isn't the *estrogen* that is typically the culprit in weight gain at midlife. There are several bigger culprits in weight gain for women:

- ◇ the changing *ratios* of the ovarian estradiol and estrone
- ◇ the changing ratio of estradiol, DHEA, and testosterone
- ◇ taking excess progesterone relative to estrogen
- ◇ the effects of excess adrenal androgens and cortisol relative to estradiol

⋄ increased insulin levels as we age and lose the beneficial
regulating effects of estradiol

⋄ the gradual decline in thyroid function as we age

All of these hormone changes combine to give us a slower metabolism. Slower metabolism adds up to excess pounds of fat. Slower metabolism plus loss of muscle mass as testosterone and estradiol decline, plus more stress, plus less physical activity when we are tired and sluggish, plus more food intake than we need as we get older: they all add up to excess pounds of fat. In addition, once you start gaining weight, there is more insulin production. Increased insulin promotes more fat around the middle of the body. So there's an added wallop packing on the fat pounds! In order to keep your *pre*menopausal body shape, you need the *pre*menopausal balance of estradiol, testosterone, DHEA, thyroid hormones, cortisol, and insulin. Otherwise, you keep moving inexorably into more apple shape or paunch-pot.

The midlife years may be a time of "hoppin' hormones" and other changes in the body, but this doesn't mean you should resign yourself to not feeling your best. Midlife is a time to refocus, a time to pay attention to ourselves and take care of these wonderful gifts of our mind and body. The choices you make now, whatever your chronological age, have a major bearing on your weight and health for the future. First and foremost, you need to understand what is happening hormonally in your body that is making you gain weight. Then, you can start taking the steps to help you break out of the vicious cycle, as I outline in Part Three with *Your Hormone Power Life Plan.* Keep reading and I will help you tap into the power of your hormones to lose weight and feel better than ever.

Chapter 4

DECADES OF DIETS

AND WHY THEY DON'T WORK

As we age, we get fatter. Entrepreneurs have quickly figured out that there is lots of money to be made with diet products of all types. The hype is everywhere, and there are figures to show we are buying into the hype: Americans spend close to $40 billion annually on diets and diet-related products. The sad part is, 95 percent of people who are buying all these diets will regain the weight.

Fads in diets crop up faster than the weather changes. New diets sell products: books, tapes, flash cards, videos, cookbooks, supplements, special foods, prepared meals—you name it and there will be a product designed to go with the newest "diet of the day." There's a diet to suit every taste and every food craving. High carbohydrate, low protein is in. No, it's out. High protein, low carbohydrate is in. Don't mix protein and carbs at the same meal. Don't mix protein and fat at the same meal. Eat grapefruit at each meal to burn fat. Don't eat grapefruit, it will cause acid stomach.

1980: Margarine is okay, butter's bad. 1990: Margarine's bad, butter's better. 2000: Flaxseed oil and Benecol are the way to go. How do you make sense of all this? My suggestion: Don't try. It doesn't make sense, *it just sells*. How do you sort out fads from facts and find something that works for you? You're going to learn that here.

TIMES CHANGE AND SO DO OUR NEEDS

First, let's look at the changes over the last 100 years in the way Americans eat; this plays a role in our current epidemic of obesity. Sugar and fat are two examples. In the eighteenth century, sugar was such a rare and expensive "delicacy" that it was often kept under lock and key. Today, in the twenty-first century, sugar is so cheap and plentiful, we put it in everything, including soups, canned vegetables, even ketchup! Today the average American consumes an average of 150 pounds of sugar per year. (And if you think you don't eat that much, then consider that somebody else is eating your share, too.) Much of the sugar we eat is hidden. It appears in processed foods of all kinds, including condiments, salad dressings, frozen dinners, and the obvious sources: desserts and soft drinks. It's been calculated that the average American gets 24 percent of his or her daily calories from sugars in various forms, mainly refined sugar (sucrose).

Then comes the fat. Americans get, on average, 40 to 50 percent of their daily calories from fat, instead of the recommended range between 20 and 30 percent. That means 64 percent of the calories you eat every day comes from fat and sugar. No wonder Americans have more obesity and obesity-related diseases than any other country in the world.

Since simple sugars and fat have little nutritional value except providing energy, that means that most Americans have to get the essential nutrients from only 35 percent of their food intake. Higher fat intake (*sugar* was overlooked as a culprit) has been considered to be related to the rise in heart disease in the first half of the twentieth century, as more medical studies uncover the link between excess fat and blockages of arteries that lead to heart disease and strokes. But recent research has found that it is the combination of increased sugar with the excess fat that is the real culprit in the obesity explosion, especially for women.

DIETS ARE DESIGNED BY MEN, FOR MEN, BASED ON MALE METABOLISM

While most diets today claim to be based on medical studies, do you how they did those studies? It wasn't until after 1990 that medical research began including *women* in studies on major diseases and problems like weight gain. That means our historical understandings, and medical textbook teachings on everything except pregnancy, menopause, or birth control were based on men. Studies of diets and metabolism were also based on the "normal" person's being a *male*. It doesn't take a rocket scientist to know that men and women are very different when it comes to gaining and losing fat. Ask any husband and wife who have ever gone on a diet together! Men tend to peel off the pounds quickly, while for women, the process is excruciatingly s-l-o-w and agonizingly difficult.

In the early 1980s, as an outgrowth of studies by Pritikin and Ornish (on men, remember) showing that higher fat intake increased the risk of heart disease, fat became the enemy. Although the American Heart Association never changed its recommendations to much less than 30 percent dietary fat, Pritikin and Ornish effectively promoted extremely low-fat diets with only 10 to 15 percent of total caloric intake as fat and much higher intake of complex carbohydrates. Food manufacturers rushed to create lots of new and tasty foods that were, you guessed it, low in fat. But manufactured low-fat versions of high-fat foods can taste like cardboard, so the food designers needed to find a way to boost taste so people would buy these products. The designers were pretty savvy: They turned to sugar. The "low-fat" foods replace the fat with sugar.

But all that fat is gone, so it sounds pretty "healthy" doesn't it? Well, yes and no. Researchers, mostly men, who designed these dietary guidelines overlooked a fundamental fact of biology: Females have a very different hormonal makeup, very different physiological demands to accommodate pregnancy, very different amounts of muscle and fat, and a very different metabolism! Women were the unwitting bystanders in this game, and we suffered a dramatic rise in obesity as we strived to follow diets that didn't fit our needs because they were based on the body chemistry of men.

Do the same guidelines work equally well for women, given our very different hormonal makeup? Of course not. When researchers really studied women, they found that our female bodies use carbohydrates to *store* more fat, while men's bodies use carbohydrates for immediate fuel for energy. That means that when women follow the high-carbohydrate, low-fat diets (and that included me, until I realized what was happening), we are on the wrong meal plan balance for our unique metabolic makeup. Sugar becomes one of those examples where differences between men and women can pack a wallop in triggering weight gain.

From an evolutionary perspective, it makes sense that females would be more efficient at storing (and keeping) body fat, to carry pregnancies. Now we live in a culture that esteems thinness, makes eating a dominant social activity, rewards good behavior with ice cream or candy, and puts "fast food" options on every street corner. What insanity. Our bodies have not had several million years to adapt to the sudden availability of excess food, and we pay the price with an obesity epidemic in the United States.

Despite the thousands of pages written each year about obesity, there is very little in the magazines and books about the underlying differences between men and women. What we see every day at our *HER Place* medical practices is that women are struggling with weight gain while the unrecognized female *hormonal* factors are not addressed.

You can help improve the ratio of lean muscle mass to fat mass by exercising regularly and by the balance in the types of foods you eat. *But*, you cannot outwit Mother Nature and our basic male-female differences. I will explain ways the female hormones interact with appetite, weight, and fat storage to help you know how to work *with* women's biology rather than struggle *against* it using a diet based on men's bodies.

"DIETS" MAKE YOU FATTER

Have you ever lost weight on a diet? Did you lose more at the beginning and then reach a plateau where the scale seemed to taunt you by staying firmly in one place? Did you regain the lost weight? Did you find on your next diet that weight loss was even harder? If you answered yes to any of these questions, then you have experienced firsthand what I mean when I say *diets make you fatter.*

The primary problem with dieting is that your body "resets" its metabolic rate to a lower, slower one to allow for the fact that you're feeding it fewer calories. Your body then outwits you by becoming more efficient at getting and using the calories it needs to survive, and it also becomes more

WHY "DIETS" DON'T WORK
ROUND AND ROUND WE GO!

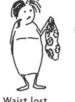

2. Eat less...
NO calories

1. Waist lost...
Upper body fat...
Hormones out of balance...
Let's go on a diet!

3. YES!
Five pounds!

10. Try the nation's #1
antidepressant to
recover

4. Then...no change
(Your rate of metabolism
has slowed)

9. No energy...
Depressed...
I give up!

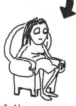

5. No energy...
Sense of failure...

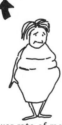

8. Slower rate of metabolism now...
Means more fat around waist...
MORE pounds

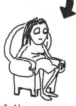

6. Vision of sweets
Food cravings
Think of food 24/7

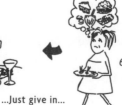

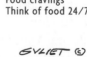

7. ...Just give in...
Overeating!

GVLIET ©

stingy about releasing its stores of fat, just in case there is a famine coming. So, your weight loss slows down, requiring you to cut calories even more. Next your body slows things again, and shifts more of your thyroid hormones into a less active, bound form to further slow your metabolism. As a result, your fat stores become even harder to use for fuel.

But since you, like most people, are unaware of all the ways your body outsmarts you, you keep cutting back on food trying to lose weight. Your thyroid becomes even less active. You feel more sluggish and tired and lack the energy to go out and exercise. But exercise is the one thing that will "rev up" your metabolism by stimulating the body to use more fuel; use its fat stores; make more muscle, which, in turn, uses more calories per minute than fat does; and improve your metabolic rate.

If you aren't eating enough calories to have the energy to exercise, or the right types of food to be able to build muscle, then your body slows down to adapt to the lower calorie intake. You know the drill: You get discouraged, depressed, angry over not losing weight, and you give up and binge on all those foods you have been craving since you cut them out. I know, I have done this a thousand times over the course of my life until I finally learned what I said at the beginning: *Diets don't work.*

What does work? Basic hormone balance + heathly eating + moving the body + being happy with yourself. These are the pieces of the puzzle that I will be exploring with you in *Your Hormone Power Life Plan.*

But first, let's look at times of hormone imbalance that cause us to gain weight.

"HORMONALLY CHALLENGED" TIMES OF OUR LIVES LEAD TO WEIGHT GAIN

Hormones. Weight gain. Women's fat-storing bodies versus men's fat-burning metabolism. Does menopause cause weight gain? Does taking hormones cause weight gain? What about those stubborn postpregnancy pounds? Is it estrogen or progesterone that makes women store fat? If estrogen, *which* estrogen is the culprit? Does testosterone cause weight gain for women, or help us burn fat? What about DHEA? Is it the culprit in all these sweet cravings that plague you, or does it help your body regulate sugars better? What's really going on with all this? And what does this mean for you as a woman? That's ultimately what this book is all about.

DR. VLIET'S GUIDE: WHEN WOMEN'S HORMONE-TRIGGERED WEIGHT GAIN IS MORE LIKELY TO OCCUR

⋄ Postpartum hormone decline if the ovaries don't come back into optimal function, particularly if the pregnancy was after age 30

⋄ Starting birth control pills with high progestin–low estrogen ratios, such as Loestrin, Mircette, Alesse, and others

⋄ 3 to 5 years after tubal ligation that causes disruption in ovarian blood flow and subtle declines in ovarian hormone production

⋄ Perimenopause, with our declining estradiol, declining thyroid function, increasing cortisol, and increasing "free" androgens

⋄ Postmenopause, particularly if *not on* hormone replenishment (HRT)

⋄ Using horse-derived estrogens (Premarin) and synthetic progestins (Provera and others)

⋄ Initial early (or prodromal) phase of a developing hypothyroidism, or thyroiditis, before TSH goes up to "abnormal" levels

⋄ 2 to 3 years after hysterectomy, especially if the ovaries were removed, but *weight gain may occur even if the ovaries were not removed* in the surgery, for similar reasons as given for tubal ligation

⋄ A period of sustained major stress or illness that interrupts menses for several months or longer and causes higher cortisol production

⋄ Starting corticosteroids, such as for asthma or arthritis

⋄ Viral illnesses that may affect the ovaries and interfere with normal hormone production, similar to what happens in viral thyroiditis

In chapter 3, I reviewed the hormones involved in regulating fat loss and gain in women, ones like estrogen, progesterone, testosterone, cortisol, insulin, thyroid (T3 and T4), leptin, GH, cholecystokinin (CCK), and many others. You will learn more about this hormone cast of characters as we journey together through the following chapters. But the ovary hormones are by far the biggest overlooked component in medical evaluations and therapies for weight loss in women. How do they fit with all the other fat-regulating hormones?

Contrary to popular belief, and contrary to many doctors' comments to women, there are some major shifts, changes, and imbalances in the hormones produced by the ovaries that contribute to more weight gain for women than men have to deal with. These powerful hormones from the ovary in turn have a major impact on every other system in the body, including your metabolism. This is very rarely addressed as a contributing factor in weight gain or loss for women.

You aren't imagining it. You do have a tendency to gain body fat at certain "hormonally challenged" times of your life, in spite of what your doctors may tell you.

All of these times in a woman's life are ones that can trigger hormone imbalances, hormone decline, and the onset of "menopausal" endocrine conditions that slow down our metabolism, make us store more fat, and change our body from the female "hourglass" (pear) to the male middle spread pattern (apple) of "toxic" weight gain.

A critical, but overlooked, factor in our gaining excess middle-body fat when we hit midlife is the loss of optimal levels of our premenopausal estrogen, 17-beta estradiol. Estradiol, which is more metabolically active, also tends to be lower in women who have experienced a surgical procedure that affected blood flow to the ovaries, such as a hysterectomy (even when the ovaries were left in place) or the bilateral tubal ligation (BTL) procedure. This "post–tubal ligation" syndrome (i.e., women having lower hormone levels after the surgery) has been well published in the medical literature, particularly in Europe. Yet, many doctors in the United States still tell patients there is no such thing.

Finally, in the year 2000, a group of researchers in this country decided to measure hormone levels and evaluate whether a "post–tubal ligation" syndrome exists. You guessed it. They found the same thing the European researchers had described over twenty-five years ago: lower estradiol; less regular ovulation; and an increase in perimenopausal-type symptoms such as insomnia, mood swings, headaches, and so forth in women following BTL.

Other factors that can contribute to these "middle-spreading" hormone imbalances are: overuse of progesterone creams to treat PMS or menopause symptoms, use of high-progestin birth control pills, use of "mood stabilizers" like Depakote and Tegretol that make you hungrier and eat more, use of beta blockers (such as for migraines or high blood pressure) that make you sluggish and more glucose intolerant, use of a variety of other medicines (such as antihistamines for allergies, tricyclic antidepressants, or steroids for asthma) that slow down your metabolism or increase your appetite . . . or worse yet, *do both.*

FROM THE STONE AGE TO THE COUCH POTATO AGE

Stone Age women and men were hunter-gatherers and burned a lot of calories hunting and gathering their food. They also ate more grains, nuts, berries, and fiber than we do, and ate meat more occasionally. Our enzyme systems evolved from this background—not from one with high-fat, high-sugar food on every corner. Because of our Stone Age ancestors, we were given the ability to store fat and draw upon it if food isn't available every day. Women, in particular, needed to effectively store fat in order to nourish a growing baby for nine months. Our primary female hormones help us with this task of "energy (fat) storage." Estradiol helps to regulate blood sugar to keep glucose levels steady, and it also enhances storage of fat around the hips, thighs, and buttocks, which provides "fuel" to help sustain pregnancy. Progesterone also helps with the pregnancy process by increasing our appetite so we will eat more to sustain mother and baby, and by promoting more storage of body fat through alterations on glucose-insulin pathways that increase our cravings for food (especially sweets). This effect of the "pro-gestational" hormone makes sense when you consider that an average pregnancy needs about 50,000 additional calories, and breastfeeding requires an added 1,000 calories a day. You don't want to try pregnancy or breastfeeding without some extra fat stores tucked away.

The plight of the Pima Indians (southwestern United States) today is an illustration of the disastrous consequences when people have evolved in environments of scarce food and are genetically more efficient at storing fat. When food is more plentiful, people genetically more efficient at storing fat will gain weight faster than others. Now that more food, and the wrong types, is available, Pima Indians have a staggering incidence of diabetes with all its complications, the highest of any ethnic group in the United States. But the rest of us aren't far behind. In the "land of plenty," more than half of all Americans are now overweight (more than 20 percent above desirable body weight), and 25 percent of adult women are obese (defined as more than 30 percent above desirable body weight). Obesity rates are rising dramatically in children as well, leading to the next generation of obese adults.

VICIOUS CYCLES: FOOD CRAVINGS AND THE MENSTRUAL CYCLE

Over my years of clinical practice, I would say that about 75 to 85 percent of women patients have described cyclic food cravings that are clearly related to the second half of the menstrual cycle. And these cravings are the kind of intense urges that override rational awareness that junk foods aren't healthy! Women have often described going out late in the evening just to buy chocolate (or something salty or whatever) because the craving was so strong. I have to admit, I did that myself on occasion when the premenstrual "have-to-have-chocolate" urges hit! Why is this? And why is it that I have never had a male patient describe cravings for chocolate the way women do?

Recent research has confirmed what women have always suspected: we get hungrier the week before our periods, due to the rise in progesterone. Appetite increases about 12 to 15 percent in the second half of the menstrual cycle. If you ignore this increase in appetite because you are dieting, you may find that the sweet cravings become uncontrollable, leading to the binge-on-sweets-feel-guilty-starve-again-then-binge-again cycle. It has been described since the 1930s, and perhaps even earlier, that women have altered glucose regulation in the luteal (progesterone-dominant) phase of the menstrual cycle.

I will go into more detail later in the book. For now, you need to know that there is a key hormonal factor that affects women and contributes to these cravings: the rise and fall in progesterone during the second half of the menstrual cycle. Progesterone makes you *less* sensitive to your insulin, the hormone that regulates blood glucose (sugar) levels. After eating simple

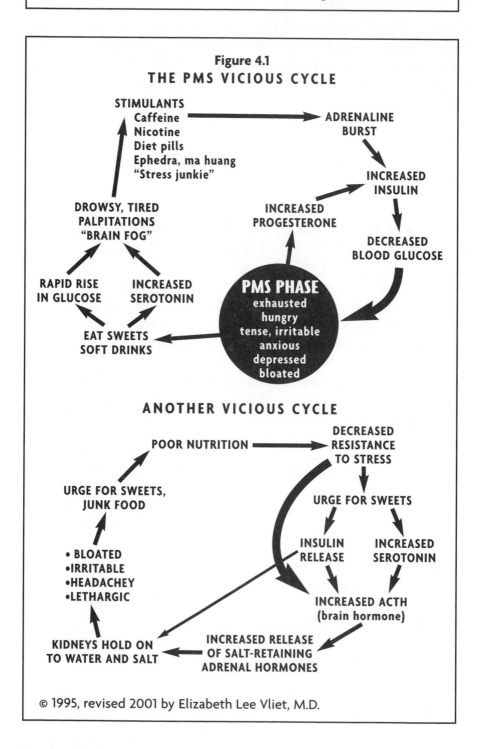

Figure 4.1
THE PMS VICIOUS CYCLE

STIMULANTS
  Caffeine
  Nicotine
  Diet pills
  Ephedra, ma huang
  "Stress junkie"

ADRENALINE BURST

INCREASED INSULIN

INCREASED PROGESTERONE

DECREASED BLOOD GLUCOSE

DROWSY, TIRED PALPITATIONS "BRAIN FOG"

RAPID RISE IN GLUCOSE

INCREASED SEROTONIN

PMS PHASE
exhausted
hungry
tense, irritable
anxious
depressed
bloated

EAT SWEETS SOFT DRINKS

ANOTHER VICIOUS CYCLE

POOR NUTRITION

DECREASED RESISTANCE TO STRESS

URGE FOR SWEETS, JUNK FOOD

URGE FOR SWEETS

INSULIN RELEASE

INCREASED SEROTONIN

• BLOATED
•IRRITABLE
•HEADACHEY
•LETHARGIC

INCREASED ACTH (brain hormone)

KIDNEYS HOLD ON TO WATER AND SALT

INCREASED RELEASE OF SALT-RETAINING ADRENAL HORMONES

© 1995, revised 2001 by Elizabeth Lee Vliet, M.D.

sugars at this time of the month, when blood sugar levels tend to be low, you are more likely to have a "reactive" drop in blood glucose, creating the desire for more sweets. On the other hand, if you eat more protein—balanced with fruit, vegetables, and whole grain breads high in complex carbohydrates—during the progesterone-dominant second half of the menstrual cycle, you provide the fuel needed to sustain blood glucose during this time. The result is that you are less likely to give in to the cravings for sweets that lead you to overeat, the main culprit in adding excess pounds. I explain this in more detail in the chapter on progesterone. Take a look at "The Vicious Cycles" (fig. 4.1) and see if you recognize yourself!

THE VICIOUS CYCLE AND ANOTHER VICIOUS CYCLE

Eating sweets not only causes a rapid rise in blood sugar that gives you a brief "energy boost," it also causes an increase in serotonin in the brain. However, if there is too rapid a rise in brain serotonin from a big load of sweets, it causes drowsiness, palpitations, and nervous/anxious feelings. Then when you're feeling drowsy, you often turn to what's quick and readily available: caffeine, sweets, or maybe the nicotine in cigarettes. These all trigger release of the chemical messengers that affect insulin, which in turn drops the blood sugar, and there goes the cycle again. Sound familiar?

A more gradual rise in serotonin can cause a sense of calming, much like a tranquilizing medication. Actually, sweets are nature's original "tranquilizing drugs." Women who binge on sweets are actually using food as a drug in terms of its effect on the brain. I've had patients say to me, "I don't want to take an antianxiety medicine or antidepressant. I don't want to take any drugs. I want to use natural things." But they don't realize they are using food as a drug. They are stunned when I point this out.

Alcohol also is digested to a simple sugar, causing a rapid rise in blood glucose and a surge in insulin. This makes women alcoholics particularly vulnerable to intensified alcohol cravings the week before their periods when progesterone is high, especially if estradiol is declining. Over the course of my career, I have consistently found that it is the progesterone-dominant (luteal) phase of the menstrual cycle when women alcoholics tend to "fall off the wagon."

FIT DOESN'T MEAN SKINNY

Most women are obsessed with the scale and what they weigh, certainly in large part due to the cultural brainwashing that to be thin is to be desirable and acceptable as a woman.

I would like to introduce you to the concept that *body composition*—the relative proportion of fat to muscle, bone, and other lean tissue—is more important than body weight. Body weight can vary immensely depending upon how much muscle mass you have built up and what your build is. Body composition can be measured as weight is, but a body composition measurement is a much better picture of good health than how much you weigh. One patient of mine is a young, petite, thin woman (size 4) who is sedentary. Her body composition showed that she had 34 percent body fat. For women over thirty, healthy ranges are about 25 to 30 percent body fat. This woman is in an unhealthy "at risk" range, although she looks terrific as a size 4, by societal standards. Another patient, who wears a size 14 and appears "heavier," is actually healthier at 25 percent body fat, achieved by regular exercise and weight training three times a week. The second patient isn't "thin" by today's images, but she is fit, strong, and healthy. The size 4 woman isn't. Fit doesn't mean skinny.

The way to really determine your optimal weight is to have a body composition test to measure percent body fat. For women, the optimal ranges are between 22 and 30 percent body fat. If you are over thirty, you lose less bone if your body fat is about 25 percent. Body fat greater than 33 percent increases health risk. If you're over age thirty and aiming for less than 20 percent body fat, you increase your risk of osteoporosis. But a woman of any age who stays below 20 percent body fat loses bone rapidly, risking her health. This happens because you lose the natural estrogen "reservoir" in body fat tissue, leading to negative effects on your health.

Even though you've hit forty and still wear the same size that you did in your twenties, your body shape may be quite different. You may notice larger breasts, larger upper arms, larger waist, and smaller hips than you used to have. This happens because, as we age, our body fat is stored in different places and our body composition changes. The ongoing Fels Longitudinal study on aging shows that both women and men had age-related increases in weight, total body fat, and percentage of body fat during the period from 1976 to 1996. Those who had the higher levels of physical activity predictably had lower percentages of body fat. Women generally experienced a *change in body composition* rather than a *loss of weight*. In other words, women who exercised didn't necessarily lose weight. They lost body fat and gained lean muscle for an overall better appearance, improved energy level, and sense of well-being. The women who did not exercise ended up gaining weight, gaining body fat, and *losing* lean muscle mass—the opposite of what you want to feel well and maintain your ideal weight.

Menopause also made a difference. The longer a woman had been postmenopausal, the higher the proportion of body fat to lean body mass. This is due to the gain in body fat as we lose our metabolically active hormones from the ovary after menopause. *Those who took estrogen, however, lost* less *lean body mass, and had* lower *body fat percentage.* Many studies have shown that women taking hormones after menopause actually have lower percent body fat, on average, than women who don't take hormones. And keep in mind, if you are a postmenopausal woman who wants to maintain a healthy body composition, the equation seems to be

E2 (the proper estrogen) + Ex (exercise) = a healthy body

If you *weigh* a little more after beginning hormone therapy, it is usually *not* due to a gain in body fat; it is due to the muscle-and-bone-building effects of estradiol (and testosterone, if you take this hormone, too). You will have a lower percentage of body fat due to the increase in lean body mass. If you are starting on hormones, or are beginning to exercise regularly again, *don't weigh on a scale!* Your body *weight* is not going to be an accurate indicator of the loss of fat tissue because fat weighs about one sixth as much as muscle tissue. It is much more accurate, and helpful, to do body measurements to show the changes. Loss of inches will give you a much better picture of the amount of fat loss. When you increase the lean body mass by taking hormones or starting to exercise, you won't realize that you're losing "lightweight" body fat as you build up heavier muscle mass if you only step on the scale to check your progress. I usually recommend that you ignore the scale, and just take your body measurements about once a month. Throw the scale away! Focus on what's happening to the health of your body, not on the number of pounds.

THE PERFECT DIET

This book is not another diet book to perpetuate the compulsion to be thin. It is the missing link to explain weight loss connections for women that other diet programs simply are not addressing adequately. *Taking* hormones does not cause weight gain, but hormonal *imbalance* does. What works, plain and simple, is a three-pronged approach: balanced eating throughout the day + optimal hormone balance + regular exercise.

If you don't have stable food intake, a fall in blood sugar sets off the brain alarm center, ramps up the stress response with cortisol release, and amplifies the hunger signals. Your body won't start burning fat effectively unless you give it the right kinds of foods in the right amounts throughout the day. This approach also provides a steady supply of fuel and helps prevent the insulin overshoots that make you store more fat. So all the way around, you will feel better, have more energy, and lose weight more effectively if you eat smaller portions at regular intervals. Then, hormone balance is the second leg to your diet stool. I'll show you how to achieve that in a later chapter. Regular exercise is the third leg to balance your program.

Once all the "legs" are in place, start building your "seat" of self-esteem. Rather than listening to external noises, listen to your internal voice. What matters to you most? Focus on changes that will make you feel better first. When you feel better you are better equipped both physically and emotionally to make further changes. Slowly, with each small step of success, you will see and feel a big difference. Compare yourself with *your* desired goals, appreciate *your* accomplishments, and celebrate *your* magnificent body. Don't be swayed by pressures around you. Go for what is right for *you*. You will be successful, and remain successful, because you did it for the right reason: for *you*.

Part Two

The Hormone Cast of Characters:

WHAT YOU NEED TO KNOW ABOUT YOUR HORMONES AND WEIGHT LOSS

Hormones are the chemical messengers that are secreted by the endocrine-reproductive organs in our body and then travel via the blood to organs and tissues of the body where they stimulate a specific activity or response. In short, hormones make our entire body function properly. It is important to understand just what the various hormones do, and their role in healthy weight regulation if you want to lose excess fat, or if you have been struggling with other troubling hormone-triggered symptoms. We all take our health for granted when we feel well and energetic. But, you would not be reading this book if you did not have some health concerns that you want addressed . . . am I right? So I want to help you become your own "health detective" to unravel these elusive hormone connections in your problems.

When our hormones are in balance and everything is operating optimally, we feel good, have the energy we desire, and are able to keep an active lifestyle as well as maintain our ideal weight. I have designed this section of the book to help you understand what is happening to your hormones as you hit midlife (or run into *any* of the "hormone challenges" I described in chapter 4), and how these hormonal changes affect your weight and health. This section helps you see the role each hormone plays in your body. It helps you use symptoms like weight gain, insomnia, low energy, and others to give you clues to the presence of hormone imbalances that sabotage your weight-loss efforts. With this information, you will be able to have a knowledgeable conversation with your doctor. You will need an open-minded physician, one who will work with you as a partner in finding constructive solutions. You will also need a physician who is willing to order the proper tests to clarify what is happening with your body, work with you to fine-tune medication prescriptions, and help you find the right balance for your body. Finding the right doctor, and getting your hormonal balance "fine-tuned," is not always easy or quick. I give you pointers on how to do that later in this section. This is a journey of many small changes along the way to your destination of a healthy, fit body and mind. This journey is well worth the trip!

Chapter 5

ESTROGEN AND YOUR WEIGHT

Have you been told that estrogen causes weight gain? Have you been told that taking estrogen makes you fat? Most of us have heard these statements. But are they really true? Why is it that *young* women with *higher* estrogen levels tend to be less fat than older menopausal women? Is there more to this picture than you may have realized? The answer is *yes.* I want to help you understand the new research that shows how our premenopausal estrogen, estradiol (E2), actually helps us keep a leaner body and improves our metabolism. I want to clarify the confusion about types of estrogen and which ones do what in your body. There is so much negative, misleading, and incorrect information in the media and other women's health books about estrogen and weight gain, I want you to forget what you may have heard before, and focus on what is presented here. If you begin to wonder who to believe, trust your instincts and your life experience. When in your life as a woman did *you* have less difficulty maintaining your weight? Trust what makes sense to you.

WOMEN'S THREE TYPES OF
ESTROGEN AND WHAT THEY DO

Women have three types of estrogen: estrone (E1), estradiol (E2), and estriol (E3). The relative amounts of each of these estrogens is determined by many factors: genetic makeup, age, amount of body fat, pregnancy, type of diet, and the presence of medical conditions or lifestyle habits that interfere with healthy hormone production. Estradiol is the form we lose at midlife making us more likely to get fatter, for all the reasons we shall see as you read further. Since there are three very different types with different actions, it becomes confusing to use the same term *estrogen* to refer to all three. Throughout this book, I will use primarily *estradiol* (or *17-beta estradiol*) to refer to the premenopausal form that is more metabolically active and more critical for all the health benefits we associate with *estrogen*. To make all this easier to remember, think of your estrogen as a cast of characters that I will refer to as the Good (E2), the Bad (E1), and while "the Ugly" isn't quite appropriate for E3, this reference may still help you remember that E3 doesn't do the "good" things that E2 does.

17-beta estradiol (E2; "the Good")

This is the primary biologically active estrogen and the major functioning estrogen for our bodies from puberty until menopause; it is responsible for over four hundred functions in the female body—everything from healthy eyes to youthful skin, strong bones and muscles, as well as our normal sexual responses and reproduction. After menopause, when the ovary no longer has follicles to make hormones, we lose our source of 17-beta estradiol. Loss of E2 causes the postmenopausal changes in skin, bone, hair, heart and blood vessels, brain, and other organs. Other hormone-producing body tissues can't make up for this loss of E2, and we are left with only the estrone (E1) made in fat tissue. E1 is a poor substitute for our E2—you'll soon read why. Ideally, if you decide to take estrogen therapy after menopause, it's best to choose a form of 17-beta estradiol to provide exactly the same chemical molecule your ovary has been making since puberty.

Estrone (E1; "the Bad")

This is the predominate estrogen found in postmenopausal women because it can still be made in the fat tissue when our ovaries are no longer producing E2. Estrone (E1) is the form of estrogen that many researchers think may be related to the higher risk of endometrial and breast cancer seen in older women who are obese. Before menopause, estrone is made by the ovary, the adrenal glands and liver, as well as in body fat. Estrone serves primarily as a reservoir (storage pool) for the body to make more estradiol, but most of this conversion takes place in our ovaries before menopause. *After menopause, very little estrone is converted to estradiol because the ovaries cease to function.* Estrone does continue to be produced in the body fat, and to a much smaller extent the liver and adrenal glands. The more body fat a woman has (before or after menopause) the more estrone is present.

Estriol (E3)

The weakest of the human estrogens, estriol is produced by the placenta during pregnancy and is not normally present in measurable amounts in nonpregnant women. Several thousand studies on estriol over the last thirty to forty years have confirmed that it does not preserve normal bone; does not improve memory, cognitive function, mood, or sleep; and does not give us the cardiovascular benefits we achieve with estradiol. In spite of what you may have read in other books implying that estriol will do all you need, there actually are hundreds of well-done scientific studies showing that you don't have the same positive results using estriol as we see with estradiol. Makes sense, since estradiol was Mother Nature's gift to make our bodies work the way they were designed!

ESTROGEN RECEPTOR BASICS

Hormones are part of the body's great communication system to make our body work properly. When a hormonal message is sent, there have to be "receptors" throughout the body so that our organs can receive and act on the message. Your body has estrogen-receptor sites everywhere: the brain, heart, lungs, blood vessels, muscles, bone, intestinal tract, urinary bladder, uterus, ovaries, breasts, vagina, skin, and even your eyes. Different organs have varying types and concentrations of estrogen receptors, so the picture is actually quite complex. But one of the critical requirements to get the right message through is having enough 17-beta estradiol available as needed at the receptor site. E2 is the most effective "estrogen" key to activate the estrogen receptors to do this. Think about it. If estrone could activate the estrogen receptors in the same way as estradiol, you wouldn't have all these unwanted changes in your body at menopause!

ESTROGEN AND YOUR BODY

With four hundred bodily functions affected by estrogen, you can see that it is a vital part of almost everything that our bodies do. Recent studies, too detailed to describe here, indicate that estradiol has a major role to play in maintaining a healthy weight and normal metabolism. What are some of the effects when our premenopausal estrogen declines during all of those times I described in chapter 4? Let's take a look:

- ⋄ Loss of E2 means more fat in the abdominal and internal "visceral" fat deposits. These "toxic" fat deposits produce more estrone, more androgens, and higher cortisol, which, in turn, increase the risk of diabetes, heart disease, and breast cancer.
- ⋄ Lower E2 means less fat around the hips and thighs, a healthier place for women to carry fat.
- ⋄ Loss of E2 means we don't build muscle tissue that is as healthy and resistant to daily "wear and tear."
- ⋄ Declining E2 is a stress that makes cortisol rise, causing more fat storage.
- ⋄ Rising cortisol and falling E2 interfere with normal thyroid function.
- ⋄ Loss of E2 makes insulin *less* effective at lowering glucose, *more* effective at storing fat, leading to increased insulin resistance.
- ⋄ When insulin resistance increases, we get fatter around our middle.

⋄ Increased insulin causes more androgen production, which in turn also causes more middle-body fat.

⋄ Falling E2 disrupts our sleep, leading to *less* GH secreted during sleep, and more cortisol release, which results in more fat storage.

⋄ GH decreases means more *loss* of lean muscle, more body fat.

⋄ More sleep disruption and less estradiol means less muscle repair at night, adding to loss of muscle mass.

And this list isn't comprehensive, just some of the most important metabolic effects that occur when we lose this crucial hormone. Now that we are living longer, you can see why it is so important to maintain a healthy level of estradiol since it has so many functions that are important in maintaining good health. Remember what I said earlier:

$$E2 + Ex = HB \text{ (healthy body!)}$$

Then, of course, you can add a healthy meal plan to complete the equation!

ESTROGEN, BODY COMPOSITION, AND WEIGHT

As you know, I don't believe in scales. I'd rather have you feel good about how you look, about how your clothing fits, and about your muscle tone. Unfortunately, muscle tone and muscle mass are quickly lost when our estradiol declines. It has been known for many years that estradiol has marked positive effects in heart muscle and smooth muscle (such as in the intestine and bladder) to improve contraction strength, improve tone, and help develop new muscle mass. Estradiol's effects on skeletal muscle have been researched more fully over the last two decades in both menopause and sports medicine centers. We are finding that estradiol enhances several aspects of skeletal muscle function in women: force of contraction, how long before the muscle is fatigued, and how quickly the muscles relax.

For example, Cauley, et al., compared hand-grip strength, physical activity, estrogen use, and body composition measures in women with or without hormone therapy at menopause. This study showed a decrease in hand-grip strength as estradiol declined. Notelovitz (1991) further confirmed this connection: Women working out with variable resistance weight training had greater improvements in muscle strength if they were taking estrogen compared to women using similar weight-training programs but not taking estrogen. Jensen (1986) and Kyllonen (1991) found that high-dose post-menopausal hormone therapy improved body composition by increasing muscle mass and proportionately decreasing body fat. Overall body weight remained unchanged (explained by the fact that muscle tissue weighs about six times as much as fat). In addition to the improvement in muscle strength, women who combined estrogen with weight training also had greater increase in bone mass than did women who used weight training alone. These studies also found that women with higher body weight (and there-fore more hormonally active muscle and fat) had greater muscle strength and bone density. These are added reasons not to be too thin as we get older!

Hormone changes during the menstrual cycle also affect our muscle strength and contraction ability. In young women twenty to thirty years old, Phillips, et al., (1993) showed that muscle strength was highest around the time of ovulation when estradiol levels were at their peak. Muscle strength declined at other times of the menstrual cycle when estradiol was lower, such as bleeding days or the progesterone dominant week before the period. In another study, Phillips, et al., (1993) found that muscle strength declined at menopause, but there was no decrease in strength if women were taking estrogen therapy. Sarwar (1996) found that the menstrual cycle hormone changes caused significant variation in muscle strength, fatigability, and relaxation times for the forearm and thigh (quadriceps) muscles in young women. The greatest muscle strength and least fatigabil-ity corresponded to the cycle phase with highest estradiol levels. Women taking oral contraceptives with steady hormone levels did not have this variation in muscle function through the menstrual cycle.

Collectively, these and other studies show that we lose muscle when our estradiol decreases, and muscle strength and mass increase when we restore estradiol to optimal levels. Other studies have shown additional estradiol effects on muscle: as a membrane stabilizer and antioxidant, two effects that help prevent muscle damage from the buildup of free radicals during exercise or after-exercise inflammatory response. This means if we lose estradiol, our muscles are more easily damaged during our daily activ-ities or exercise and don't repair as quickly as they do if our estradiol levels are optimal.

Remember, muscles burn more calories than other tissues. If we lose muscle mass, we are losing our most effective fat-burning machinery, so our metabolism slows even more. To maintain a healthy body weight, it is critical to have optimal hormone levels along with exercise to maintain our muscle mass.

OTHER METABOLIC EFFECTS OF ESTRADIOL

Aloia, et al., (1991) found an increased rate of potassium loss as women lost estradiol when approaching menopause. When estradiol is optimal before menopause, there is very little potassium loss. As we know, potassium balance is crucial for healthy muscle function as well as multiple metabolic pathways. Estradiol also helps absorption of calcium, magnesium, and zinc. All of these minerals are needed for our body's enzymes to work properly in metabolism as well as for making healthy bone and allowing our muscles to work properly.

Estradiol also improves the "good" cholesterol, HDL, and lowers both the "bad" cholesterol (LDL) and total cholesterol. High total and LDL cholesterol are often found in people who are overweight, so this is another positive metabolic benefit of restoring estradiol to optimal levels. The "patch" form of estradiol also lowers triglycerides, a blood fat that is often increased in overweight women and leads to a higher risk of becoming diabetic. Estradiol improves platelet function, leading to less platelet "stickiness," which can cause blood clots, another problem that occurs at higher frequency in overweight women. All of these metabolic problems that are more common in overweight women lead to higher rates of both diabetes and heart disease, so these are additional reasons that estradiol needs to be optimal if you are struggling with excess weight at midlife.

Estradiol facilitates the release of GH during Stage IV sleep. Progesterone, on the other hand, suppresses GH production. Why is this important if you are trying to lose weight? GH stimulates muscle growth and repair, and overweight women often have lost a great deal of healthy muscle mass. GH decreases as we approach menopause, in part triggered by the decrease in our ovarian estradiol. If your estradiol and GH are lower than optimal, it means you don't get the full benefit of exercise to build muscle. I describe these hormone effects on GH in more detail in chapter 6, where I will compare the estrogen and progesterone effects.

We have often been told that only testosterone helps build muscle in men and in women. But these new studies illustrate the many ways that estradiol also helps us maintain healthy muscles that, in turn, help our body burn excess fat. So let's now revise my equation:

E2 (estradiol) + Ex (Exercise) = *Lean* HB (healthy body!)

There are many, many other brain-body functions and benefits of our estradiol that I do not have space to describe in this book. I have just focused here on those that are most directly involved in weight regulation. If you'd like to read more about this critical hormone, I suggest you turn to *Screaming to Be Heard.*

ESTROGEN EFFECTS ON SEROTONIN AND OTHER MOOD REGULATORS

Some of you may remember that we use serotonin-boosting medicines to help reduce appetite and make weight loss easier. Studies over the past three decades have shown that reduced serotonin levels are related to excess weight gain as well as to other problems such as depressed mood, increased irritability, increased generalized anxiety, increased pain sensitivity, eating disorders, obsessive-compulsive disorders, and disruption of normal sleep cycles.

Did you know that Mother Nature gave you a natural "serotonin booster" in the estradiol made by your ovary? Many factors affect serotonin balance. The loss of estradiol at the times I outlined in chapter 4 is a key gender difference and leads to women losing optimal serotonin function and then having greater susceptibility to weight gain as well as depression and suicide. Other factors that decrease serotonin production and increase serotonin breakdown are aging, the effect of prolonged stress, chronic alcohol overuse, regular use of certain medications (decongestants for allergies, some asthma medicines), and cigarette smoking.

In women who have not had a hysterectomy or tubal ligation, the gender difference in rapid weight gain and depression is most marked in those aged forty-five to forty-nine, when estradiol is typically decreasing most rapidly. While these changes are occurring, women often tell me they feel like they are on an emotional roller coaster ride. Most of us don't like to feel so out of control, especially when we can't seem to explain what is happening to us. You aren't being a hypochondriac. Your body *is* changing, and it affects not only your mood, but also your metabolism and your fat-storing pathways.

Ovarian hormones also have been found to have effects on several other mood-altering brain chemicals: endorphins (the "morphine within" pain reliever), oxytocin, vasopressin, and prolactin. All of these brain hormones are involved in appetite, metabolism, and body weight set-point control. So when your estradiol declines, it is also affecting these other weight-regulating hormones in undesirable ways.

High estradiol levels in late pregnancy contribute to high levels of endorphins in human females. We eat less when the endorphins are high. Lower endorphin levels make us more anxious, irritable, or depressed; then we eat more to feel better, and we gain weight. When the baby is delivered, there is a sharp drop in both estradiol and progesterone, and this triggers a rapid drop from the high endorphin levels of the last few weeks of pregnancy. This "withdrawal" from our endorphins is similar to withdrawal from morphine, causing irritability, tearfulness, anxiety, stomach upset, diarrhea, and sweating. I think the drop in endorphins triggered by the abrupt hormone "crash" plays a role in women's difficulty losing weight after delivery . . . unless we work hard to increase endorphins, for example, with exercise.

SLEEP DISORDERS AND WEIGHT GAIN

Almost all overweight people have some degree of sleep disturbance, in part related to a heavier upper chest that makes it harder to breathe deeply during sleep and adds to the possibility of sleep apnea. It is sometimes hard to say which comes first, a chronic sleep disturbance or being overweight, so I prefer to view it as an integrated problem and try to identify ways of constructively breaking the cycle. For example, in women, estradiol plays a key role in overseeing normal sleep patterns, so when it declines, our sleep gets quite disrupted. Simply taking sleeping pills doesn't get to the underlying cause. Besides, sleeping pills don't improve all the other metabolic changes that occur when estradiol declines.

We now know that sleep disorders play a very big role in weight gain, based on studies from sleep laboratories. Here, patients sleep in a laboratory "bedroom" wearing monitors that keep track of brain wave patterns, muscle activity, eye movements, heart rate, breathing rate, oxygen concentration in the blood, and a number of other measures of the quantity and quality of sleep. Obese women typically show a marked degree of fragmented sleep. They have more overall waking episodes at night, and more interruptions of the deepest or most restful stage of sleep (Stage IV). Stage IV sleep is important in repairing tissue damage and feeling physically and psychologically rested when you wake up. If Stage IV sleep is reduced, it can contribute to loss of energy as well as decline in your muscle mass. In addition, women develop sleep apnea at greater frequency than men, and this disorder increases during perimenopause and menopause. The more overweight a woman is, the more likely she is to develop sleep apnea.

Restless, fragmented sleep along with less Stage IV sleep are additional reasons that overweight women describe feelings of daytime fatigue. Fatigue can also be due to the decline in estradiol and lower testosterone that sap your energy. Since we know that *both* sleep problems and decreased ovarian hormones lead to less muscle growth and repair, you then have even less ability to burn fat over the course of each day because you have less muscle mass. The combination of weight gain and fatigue then often limits physical activity and endurance. So you don't burn as many calories each day, and the resulting lack of physical exercise contributes to the unfit muscles . . . leading to more weight gain. It is an awful trap, leaving you feeling like you are stuck in quicksand and can't get out.

If you have trouble going to sleep, you may find yourself turning to alcohol thinking it will help you sleep better. The problem with alcohol, especially for women with midlife middle spread, is that alcohol makes your sleep *more* fragmented and causes more *loss* of Stage IV sleep. Alcohol is also metabolized as a simple sugar, which stimulates excess insulin and makes your body store more fat. This effect is even worse if you drink alcohol at night, which of course is what you do if you are using it to help you sleep!

Daily alcohol use also further suppresses ovarian hormone levels and shifts your estrogen balance toward more *estrone.* Alcohol diminishes production of endorphins, the brain chemicals that help regulate appetite and lift mood and are natural painkillers. When alcohol is wearing off, it creates an adrenaline rebound, which leads to more disrupted sleep, increased muscle tension, and more damage to muscle fibers. Another problem is that drinking alcohol makes you *hungrier,* and it is giving you nutritionally "empty" calories. As if all these bad effects aren't enough, alcohol significantly increases your risk of breast cancer if you drink more than one drink a day on a regular basis. If you want to lose excess body fat, sleep well, be energetic, have a healthy sex drive, and do all you can to reduce your risk of breast cancer, a helpful strategy is to cut out alcohol.

TESTS FOR ESTRADIOL LEVELS

The blood test for estradiol is highly reliable and commonly used in infertility evaluations today. While there is some variation over the course of a day, and throughout the menstrual cycle, the variation is no greater than other tests, such as cholesterol, that we use regularly. We simply learn how to take this variation into account in our interpretations. I use the estradiol blood test to help in both evaluation and treatment for women with hormone-related problems. If you are still menstruating, I check these levels on Day 1–3 (early follicular phase), and again on Day 20–21 (luteal phase peak). Make sure that your doctor checks *estradiol*, not "total estrogens."

In my clinical work with women, I find that we typically have our best energy level, mood, sleep, and memory when serum (blood) levels of estradiol are *above* 90 to 100 pg/ml. This is the *lower* end of the range for healthy menstrual cycle levels. Levels up to about 200 or so are the *normal estradiol levels* reached in the first half of the menstrual cycle before ovulation. At ovulation, estradiol levels are typically in the range of 300 to 500 pg/ml, and then in the luteal phase of the cycle (when progesterone is produced), a healthy level of estradiol is generally in the range of 200 to 300 pg/ml. After menopause, women typically have estradiol levels of only 10 to 30 pg/ml, a far cry from the levels we have been used to our entire adult life.

Estradiol levels below about 90 pg/ml are generally too low to provide adequate relief of symptoms from hot flashes to muscle/joint pain, insomnia, memory loss, and middle spread, not to mention helping us achieve our usual energy and zest and having our normal feeling of well-being. International research has found that bone loss continues to occur with estradiol levels *below* about 80 to 90 pg/ml. Cardiovascular benefits of estradiol have been found to occur at levels *above* about 80 to 90 pg/ml as a starting point. Memory, sleep, and concentration typically improve the most if estradiol levels are above 100 pg/ml. Therefore, I suggest you look for a level of about 90 or better and then correlate this with your symptoms to see whether you have reached an optimal level for your body. It's fairly straightforward to know if you are getting too much estradiol—your breasts feel uncomfortably full and tender. Your blood tests are a guide, but *how you feel* is also important in deciding what dose or type is best for you.

SUMMARY

We have only begun to scratch the surface of appreciating how widespread are these estrogen connections in weight management. You may have been told that estrogen *causes* weight gain, but I hope this chapter has helped you to see clearly that there are many ways that healthy levels of our premenopausal estradiol actually help our metabolism work *better.* You aren't imagining it—we do tend to get fatter as we approach menopause. And, there is something you can do about it, now that you understand some of these connections between our estradiol and the brain's own weight-regulating messenger molecules. Certainly, it is straightforward to check estradiol levels and consider this hormone a part of an overall treatment approach.

As you have seen, there is a wealth of clinical and basic science research that shows the many ways loss of estradiol affects change in body fat deposition, metabolic rate, muscle metabolism and function, along with estrogen's effects on mineral absorption, serotonin production, and other hormones involved in weight regulation. And I haven't even discussed all the other known crucial ways estradiol helps maintain our health as we get older. You may want to read about all those in *Screaming to Be Heard.* I realize that this is complex, but I hope I have helped you see that new insights and approaches are available if you have been struggling with unrelenting weight gain.

ESTRADIOL EFFECTS THAT HELP WEIGHT LOSS

◇ improves insulin sensitivity, which improves fat burning

◇ improves muscle mass, strength, and metabolism

◇ better muscle mass = increased metabolic rate, and you burn more calories every day

◇ increases serotonin function, which helps decrease food cravings and desires for sweet binges

◇ increases endorphin activity, which decreases appetite

◇ inhibits MAO enzyme activity, which prolongs activity of serotonin, dopamine, and norepinephrine and helps to decrease appetite

◇ restores normal sleep stages, which lowers cortisol, increases GH, and improves nighttime muscle repair

◇ helps reduce excess cortisol production and restores the normal daily rhythm of cortisol release, which helps reduce excess fat storage

Chapter 6

PROGESTERONE:

YOUR PREGNANCY/
FAT-BUILDING HORMONE

"Doris," a fity-one-year-old attorney, came for her consult, distraught about a weight gain of over fifty pounds in the last one and a half to two years. She couldn't figure out what was happening, since she was a vegetarian eating a healthy diet. She made sure she took all her supplements and did her regular exercise four or five days a week, in spite of her busy work schedule. About two years ago, she had started having occasional hot flashes along with PMS mood changes, even though she was still menstruating. Her periods had become lighter in flow and shorter in length. She had no other changes to suggest she was menopausal.

She was not been on any estrogen replacement therapy or birth control pills. Two years earlier, she saw a "nutritionist" who suggested she use ProGest body cream for PMS-type symptoms. This "nutritionist" had no formal training or credentials in nutrition. Doris faithfully used her progesterone cream for fourteen days a month, a quarter-teaspoon twice a day as directed. She initially thought her PMS was better, but after about six months, she could no longer tell much difference. She did notice that a few months after starting the progesterone cream, her weight began "ballooning up." The "nutritionist" told her that progesterone cream would *help* her lose weight. She continued to use the progesterone cream, even though her weight gain really upset her. She cut calories in her attempts to lose the excess weight.

By the time I saw her, she felt sluggish, tired, and had difficulty with her mental concentration at work. She was having much worse mood swings and irritability for the two weeks before her periods, her bleeding had gotten heavier with more cramping, she felt bloated and miserable, and was tired of feeling so fat and out of sorts. She was also worried that she might be developing diabetes, because she felt her "blood-sugar swings" getting out of control the ten days before her period. At times she felt hypoglycemic and shaky; at other times she was so sleepy after eating that she fell asleep at work. She felt like "a disaster had struck." She did not realize that her problems, especially the marked weight gain, all began *after* she started using progesterone cream.

Her hormone levels helped clarify the picture: Her Day 20 estradiol (E2) was far too low at 70 pg/ml (it should be about 200–250 at that time of the cycle), and her progesterone (P), while using the progesterone cream at that time of the cycle, was 24 ng/ml. This is at the top of the range for an ovulatory cycle. Her E2:P ratio was quite imbalanced as a result of the added progesterone at a time when her own estradiol was declining. The progesterone dominance had shifted her metabolism similar to pregnancy: more storage of fat, less ability to tolerate glucose, higher cortisol, and less responsiveness to her body's insulin. The cream she thought was to *help* weight loss had actually made her fatter and triggered early diabetes. Needless to say, she wasn't very happy about all this. Two years later, she is on the right combination of estradiol and natural progesterone, feels dramatically better, and has lost the excess weight.

There has been an exponential increase in over-the-counter progesterone creams and multilevel marketing schemes today, with incredible claims touting progesterone as a "wonder hormone" to prevent osteoporosis, lose weight, increase sex drive, and solve all of women's other problems. Based on reputable scientific research, most of these claims simply are not accurate. I have seen too many women have serious complications from overuse of these progesterone creams. People who recommend such broad use of progesterone have done a disservice when they forgot that women have a variety of hormones with different functions, and each one has to be in proper balance.

Let's explore how progesterone is involved in regulating body fat, appetite, and weight. My goal is to give you a reliable "road map" through the maze of conflicting information out there.

WHAT IS PROGESTERONE AND WHAT DOES IT DO?

Progesterone acts in a variety of ways to produce the metabolic and physical changes that prepare the female body to adapt to and nurture a pregnancy. As a result of its pregnancy-promoting effects, it was given the name *progesterone* ("pro-gestation-al" hormone). During pregnancy, progesterone levels are about fifteen times greater than in our menstrual cycles. In the first half of the menstrual cycle (follicular phase) there is no significant amount of progesterone produced, and levels in women are about 0.3 to 0.9 ng/ml. When ovulation occurs, the egg is released and becomes the corpus luteum, which begins to secrete progesterone. Levels of progesterone in the second half of the cycle (luteal phase) rise to about 15 to 30 ng/ml, or up to *thirty times* the level of the first half of the cycle.

The progesterone secreted by the corpus luteum stimulates the lining of the uterus to thicken and become secretory so it can receive a fertilized egg and help it grow. If there is fertilization and pregnancy, the placenta becomes a hormone-producing factory, and begins pumping out increasing amounts of progesterone throughout pregnancy. With so many changes needed in a woman's body for her to sustain a pregnancy, it is not surprising that progesterone has a wide range of metabolic effects on the whole body, not just the reproductive organs.

Progesterone has a number of effects to increase storage of body fat, which I will explain a little later. This occurs in many different species, not just humans. This fat-storing effect has an obvious evolutionary advantage for survival of mother and baby, since it ensures that pregnant women have adequate fat stores to survive nine months of gestation should food become scarce. Over the millions of years of human evolution, the women who were able to survive and reproduce in times of food scarcity were the women who could extract nutrients from food and store fat efficiently. As a result, our bodies—directed by progesterone—have become remarkably efficient at pulling maximum nutrients from what we eat, even when food resources are meager. It stimulates our appetite and our desire for carbohydrates, which are, in turn, used for fuel and stored as fat. But ah, now that we live in a time of food being ever-present and abundant, our fat-storing efficiency has become a curse!

In addition to its fat-storing effects, progesterone also relaxes the smooth muscles of the intestinal tract. This slows down the movement of food through the stomach and intestine, allowing for even greater absorption of nutrients. For a pregnancy, better absorption of nutrients is a beneficial effect. If we are not pregnant, we experience this "slowing down" of the intestinal tract as bloating, fullness, and constipation (especially if you don't get enough fiber), and it may contribute to a sluggish gallbladder, which increases your risk of developing gallstones. The "slowing down" also means more calories are absorbed from every single bite you eat, unlike with men, who pass food more quickly through the stomach and intestines and don't absorb every last little calorie!

PROGESTERONE AND PROGESTINS: UNDERSTANDING THE IMPORTANT DIFFERENCES

We know that the function of steroid hormones is significantly affected by even small changes in the molecule. The number of carbons, side chains, unsaturated chemical bonds, other atoms added—all can make an enormous difference in the way that molecule works in the human body. These small molecular changes alter the desired effects and may cause unwanted side effects. It is crucial, therefore, to understand the important differences among the progesterone and progestin options available to you. I explain this in more detail in chapter 13, but I want to clarify these terms for you now.

Progestogen is the broad term used to describe any substance that has biochemical effects to sustain a pregnancy, called "progestational" activity.

Progesterone (found in humans and all vertebrate animals) is a biologically natural progestogen. Human progesterone is produced primarily by the corpus luteum after ovulation and by the placenta during pregnancy.

Tiny amounts of progesterone are made by the adrenal glands, but this is not sufficient to prepare the body to sustain a pregnancy. When made in the laboratory from the building-block molecules found in wild Mexican yams and soybeans, and then purified to meet FDA standards for use as a medication, it is called USP progesterone. An injectable form of USP progesterone has been available in the United States since the 1940s, made by Upjohn, the company that also invented Provera (medroxyprogesterone acetate, or MPA) tablets that could be taken by mouth.

Progestins are man-made chemical molecules that have a different chemical structure from the molecules naturally found in the human body. They have many properties and actions *similar to* progesterone but because their molecules are "rearranged" slightly from progesterone, they have a number of *different* actions as well, and are many times *more potent* than natural progesterone. As a result, progestins can produce different effects in the body. At times these are desirable and needed; at other times they are quite bothersome or problematic.

Synthetic progestins, especially MPA, are the most common cause of unpleasant side effects associated with "hormone therapy," in particular *weight gain*. There are two major factors important in determining the balance of desirable versus undesirable side effects: the balance of progestin relative to estrogen in the preparation, and the relative balance of progestational and androgenic activity. Progestin-only products that contain *no estrogen*, like Norplant and Depo-Provera, typically have the worst side effect profile of all, because you get all the negative effects of the progestin without any compensating benefits of the estrogen.

Why even use the synthetic progestins if they tend to cause so many side effects? There are some situations and some women for whom the synthetic progestins actually work better or have fewer side effects. Some women feel excessively hungry when taking natural progesterone, and don't have this problem when they use norethindrone (found in Micronor and some birth control pills). So it is a very individual response. We must take this into account to find one that is right for each woman. I describe in chapter 13 how to work with your physician to do this.

HOW PROGESTERONE AFFECTS THE BODY

Progesterone's Effect on Metabolism

The menstrual cycle's ebb and flow of hormones, and balance of progesterone relative to estradiol and testosterone, has effects on multiple metabolic pathways that are involved in weight regulation: carbohydrate and fat storage and breakdown, rate of stomach emptying, insulin release, cortisol production, caffeine metabolism, protein metabolism, food cravings, and hormones affecting the gallbladder and immune system, to name a few. Progesterone and estradiol work together to regulate your body fat stores, muscle growth and repair, as well as body composition. They do this in part by altering the enzyme lipoprotein lipase (LPL) activity in fat cells (adipocytes). Estradiol acts to lower body fat (adiposity) by lowering LPL activity, while progesterone increases body fat storage for a possible pregnancy by increasing the activity of the LPL enzyme. And you wondered why it is harder for women than men to lose weight, even with a good exercise program!

Estradiol and progesterone act in concert to oversee our body's insulin release in response to glucose. In animals and humans, both hormones increase the release of insulin from the pancreas after you eat, but estradiol and progesterone have very different effects on insulin sensitivity in other body tissues. Insulin sensitivity refers to how well insulin is able to work at its receptors, thereby preventing excess insulin surges in response to glucose in the bloodstream. Progesterone *decreases* insulin sensitivity and causes resistance to the way that insulin is supposed to work to regulate glucose. Progesterone's effect on insulin is quite rapid and can be detected within ten minutes of administering the hormone. It appears to be a direct effect of progesterone on the pancreas itself. This is one of the reasons women often experience increased cravings for sweets in pregnancy, or during the second half of the menstrual cycle when progesterone rises. Women with diabetes are especially vulnerable to this blood sugar–elevating effect of progesterone and need to use the least amount of progesterone possible.

Estradiol, on the other hand, *increases* insulin sensitivity and improves glucose tolerance in humans and animals. The beneficial effect of estradiol to improve our body's glucose handling occurs both in premenopausal menstruating women and postmenopausal women if they are using the patch form of estradiol. Diabetic women also experience this beneficial effect of transdermal ("the patch") estradiol on glucose control. Both your fat cells (adipocytes) and your muscle cells respond to estradiol with improvement in insulin sensitivity. The improvement appears to occur by multiple pathways rather than a direct effect on the pancreas.

In a normal menstrual cycle with optimal hormone ratios, the opposing actions of estradiol (E) and progesterone (P) on insulin tend to offset each other. This suggests that the *E:P ratio* is more influential in determining the net metabolic effect. In the women I see in my practice for evaluations of hormone levels, the E:P ratio has been one of the key factors in determining degree of symptoms and when they feel better. When the luteal phase hormone ratios show lower-than-optimal estradiol with a normal progesterone rise, women usually have more intense sweet cravings and more weight gain.

Prolonged use of progesterone without adequate balance of estradiol makes insulin resistance worse, which causes weight gain around the middle of the body, increased total cholesterol, lower levels of good cholesterol (HDL), and higher levels of bad cholesterol (LDL) and triglycerides (TG). Insulin resistance also causes high blood pressure and significantly increased risk of heart disease from plaque building up in the arteries. Because the complications of insulin resistance can be so severe, it means this is a crucial factor to consider in evaluating women who are gaining weight, determining which hormones are given, and deciding whether hormones are given orally or absorbed through the skin. I will talk more about insulin resistance in chapter 10. In chapters 14 and 16, I will explain how to help reduce this problem with the types of hormone and dietary approaches you select.

Progesterone's Effects on Muscle and Connective Tissue

Muscle protein metabolism and the rate of muscle breakdown are affected by the hormone changes of the menstrual cycle, as I described in chapter 5 for estradiol. This can be determined by measuring protein breakdown products such as urea in the urine during the phases of the cycle: mid-follicular (high estradiol) or mid-luteal (high progesterone). The highest levels of urea in the urine indicate more muscle breakdown, and this occurs during the mid-luteal, high-progesterone phase of the cycle. If there is an elevated progesterone-to-estradiol ratio, there is more breakdown (catabolism) of body muscle proteins. Women with more body fat and lower muscle mass, as well as women with muscle pain syndromes, should be cautious about using progesterone without adequate balance of estradiol in order to avoid any excess breakdown of protein and muscle tissue. Remember, when you lose muscle, you lose the most effective fat-burning machinery in the body.

Canadian researchers found that women between twenty and thirty years old had their highest muscle strength around the time of ovulation when estradiol levels were at their peak. Muscle strength was lower at times of the menstrual cycle when progesterone was dominant in the luteal phase or when estrogen was low during the bleeding phase. Menopause resulted in a significant decline in muscle strength if women were not taking hormone therapy, but *no* decline was found in women taking postmenopausal estrogen therapy. These findings suggest that if you want to keep from losing muscle and gaining fat, you will want to avoid using more progesterone than the minimum you need to prevent excess buildup of the uterine lining.

Progesterone also has interesting effects on connective tissues that make up our body's ligaments and tendons. These effects are a special concern for women who have gained a lot of weight. For example, in pregnancy, high levels of progesterone help prepare the ligaments of the pelvis to relax and allow the mother's pelvic bones to separate enough for the baby's body to be delivered through the birth canal. This is a desirable effect of progesterone to allow the pelvic bones to separate enough for birth. But these relaxed ligaments also cause more backaches and leg aches in the last trimester of pregnancy, as you probably experienced. But if you have not been pregnant, you experience these same effects in the second half of the menstrual cycle when progesterone levels are high. This is one reason women athletes have more exercise-related injuries in the progesterone-dominant phase of the cycle compared to the first half when estradiol is higher and progesterone is low.

But what about if you are just overweight? If you have too much progesterone relative to estradiol—as a result of your own estradiol declining, or taking HRT, or from using progesterone creams for PMS or menopausal symptoms—you will also have "relaxed" ligaments. The "relaxation" of ligaments, added to excess weight being carried around all day, causes more backaches, leg aches, and aching hips. High doses of synthetic progestins also have this ligament-relaxing effect. This is another reason for overweight women to have hormone levels checked during the progesterone phase of the cycle, and to avoid taking too much progesterone in hormone therapy or taking birth control pills that are too high in progestin, such as Alesse, Mircette, or Loestrin.

I have done many consultations for overweight women who also had low back pain due to excess relaxation or looseness of ligaments in the sacroiliac joints and pelvis. Without realizing the ligament effects of progesterone, some of these women have sought out prolotherapy to strengthen these ligaments. This is a series of painful injections using a sclerosing, or scar-forming, solution to make the ligaments form scar tissue to strengthen them. Even though prolotherapy can be quite painful during the treatment, it has clearly been helpful for some people to provide stronger ligamentous support and reduce back pain. But you certainly don't want to be undergoing an expensive, painful treatment if the cause is excess weight coupled with excess progesterone!

Progesterone's Effects on the Immune System

Another important effect of progesterone is to suppress the immune system. This may be one of the reasons that women tend to have more allergies and herpes outbreaks during the progesterone-dominant phase of the menstrual cycle each month. Progesterone's immune-suppressing effects in pregnancy prevent the mother's body from "attacking and destroying" the foreign protein of the developing fetus that contains the father's genetic make-up and protein-coding systems. This is a crucial function of progesterone for a pregnant woman, but we don't want immune suppression when we are *not* pregnant. Many of the immune-regulating chemical messengers are also involved in regulating body weight and metabolism, so you don't want any negative effects here if you are trying to lose weight.

Progesterone's Effects on Sleep

I described in chapter 5 how estradiol produced before menopause is one of the primary hormones regulating the brain's sleep center and facilitating the normal stages of sleep. When estradiol declines, the normal stages of sleep, especially periods of Stage IV deep sleep, are disrupted. So it is crucial for women to have adequate estradiol to regain normal deep sleep and muscle repair. Progesterone's effect on sleep is quite different from estrogen's effects, so progesterone doesn't replace the need for estradiol to restore sleep pathways, as some books claim. There are a number of metabolites of progesterone, however, that have potent sedative effects, very similar to barbiturates and benzodiazepines. One breakdown product of progesterone, called 3-alpha-OH-DHP, is about eight times more potent than the sedative methohexital, a potent barbiturate used for anesthesia. The liver provides most of the conversion of progesterone to these sedative compounds, so the sedative effects of progesterone occur mainly if it is taken orally and goes through the liver's "first pass" metabolism.

Progesterone has effects on the brain that help sleep, by acting on the same brain receptors as medications you may already know: Klonopin, Ativan, Ambien, Xanax, Valium, and others. Since progesterone can make you sleepy like these medicines, there may be times when it can be a useful addition to hormone therapy even if you do not have a uterus. But this has to be balanced against the unwanted, potentially negative metabolic effects of progesterone, such as weight gain. If I recommend progesterone to improve sleep, I find that lower doses can be effective if estradiol has been restored to optimal levels. If you have a uterus, however, you and your doctor have to be certain that you are taking an appropriate dose of progesterone for the desired protective effects on the endometrial lining.

PROGESTERONE'S INTERACTION WITH OTHER FAT-REGULATING HORMONES

Progesterone's Interaction with GH, Insulin, and Cortisol

Progesterone decreases GH, increases insulin levels, and increases adrenal production of cortisol. This metabolic pattern is the same one seen in obese people, in Cushing's disease (excess cortisol), and after starting corticosteroid medication (such as for arthritis or asthma). This metabolic pattern makes you fatter, so it clearly isn't a very desirable one to continue. In addition, GH triggers growth of more lean body mass, such as muscle and bone, at the same time that it reduces the amount of body fat. One of the reasons that some doctors today prescribe GH to older folks is to help build more muscle mass. So anything that decreases GH, such as getting older or taking the wrong hormones, ends up making us fatter.

Higher levels of progesterone, such as in pregnancy or when taking large doses for PMS or menopause therapy, are associated with greater amounts of unbound (free) cortisol in the blood. This further decreases GH and causes higher insulin levels with more insulin resistance. This is another reason that using progesterone regularly, in doses that give blood levels similar to pregnancy, can have negative health effects on a non-pregnant woman. These changes triggered by high progesterone levels can wreck havoc with maintaining healthy production of GH, insulin, and cortisol, and, in turn, lead to excessive weight gain, blood sugar swings, increased risk of diabetes, abnormal cholesterol profiles, and many other problems.

TESTS FOR PROGESTERONE LEVELS

Current blood serum tests for progesterone are both accurate and reliable. The amount of progesterone in the serum reflects the balance, or equilibrium, between the bound and free hormone and gives a total picture of the amount available for the body to use. Since there is a constant dynamic process between the part that is "free" (i.e., biologically active) and the part that is "bound" to carrier proteins, I have found it is important to measure this total amount. I recommend checking blood level of progesterone on about cycle Day 20 or 21 to get the peak level of the luteal phase of the cycle. A Day 20 blood level should be typically between 5 and 30 ng/ml to indicate that you ovulated in that particular menstrual cycle. As I mentioned earlier, progesterone levels in pregnancy are about fifteen times higher than this luteal phase level. It doesn't take very much supplemental progesterone to create blood levels equal to those of pregnancy. For example, an *oral* dose of 300 mg micronized progesterone given *daily for one week* can produce blood levels of progesterone equivalent to the third trimester of pregnancy. This is why you need to be careful about overuse of the nonprescription creams. A good rule of thumb for converting oral to nonoral doses is that the *cream or gel should be about one tenth the oral dose*. If your cream prescription has more progesterone than this amount, and you are gaining weight or having trouble losing weight, you should talk with your doctor to see whether you are getting more progesterone than you need.

SUMMARY

Progesterone has its place in our lives, and an important role in restoring hormone balance after menopause if you have a uterus. But I am concerned about the overuse of this hormone in so many over-the-counter creams that may sabotage your health and your efforts to lose weight. I want you to be an informed consumer, and not be misled by false claims. I urge you to work closely with your physician on proper progesterone doses so that it won't aggravate weight gain during midlife. There are many ways to do this in order to help you better meet your overall health needs and goals, as I describe in chapter 13.

Chapter 7

TESTOSTERONE AND DHEA:

YOUR ANDROGEN HORMONES

"Claudine," a healthy woman in her early sixties, had noticed a significant decrease in her strength, stamina, and energy on the ski slopes in recent years. She had also been getting fatter around the waist, in spite of all her strenuous skiing workouts. She wondered if the decline in her muscle strength and endurance was related to her hormones. She had been on Premarin 0.625 mg since a complete hysterectomy in her forties. She had asked about having her hormone levels checked, but her gynecologist would not agree to do it. At her consult with me, her estradiol was far too low at 40 pg/ml, and her testosterone level was barely detectable at less than 10 ng/dl. I recommended a change to the 17-beta estradiol transdermal patch, with added testosterone using a compounded sustained-release oral capsule. Since she had a hysterectomy, she did not need to take progesterone.

Within the first six months, she described a marked increase in her energy level, and said, "My old spark is back!" The next year at her follow-up visit, she gleefully told me that when she returned to the ski slopes the season after starting testosterone, her ski instructor commented on the noticeable improvements in her muscle strength and stamina. He asked her what her new training regimen had been over the summer. She smiled and said, "I never told him what really made the difference, but I know it was the hormones—I had my testosterone back . . . and I had more estradiol!"

WHAT IS TESTOSTERONE AND WHAT DOES IT DO?

Testosterone? That's the male hormone isn't it? No, it's not just for men. Women's ovaries also make testosterone before menopause, and our testosterone production is actually greater than our estrogen, when you compare them on the same units. More about this later. Women lose, on average, more than 50 percent of their normal testosterone with the decline in hormone production around menopause. Testosterone is one of a group of hormones called *androgens,* from the Greek *andros,* meaning "male-like." All of the androgens are made from cholesterol, by the ovary in the female, the testes in the male, and, to a lesser extent, by the adrenal glands in both men and women. Androgens are also made from chemical "building blocks," or precursor molecules, in body fat tissue, muscle, liver, skin, and brain. This is why overweight women typically have higher androgen levels, which can further adversely affect weight. But then these precursor molecules are further changed in the ovaries and adrenal glands, so it really ends up that the ovaries and adrenal glands together are responsible for either directly or indirectly making all of a woman's testosterone.

Women need testosterone, too—it is the hormone that activates the sexual circuits in the brain for men and women and promotes healthy sexual desire. But did you know that it is also an important hormone involved in regulating your amount of body fat versus lean muscle mass? This interesting hormone has a lot of positive effects on women's bodies, particularly to improve your muscle mass and decrease your percent body fat. This is why testosterone is called an anabolic hormone, because it stimulates the building of lean mass (muscle and bone) and uses fat for fuel to do so, which decreases the amount of body fat. Remember, muscles are your best and most efficient fat-burning machinery, so if you are getting fatter as you get older, one way to help that is to improve muscle mass. And that means checking your testosterone quotient!

There is a myth perpetrated by the sellers of over-the-counter hormone and wild yam creams that you can use these progesterone creams to give the body the building blocks it needs to make more testosterone and estrogen from progesterone as a presursor. This is false. This process requires enzymes and reactions that take place in *functioning* ovaries in women and testicles in men. If you have had menopause or a hysterectomy or tubal ligation or other factors that cause loss of ovarian function, then you don't have the pathways working properly to convert progesterone to testosterone and estradiol. You end up having a load of progesterone and no way to effectively convert it to testosterone. This is a crucial point for women with weight problems, as I described in chapter 6.

This loss of ovarian testosterone production doesn't just happen with natural menopause, although that is the cause most of us know more about. Even *before* menopause actually occurs, women's adrenal glands have already decreased androgen production by about 50 percent and the ovary levels of testosterone have already started to decline. One reason there is *less* of the active form of testosterone after menopause is that the precursor molecule, *androstenedione*, decreases more than 50 percent when the ovary ceases its hormone production. So, you lose the precursors usually made by the ovary, as well as the ovarian enzymes that make these chemical processes work. Many doctors do not realize that women's decline in *estrogen* production also results in a decrease in *testosterone* production due to this loss of precursors and enzymes from the ovary.

All these changes mean you begin losing muscle mass and getting inexorably fatter several years before you actually stop menstruating at menopause, not to mention that your sexual desire and ability to become sexually aroused are also dampened considerably! Women now live on average about thirty to forty years beyond the ending of ovarian hormone production, and that's a long time to live without the benefit of these critical metabolic hormones. Ever heard of a *man* who wanted only half of his normal testosterone?

If you have a hysterectomy *with* removal of the ovaries before you are actually at menopausal hormone levels, the change is even more drastic. Concentrations of testosterone in the bloodstream fall markedly *within twenty-four to forty-eight hours* after surgery. Since you no longer have the ovaries to make more testosterone, or to efficiently convert adrenal

DHEA to testosterone, there is an abrupt loss of this energizing hormone. That's a big shock to the body, and one of the additional reasons women frequently gain weight after hysterectomy.

Even if one or both ovaries is left in place and you are only in your thirties when you have a hysterectomy, we now known that about 60 to 70 percent of women experience decline in their hormones to menopausal levels within three to four years of surgery. That's a scary thought if you are thirty-four when you have a hysterectomy and are thinking (or have been told) that your ovaries will work just fine until you hit your fifties! This more rapid decline in hormones after the uterus is removed is thought to be due to decreased blood flow to the ovaries as a result of having to cut and tie off the uterine artery during surgery.

In addition, if you are then started on just estrogen therapy, the amount of free, biologically active testosterone falls even further, since estrogen increases *sex-hormone binding globulin* (SHBG), which "binds up" more of the testosterone molecules. This is one reason that many women lose muscle mass, gain fat, and lose sex drive and energy after hysterectomy. They think these losses are due to the surgery, but it isn't usually the *surgery* that caused the problems. You need optimal hormone replenishment with both estradiol and testosterone to restore the levels you had before surgery.

In a Gallup poll of American women, conducted for the North American Menopause Society in 1993, only 5 percent of the women polled knew that their bodies make "androgens" and that this amount declines after menopause. Doctors used to think that testosterone isn't very important for women, and many are still unsure of how to prescribe this hormone, so the whole issue of testosterone therapy for women is relatively new. The amount of circulating active androgens in women is obviously much lower than in men, but these compounds are important for quite an array of vital functions in women. Fortunately today, more women are aware of the importance of androgens like testosterone and DHEA and are asking physicians for more information about how to measure them and what options there are for adding back what the body formerly made. In this chapter, I will primarily focus on how testosterone and DHEA affect your weight, even though both hormones have many other functions.

HOW DOES TESTOSTERONE AFFECT YOUR WEIGHT?

Testosterone has primarily been associated with sexual desire ("libido") in men and women; yet, it has many effects on other body systems, including how much body fat you have and where it gets deposited on your body. The changing hormone balance during the climacteric or midlife years takes many forms, but two are particularly important as they affect testosterone: lower estradiol, higher estrone and lower estradiol *relative* to the amount of testosterone present. These changes cause the testosterone effects to be "unmasked," so that you experience more of the male-like androgen effects on distribution of body fat, muscle mass, facial hair, voice, sex drive, and energy level.

Decrease in estradiol at midlife leads to a decrease in SHBG. Since this carrier protein "binds" the sex hormones, having less of it means more androgens are now in the "free" or biologically active portion in the bloodstream. At midlife, even if you have less testosterone and DHEA present than you did earlier, more of it is now in the active (free) form at the same time you have less of the feminizing estradiol effects . . . so you watch your body morph from a "pear" (gynecoid, or female) pattern to an "apple" (android, or male) pattern of body fat around the waist and "trunk" or upper abdomen/chest, grow more facial hair, and lose hair on your head. It isn't just that you don't have the "willpower" to lose that middle spread; it is that your hormone ratios are now working against you.

When estradiol declines, the dominance of androgens from the adrenal gland and fat tissue begin to produce even more unwanted metabolic changes for women: increasing blood pressure, increasing total cholesterol, decreasing HDL (good) cholesterol, along with increasing LDL (bad) cholesterol, and higher insulin and cortisol. All of these changes contribute to the increasing risks of heart disease, hypertension, and diabetes in women in over thirty-five.

At first, we thought that testosterone itself was responsible for these negative effects on the cholesterol ratios. Newer studies have shown, however, that testosterone actually helps maintain the normal mechanisms involved in dilating blood vessels to help lower blood pressure, *if* it is given with the right balance of estradiol. If given *alone* to women, testosterone and DHEA promote buildup of artery-clogging plaque (atherosclerosis). If the androgens are *given with* estrogen, however, they have the opposite effect on the arterial wall and actually help prevent buildup of plaque in the arteries.

Throughout a woman's life, testosterone has important functions in maintaining muscle tissues in women, that wonderful "fat-burning" machinery. Lower testosterone levels mean less ability to build muscle, even if we are exercising several times a week. Testosterone also plays a key role to help build bone and prevent osteoporosis, even more as women lose the bone-preserving effects of estrogen. Furthermore, testosterone helps keep our energy level optimal. Decline of testosterone is one of the frequently unrecognized factors in "chronic fatigue." Many women have multiple medical evaluations and spend hundreds or thousands of dollars on tests and therapies to diagnose and treat CFS and never have a proper blood-level test for testosterone.

TESTOSTERONE'S EFFECTS ON MUSCLE TISSUE

At menopause, when women lose both estradiol and testosterone, we begin to lose muscle and bone faster than men because we experience a more dramatic and sudden loss of testosterone. Men's testosterone falls much more slowly over many years, so they lose muscle mass and bone more gradually and later in life. Women's loss of testosterone also contributes to excess upper-body fat in midlife, in part because testosterone builds new muscle and keeps our muscles healthy and strong. Loss of muscle slows our metabolic rate. Our body composition shifts toward more fat. You need adequate testosterone levels as you get older to keep your metabolic engines revved up and hang on to your muscles! But it must be balanced with the right amount of estradiol or you will start packing on pounds around your middle!

TESTOSTERONE'S EFFECTS ON THE BRAIN

There are some important reasons I talk about this in relation to your weight management in midlife. Not only does testosterone activate the brain "sexual circuits" in women and men, it also has a mood-lifting or antidepressant effect to enhance our psychological sense of well-being. Testosterone also significantly increases performance on cognitive tasks.

And, it is involved in stimulating the brain chemicals that are crucial in weight regulation! In some women, what appears to be depression turns out to be a deficiency of testosterone. But as testosterone levels get too high (whether from overproduction in the body or from taking excess supplemental hormones), women have restless sleep, intense dreams and/or nightmares, aggressive or violent dreams, and sometimes experience unpleasant, intense sexual urges. Excess testosterone relative to estradiol also causes marked increase in appetite and more body fat around your waist. Testosterone abuse, such as used for muscle building, causes both men and women to develop toxic behavioral effects such as extreme irritability, volatile/explosive moods, aggressiveness or assaultiveness. When other androgenic steroids such as DHEA and "andro" (androstenedione) are abused, the same toxic behavioral effects occur. Obviously, the key is to have the right balance.

How do these brain effects make a difference for you if you have been struggling with weight gain? Think about all the times a physician has recommended a tricyclic antidepressant to help improve your energy and mood, thinking depression was causing you to overeat. It turns out, however, that you have a natural "antidepressant" hormone in testosterone. Testosterone has significant "activating" effects on the brain, mainly by elevating brain levels of norepinephrine. These are the *same* type of brain activation patterns seen with the tricyclic antidepressants like desipramine (Norpramin) and imipramine (Tofranil). But a hidden problem with these medicines is that they increase your appetite and lead to more weight gain. Did anyone check your testosterone level before suggesting an antidepressant? It seems that in our current focus on medications, we have overlooked the antidepressant effects of our natural hormones testosterone and estradiol that Mother Nature gave us eons ago! Not to mention their crucial fat-burning effects.

New research has shown that for testosterone to work properly in women, an optimal level of estradiol (estrogen) must be present. The brain testosterone receptors seem to be *created* by the presence of estradiol. Without enough estrogen to "prime the pump," even the testosterone produced by our own bodies cannot attach properly in brain centers. So, your level of estradiol becomes important here as well, since it also plays a role in how well your body's testosterone can work.

TESTOSTERONE'S EFFECTS ON SLEEP

I explained in earlier chapters that sleep disorders can make you fatter by disrupting the normal cortisol patterns and by increasing insulin release. Excess levels of testosterone, particularly when estradiol declines, may further aggravate sleep disorders, since testosterone is a significantly stimulating hormone. If testosterone is given to men *or* women at bedtime, it will interfere with sleep, leading to fragmented sleep and/or violent or aggressive, disturbing dreams. Then you wake up feeling like you have been in a battle all night long. Patients tell me that other physicians suggested testosterone be taken at night to help improve muscle repair. This theory isn't completely accurate. The activating brain effects of testosterone will disrupt Stage IV deep sleep, especially in women. This is the sleep stage for muscle growth and repair and for release of GH, which also affects muscle formation. If you don't get good Stage IV sleep, you won't have much muscle repairing and building going on, no matter how much testosterone you have. It is best for women, and men, to take testosterone in the morning to give you the desired boost to your energy over the course of the day, yet allow you to sleep at night.

CHECKING TESTOSTERONE LEVELS

I regularly use serum hormone levels to monitor need for and response to hormone therapy, and I have consistently found these to be reliable and cost-effective approaches. I usually check the total, free, and weakly bound forms of testosterone circulating in the bloodstream so I can better help my patients make the best decisions on the right dose. What should you be looking for as a desirable target range for testosterone?

In my clinical experience, women typically experience their optimal normal energy level and libido when serum (blood) levels of total testosterone are between 40 and 60 ng/dl, with the percent of free testosterone at about 1 to 2 percent of the total. For comparison, using the same pg/ml units we use for estradiol, 40 to 60 ng/dl would be 400 to 600 pg/ml. For comparison, men's testosterone levels run about 450 to 1,200 ng/dl (or

4,500 to 12,000 pg/ml). Most men don't experience a loss of libido until testosterone drops down to around 600 ng/dl (6,000 pg/ml) or less. Women are more sensitive to small amounts of testosterone, so a drop of only 10 to 15 units can make an enormous difference in whether a woman will feel her usual energy level and sexual spark. For women, levels above 60 ng/dl (600 pg/ml) or so may cause more middle-spread weight gain, excess facial hair, acne, irritability, restless sleep, and other signs of androgen excess. Levels below 20 ng/dl are generally too low to maintain your usual libido, intensity of orgasm, energy level, and bone mass. The majority of menopausal women I have evaluated, particularly those who have had surgical removal of the ovaries in their thirties and forties, have had testosterone levels of less than 10 . . . with unmeasurable amounts of free testosterone. No wonder they don't have any sexual desire left! This is also a significant factor in fatigue and low energy.

When your testosterone levels are too low, we have a number of effective options to restore a healthy balance for you. I will discuss testosterone replacement in chapter 13.

WHAT TO DO IF YOU SUSPECT YOU HAVE TOO MUCH TESTOSTERONE

High androgens for women can cause serious medical problems and marked middle-body weight gain. It is crucial to properly check all these hormone levels if you suspect excess levels of the male hormones. What are the clues to watch for? Women with upper-body obesity, excess body hair, scalp hair loss, and/or severe acne need to have serum levels checked for testosterone, dihydrotestosterone, DHEA, DHEA-S, and androstenedione. If these are too high, further evaluation is needed to determine the cause. You may have PCOS, or you could have an androgen-producing tumor of the ovary or adrenal gland. These kinds of problems are usually found with special imaging studies of the abdomen and pelvis, such as ultrasound, MRI or CAT scans. The type of treatment you would need depends upon the specific cause that is found.

SUMMARY OF TESTOSTERONE EFFECTS

TOO LITTLE	JUST RIGHT	TOO MUCH
low energy	normal energy	hyper feelings
loss of sex drive	normal libido	increased libido
slowed down	alert, interested	"scattered" thoughts similar to ADD
loss of muscle, increase in body fat	normal body composition	apple-shaped weight gain
mildly depressed mood	positive mood	irritable, anxious, edgy, tense, aggressive mood
fewer dreams	normal dreams	intense dreaming, aggressive dreams, violent dreams, disrupted sleep
thin, fine hair	hair thicker	facial hair
scalp hair loss (alopecia)	normal hair growth	scalp hair loss (alopecia)
dry, thin skin	normal skin	acne, oily skin

© 1995, revised 2001 by Elizabeth Lee Vliet, M.D.

DHEA: OUR "OTHER" ANDROGEN

DHEA, and its sulfated form (DHEA-S), are androgens made in the adrenal glands and ovaries in women. Levels are high during fetal development, then drop for most of early childhood, until about ages six to eight when the adrenal glands begin producing more androgens in both boys and girls. Our levels reach their highest from puberty until our thirties. Both men and women lose DHEA as we age, and by the time we reach age seventy, DHEA levels are only about 10 percent of what they were in our earlier reproductive years. We don't yet know for certain whether this decline in adrenal androgens, called "adrenopause," represents just an effect of getting older, or whether the decline itself causes the problems we thought were due to aging, such as loss of muscle strength, loss of optimal immune function, loss of cognitive "sharpness," loss of bone, and many other effects.

In women, the production of DHEA requires enzymes found in healthy, functioning ovaries for DHEA to be changed into testosterone or estradiol by the body. If for whatever reason, your ovaries are not functioning optimally, you won't be able to adequately convert DHEA to the other hormones further down the pathway. That's why it is not a good idea to take DHEA supplements without knowing your blood levels of other hormones. Too much DHEA can cause exactly the same side effects as too much testosterone.

Since women's testosterone receptors need to be "primed" with estradiol in order for the androgens to have optimal effects, if you are given DHEA and your estradiol levels are too low, you risk excess androgen effects such as middle-spread abdominal fat gain, hair loss, increased irritability, and restless sleep seen with excess testosterone. Obviously, this is a serious problem if you are already struggling with unwanted weight gain. If you have fibromyalgia, the impact is even worse: Women tend to experience worsening muscle pain and spasm if androgens such as DHEA or testosterone are boosted prior to having optimal estradiol. It is a balancing act, as I have emphasized throughout my career. Remember your basic body chemistry and the differences between men and women . . . you need a *woman's* balance restored.

DHEA'S EFFECTS ON WEIGHT, INSULIN RESISTANCE, AND LIPIDS

Before you rush out to buy DHEA in hopes it will help you lose weight, as the ads claim, you need information based on studies of *women,* not men. You also need information on DHEA benefits from *human,* not animal, studies. The effects are quite different. The current hype about DHEA and its report-ed benefits as an "antiaging" miracle hormone came from studies in animals, primarily rats. Rats' bodies function differently from ours, particularly where DHEA is concerned. Most of the popular books that report DHEA *benefits*—anticancer, antiobesity, insulin-sensitizing, bone-preserving, heart-protecting, memory-enhancing, immune-enhancing effects—are based on *animal* models with doses that were hugely in excess of what is natural or nor-mal for that animal or for the amounts humans normally produce. The human studies so far *do not* show these same beneficial effects, especially when done in *women.*

There are a number of problems with trying to generalize the animal results to humans: Most of the animals used had *natural* adrenal androgen levels that were *negligible,* so DHEA given to them created a very artificial state. Mice and rats show a dramatic and consistent positive response to DHEA, while other animals such as dogs and monkeys don't show such a positive response. The doses used are so much greater than what would be appropriate "replacement" for humans that we can't compare the results (e.g., animal studies routinely use 50 to 400 mg/kg body weight to demon-strate effects on obesity, while human studies seldom use more than 20 mg/kg body weight, and even at this lower level, women developed serious androgen side effects). There are major differences in effects based on whether the DHEA is given orally, or whether it is given nonorally as a cream or vaginal suppository. Most of the studies to date have used *male* laboratory animals. The animal model itself is flawed, since animals don't go through the same "adrenopause" as humans do.

But, in spite of all these limitations and problems, sales of over-the-counter DHEA supplements have skyrocketed in recent years, as more and more men and women use it thinking they can stay youthful and lose excess weight. Many women who are taking it have no idea that this sup-posedly innocuous over-the-counter "supplement" can be causing them to eat more sweets, gain more waistline body fat, lose hair, feel irritable, and have restless sleep! Adverse effects with DHEA are even worse if you are already overweight, or have elevated cholesterol and high LDL cholesterol along with lower-than-optimal estradiol. Taking DHEA also causes the symptoms of PCOS to get markedly worse.

The problems are more serious for women since we have such a narrow *normal healthy range* for our androgens. High-dose DHEA (50 mg or greater) causes women in most studies to become "androgenized," with increased abdominal weight, increased facial and body hair, acne, decline in good (HDL) cholesterol and increase in bad (LDL) cholesterol, decreased SHBG (which frees up more androgens to exert negative effects), and *increased* insulin resistance. These findings mirror exactly the metabolic abnormalities found in women with PCOS who typically have high DHEA-S levels.

If women use DHEA at all, they need lower doses than we had previously thought, usually no more than 5 to 15 mg (oral) a day. In *women,* DHEA doses higher than this over time have consistently resulted in more abdominal body fat, unwanted middle spread, and increased insulin resistance with glucose intolerance. Most researchers have now concluded that any beneficial effect of DHEA on obesity in humans is seen only in men, and even in men, it is a very modest effect.

Initial studies suggested a cardio-protective effect of DHEA, but these studies were also done in *men.* When the studies were repeated in women, the positive effects were not seen. In fact, a three-month study of DHEA 50 mg/day in perimenopausal women found that this dose caused negative changes by *decreasing the "good" cholesterol.* This is another negative for women who are already overweight, since many of these women will already have high cholesterol, high LDL, high triglycerides, and lower-than-optimal HDL.

DHEA'S EFFECTS ON BONE

We have observed that bone loss in humans follows the patterns of decline in adrenal androgens such as DHEA in both men and women, which led to speculation that DHEA may help prevent osteoporosis, but so far the results in human studies have been disappointing. Dr. Casson's group at Baylor College of Medicine in Houston measured the effects of DHEA replacement on various markers of bone breakdown and found no benefit to decrease the rate of these breakdown products being excreted in the urine and no benefit on bone mineral density (DEXA) testing at the six-month point. Only one study in women has shown some promise in improving bone density using a 10 percent DHEA cream applied daily for one year, but this dose is so high that most women would have very unpleasant androgenic side effects (and probably be screaming about how fat they are getting!).

DHEA'S EFFECTS ON THE BRAIN, SLEEP, AND COGNITIVE FUNCTION

DHEA has been promoted as the "feel-good" hormone, improving one's sense of well-being, energy, memory, and mental sharpness, but objective data in humans is very limited. There is one placebo-controlled, double-blind randomized trial that showed DHEA improved rapid eye movement (REM) sleep when compared to placebo, but *no women* were included in this study. Since improvements in REM sleep are known to correspond with overall better sleep quality, this could be a way that DHEA seems to help men's feeling of well-being in the few studies that showed improvement.

Unfortunately, the few carefully done, placebo-controlled studies of possible cognitive benefits with DHEA have been disappointing. To date, there is no clear evidence of improved mental function or memory enhancements.

DHEA—SOME CAUTIONS

To date, there is no good evidence to support DHEA being given *routinely* to healthy menopausal women for hormone replacement. In addition to the possibility of weight gain with excess DHEA, there is a concern emerging from animal studies about possible adverse liver effects of long-term oral DHEA use, such as increased liver size and increased development of liver cancers. There is also conflicting data about the effects of DHEA on breast cancer in women, with some studies showing that it increases the risk of developing breast cancer. These problems are particularly a concern with the high doses being promoted for women in the over-the-counter products and some of the compounded cream prescriptions. In summary, there really are not many reasons to take DHEA, and a lot of reasons for women with weight problems to *avoid* it.

SUMMARY

We know more today about the important effects of testosterone on our total health, and we have safe, reasonable options to restore this hormone to healthy levels. On the other hand, there is still a lot of fear about testosterone for women, and doctors sometimes scare women with horror stories about it: "You'll have a moustache, develop a beard, your voice will get deep, you'll have liver damage, you'll lose your hair," and so on. Then, to make it all more difficult, we are surrounded by ads that exhort us all—men and women—to stay young by taking DHEA for its antiaging benefits.

I have had to treat complications that arose when women had been given androgenic hormones (prescription or over-the-counter) in too high a dose. I have also seen women develop androgen excess from taking pregnenolone supplements, and this has been reported in the medical literature as well. Pregnenolone may be converted to DHEA, which then produces the typical unwanted "male" side effects and excess body fat.

Although I have said all this about the potential problems with androgens, remember that testosterone is an important compound for our bodies in our younger years. I think we need to consider that this hormone may be necessary for us to feel our best and have a healthy body as we age, especially since so many of us are living so much longer now. How do you sort it all out and make sense of the conflicting information? How do you use it appropriately, in the right dose, type, and delivery for women? How do you avoid abdominal weight gain from excess androgens?

Using natural micronized testosterone at doses designed for women, I rarely see unwanted side effects. If properly done, and appropriately monitored, restoring testosterone to an optimal level has significant benefits on metabolism, muscle growth/repair, energy level, sense of well-being, and our sexuality. There is a way to use these hormones safely, and I will describe this in more detail in chapter 13.

Chapter 8

THE THYROID HORMONES

(T3 AND T4): MASTER METABOLIC REGULATORS

Janeta was thirty-six when I first saw her. The last of her three children had been born four years earlier. Over the past three years, she had experienced a marked weight gain of forty-five pounds, a severe loss of energy, and a diminished level of concentration that made getting through her workday difficult. She was worried she might lose her job. She developed severe premenstrual mood swings and chocolate cravings that were driving her crazy. She told me that she couldn't lose weight no matter how much she exercised, and that her memory wasn't as sharp as it used to be: "my brain just won't work like it should." She thought she might have a thyroid problem, but her family doctor said her thyroid tests were normal.

When I did her thyroid tests, however, and included measures of thyroid antibodies, she had striking *abnormalities* in both her antithyroid peroxidase (anti-TPO) antibody level at well over 1,000, and her antithyroglobulin antibody at 850 (normal range for both is less than 10). She had a level of 1,500 on a later check of her antithyroglobulin antibody, even though her TSH was still testing normal at that time. Her antibodies were acting like "blocking agents," keeping the thyroid hormones from being able to work properly, which caused her diverse symptoms. I started her on a low dose of T4 initially (0.025 mg), and she felt better fairly soon. A year later, she described feeling "back to my old self" . . . and she has been successful in losing all the weight she gained with her thyroid problems.

Janeta's story shows how important it is to pay attention to both the weight gain and the changes in brain function as clues to thyroid problems, especially when a woman hasn't had such difficulties previously. Our metabolic pathways and our brain are so exquisitely dependent upon normal thyroid function for the cellular energy reactions to work properly that changes in these are often the first clues to early declines in thyroid hormone function. The "overall pattern" is what helps determine what tests to do. And, the clinical findings help us know when medication is needed, not just the lab values. As I have said for my whole career, physicians are treating *people*, not lab values.

A WOMAN'S THYROID . . . DIFFERENT FROM A MAN'S!

Thyroid disorders of all types are eight to twenty times more common in women than in men of the same age. Thyroiditis, a group of autoimmune disorders of the thyroid gland, are about *twenty-five times* more common in females than males. The incidence of thyroid disorders increases with age in both sexes, but there is a more dramatic increase in women from age forty to sixty-five. There are several different types of thyroiditis, including viral, bacterial, toxic, and postpartum, all of which usually result in production of antibodies to the gland tissue (*microsomal* antibodies) or antibodies to the thyroid hormone itself (*thyroglobulin* antibodies).

These antibodies act like pieces of clay stuck to a key, preventing it from fitting into its lock; they keep the hormones from working properly, so you begin to experience the clinical symptoms of declining thyroid gland function like Janeta did. Often, there is elevation of thyroid antibodies *before* there is a compensating rise in TSH produced by the brain in response to the gland being destroyed by the antibodies. This means a woman may experience the symptoms of thyroid disease months or years before TSH goes up.

In particular, women who are struggling with weight gain may have high levels of thyroid antibodies that cause disruption in thyroid ability to properly regulate metabolic pathways in muscle and fat cells. These pathways provide the energy to run your body and are extremely sensitive to loss of proper thyroid hormone balance and function, which also affects normal muscle growth and repair. I think this is one reason that in autoimmune thyroid disorders such as Hashimoto's, we see weight gain along with muscle pain, or myalgias, as an "early warning" symptom, long before TSH goes up. For example, women with fibromyalgia often have abnormally high levels of thyroid antibodies. A study from Norway (Aarflot and Bruusgaard, 1996) reported that elevated thyroid antibodies were found commonly in women with chronic musculoskeletal pain complaints, but this same connection was not found in men. They observed that, in women, the abnormal levels of thyroid antibodies are perhaps more important than is overall thyroid function. This supports my long-standing opinion that in women with mood, pain, and weight problems, thyroid antibodies should be checked, even if TSH is normal.

Even if the antibodies are not elevated, subtle early thyroid imbalance may lead to weight gain, long before the TSH has been affected. This is why it is so frustrating for a woman to be dismissed by her doctor when she suggests the thyroid may be a problem in her weight gain. Most of you have read that *hypo*thyroid conditions can trigger weight gain. But did you know that even *hyper*thyroid conditions, in the early stages, may cause a gain in weight? This happens due to increases in appetite and increased food intake until the excess production of thyroid hormones becomes so toxic that weight loss occurs. When the basic thyroid tests comes back "normal," you feel even more discounted and more of a failure if you are told to "just eat less and exercise more." You may have been right, and the thyroid problem just hasn't shown up yet as an abnormal TSH. So, if you are having weight problems, don't give up just because your doctor dismisses your concern. At least check into having more complete thyroid testing.

Even subclinical thyroid disease can cause menstrual irregularity, infertility, worsening PMS, atypical depression, new onset depression later in life, postpartum depression, anxiety syndromes, fibromyalgia, excessive fatigue, elevated cholesterol, abnormal glucose-insulin regulation, and a host of other problems . . . all of these, in turn, make losing weight even more difficult. Yet, all too often, women with some of these other "vague" symptoms are not evaluated adequately for thyroid disease, and are instead given a psychiatric diagnosis, perhaps started on antidepressants that may even increase appetite, and then referred to a therapist for "stress management."

Studies of patients admitted to psychiatric hospitals have repeatedly shown a high incidence of previously unrecognized thyroid disorders that were likely the causative factor in the mood disorder. At midlife, when thyroid disease rates are increasing for women due to many causes (including what you eat, as I discuss later), you need careful evaluation of thyroid function, including tests more sensitive than just a standard profile.

THYROID HORMONES AND WHAT THEY DO

T3 (triiodothyronine) and T4 (levothyronine) are the two primary hormones produced by the thyroid gland, a small butterfly-shaped gland that lies in your neck over the Adam's apple. T3 and T4 are your major metabolic regulators, governing energy use and production in every cell and tissue in your body. Thyroid hormones are to your body what the gas pedal is to your car: too little and you become sluggish and have trouble moving; too much and you feel like you are racing. It's no wonder that when these hormones go awry, weight can be greatly affected. When your thyroid balance is out of whack, you may also have myriad symptoms that can be confused with many different illnesses. That's why thyroid disease has sometimes been called "the great imitator." Both *hyper*thyroid (too much thyroid hormone, e.g., Graves' disease) and *hypo*thyroid (too little thyroid hormone, e.g. Hashimoto's thyroiditis) conditions can adversely affect your normal mood, sleep, immune system, and weight and pain regulation pathways.

The Thyroid Hormones

T4, made in the thyroid gland, is converted in the gland and in body tissues to the more active form, T3—*if* all the pathways are working properly. The thyroid gland has several important enzymes such as TPO that are critical in converting T4 to T3. Failure to convert T4 to T3 is one of the problems that can lead to symptoms of thyroid disorder even with supposedly "normal" standard thyroid profile blood tests. The thyroid gland also produces another hormone, calcitonin, that is important in regulating calcium balance in the body and plays a role in preventing osteoporosis. But it doesn't play as direct a role in weight gain as we see with T3 and T4.

The thyroid system is controlled by the brain's master control center in the hypothalamus. The hypothalamus produces *thyrotropin releasing hormone* (TRH), which stimulates the pituitary to produce and release TSH or *thyrotropin.* TSH circulates in the blood and directs the thyroid gland to make its hormones, T4 and T3. The levels of the two thyroid hormones circulating in the bloodstream give feedback to the pituitary and hypothalamus about how productive the thyroid gland is—not enough or too much or just right—so the pituitary and hypothalamus determine how much TRH and TSH to make.

As you read this chapter, keep in mind that if the thyroid gland is not making enough T4 and T3, then the pituitary puts out *more* of the stimulating hormone, TSH. This means an *underactive thyroid* gland shows up with a *high* TSH. Many patients think that a low TSH means hypothyroidism, and it is the opposite. A *low* TSH means the pituitary senses *too much* thyroid hormone in the bloodstream, and shuts *off* the stimulating hormone. If TSH is too low (i.e., less than 0.4 uIu/ml), this indicates an *over*active thyroid gland. Make sense?

What the Thyroid Hormones Do

Maybe a simpler question is what *don't* they do! Basically, these two hormones, T3 and T4, oversee about every cellular metabolic process in our body . . . two of which, fat burning and muscle growth and repair, are particularly crucial to those of you with weight problems. The thyroid hormones are also involved in the pain-regulating processes and pathways that are involved in muscle repair and growth, as well as pathways for normal brain and nerve function. Because of their far-reaching effects in the body and brain, loss of the thyroid hormones *(hypothyroidism)* or insensitivity to their actions (called *thyroid resistance syndrome*) produces a vast array of symptoms. I have shown some of the common ones in the chart below, but even this is not an exhaustive list.

As you read the hypothyroidism chart, keep in mind that most of the same symptoms are also caused by loss of the ovarian hormones, as well as many other causes, including early diabetes. *You cannot just rely on symptom lists. You need proper blood tests to have a correct diagnosis.*

To make matters even more complicated, sometimes the same symptoms may be produced by *both* hyperthyroid syndromes *and* hypothyroid disorders, or by autoimmune disorders that interfere with normal hormone action. Some symptoms may differ, depending on whether there is too much or too little thyroid activity. It can be confusing to sort it out if you are just looking at the symptoms and not putting these together with the properly done laboratory evaluations.

Dramatic and diverse effects on multiple organ systems of the body, like the ones in the chart, can also occur when there is *abnormal function* of the thyroid hormones at cellular receptors, even if the overall levels of the hormone are normal. This condition is called thyroid hormone resistance, currently being intensively researched and recognized as a "real" condition. Dr. Weintraub, from the National Institutes of Health (NIH), reported in 1991 that "thyroid hormone resistance syndrome may affect thousands of unsuspecting Americans." Weight gain is one of the symptoms of *thyroid resistance* syndrome that many doctors may not fully appreciate.

DIETING SABOTEURS OF YOUR THYROID HORMONE BALANCE

Of the two thyroid hormones, T3 is the most metabolically "potent" form and the one needed to activate the cell's receptors, so it is crucial to have optimal *amounts* of T3 available. It is also critical to have the optimal *balance* of T3 in the *free* (active) state versus the *bound* (inactive) state in the bloodstream so it can trigger the energy-generating reactions in cells throughout your body to maintain healthy metabolism and weight.

Think of T3 as like the gasoline that runs your car engine. In this analogy, the body carefully regulates the amount of T3 that's "free" (and *active*) at any given time so the cells get the right amount of T3 stimulation to produce steady energy supplies. T3 that stays in the "bound" (*inactive*) form in the bloodstream is like gas in your tank, waiting to be used when needed. Then, much like your carburetor regulates gas flow to the car's engine for it to run properly, your body has to regulate the amount of T3 that is present in each form, free or bound. Too little gas getting to the engine means it shuts off and won't run. Too little *free* T3 means your cells act like they are hypothyroid, even if the *total* hormone level is normal.

But too much T3 in the free state causes excess thyroid stimulation ("thyroid storm" or thyrotoxicosis), and your cells don't work properly.

COMMON SYMPTOMS OF HYPOTHYROIDISM

◇ Weight gain, difficulty losing weight
◇ Severe fatigue, loss of energy, feeling "sluggish"
◇ Depressed mood, usually not as severe as major depression, but may be mistaken for primary depression
◇ Menstrual irregularities, difficulty becoming pregnant/infertility
◇ Low body temperature (may also occur with low estradiol and testosterone)
◇ PMS symptoms, with premenstrual mood changes common
◇ Premature menopause
◇ Dry, scaly, itchy skin and scalp
◇ Dry, brittle hair and nails
◇ Losing hair (alopecia)
◇ Hoarseness
◇ Chronic constipation
◇ Puffiness of face, lower legs, and feet
◇ Slowed heart rate, unusually low blood pressure
◇ Diminished reflexes
◇ Difficulty tolerating cold environments, climate ("can't get warm")
◇ Sleeping much more than normal, then not feeling rested
◇ Tingling in wrists/hands, mimicking "carpal tunnel syndrome"
◇ Clotting problems
◇ Multiple joint aches (arthralgias)
◇ Achy muscles (myalgias), leg cramps, muscle weakness
◇ Diminished or lost sexual desire (libido)
◇ Decreased memory, concentration (also brain effect of low thyroid may be misdiagnosed as dementia in an older person)
◇ Worsening allergies
◇ Abnormal lab tests: high TSH, low free thyroid hormones, elevated thyroid antibodies, high total cholesterol, low HDL, high LDL, possibly elevated liver enzymes

© 1995, revised 2001 by Elizabeth Lee Vliet, M.D.

It's just like too much gasoline coming in at one time, flooding your car engine and causing it to stall. Too much free T3 can damage your cells, especially heart-muscle fibers, so your body has a number of protective responses to regulate the free versus bound balance of T3 very carefully to keep everything humming along smoothly.

What are some things that trigger these protective responses to kick in and push more free T3 back into the bound T3 form? One occurs when brain-body "sensors" pick up clues that there may not be enough energy supply (i.e., food intake) to provide adequate fuel to keep cells working at their usual metabolic rate. What are some situations to make the brain think there isn't food enough for your metabolic fuel? One is *starvation.* Obviously, if you truly are not getting enough food, the body has to conserve what it has to enhance survival; it slows down its metabolic rate to save fuel.

In starvation conditions, two things happen with T3: first, the body makes *less* of the hormone, and second, what is made is mostly present in the *bound* form. The result is that your metabolism slows down to extend the available fuel supplies. With food so plentiful, most Americans today are not really in danger of starving. But there are times that your body *thinks* it may be starving, such as when you eat a very low calorie diet (less than 1,000 calories a day). The idea is to take in less food, make the body start burning fat for the fuel it needs, and lose weight. Right? Most of you reading this have "been there, done that."

But—here's the catch that gets you into trouble with the T3 pathway when you go on a *very low calorie diet* or try a fasting regimen for more than a day or two. If you are overweight and trying to lose weight by drastically restricting calories below your resting metabolic rate (RMR, the level needed to sustain resting activity for twenty-four hours), the body thinks it is starving, even though this is not actually the case. It aggressively goes into "save and store" mode. It defiantly holds on to every last calorie it can. One of the ways it does that is to force more T3 hormone back into the bound form to slow down your metabolism.

This is a reason women feel "hypothyroid" (cold, sluggish, dry skin, hair loss, constipated, etc.) after they have been on a diet with less than 1,200 calories a day for more than a few weeks. You don't need more thyroid in the form of medication—that would just make the problem worse as the body shifts more into the protein-bound form. "Hey," you say, "I want to speed up my metabolism to lose weight, not slow it down." And you are right. A revved-up metabolism is exactly what you need, but in order to do that, *you have to give the body more fuel* (calories) so it will think it has enough to rev up the engines again. To shift more T3 back into the free and active form, you have to have enough calories coming in, the *right kind* of calories coming in, and they have to be properly spaced out over the day.

Very low carbohydrate intake, such as recommended in the Atkins Diet, is another situation that causes the body to shift more T3 into the bound form. This is one reason that the Atkins Diet doesn't usually work as well for women as it does for men. Carbohydrates are the body's source of rapid fuel (glucose) to the cells, and glucose is the only fuel the brain can use. If the brain-body sensors detect too little carbohydrate coming in, this "deficit" sends a signal that there isn't enough of the right type of fuel for the metabolic processes. This causes some of your T3 to be pushed back to the bound, inactive form to prevent overstimulating the body. Too much carbohydrate, on the other hand, triggers a more rapid rise in glucose with more insulin being produced, which in turn makes you store more fat instead of burning it for fuel. Both too much and too little carbohydrate will end up sabotaging your weight loss efforts. The right balance of carbohydrate, protein, and fat is critical to your weight loss success. That's why I designed *Your Hormone Power Life Plan* to give you a food MAP (Meal Action Plan) to work *with* your body's hormone metabolic regulators, not against them.

Vegetarian diets, particularly the true vegan diet without any diary products or eggs, can also inadvertently sabotage your T3-T4 balance. Women who are vegetarian have more menstrual irregularities than women who also eat animal sources of protein, based on a variety of studies from several countries. The menstrual irregularities are thought to occur as a result of plant compounds that act as "endocrine disruptors" of two pathways: the conversion of T4 to T3 in the thyroid gland, and the ovarian production of estradiol and progesterone. If you have recently developed symptoms of hypothyroidism after changing to a vegetarian diet, you may need to add back more animal-derived protein to normalize your thyroid function. Standard thyroid profiles with just the total T4 and T3 won't show this; you have to have a measure of the TSH along with the *free* T4 and T3 measures.

Now here is one of the T3 "saboteurs" that will surprise you: *soy*. That's right. Soy has been known for many years to have antithyroid effects, but with all the glamorization of soy as the "wonder plant" for menopause and

PMS, it isn't mentioned that there are significant ways that soy interferes with healthy thyroid function. This antithyroid effect of soy was known to the ancient Chinese. Although they did not know that this "lump in the neck" we now call goiter was due to disruption of the thyroid gland function, they could tell the adverse effects on the body: weight gain, slowed thinking, fluid retention, low energy, dry skin, and slowed pulse. Soybeans were one of the seven sacred grains in ancient Chinese culture, but the only one of the seven that was not used for food at that time. In ancient China, soybeans were used only in crop rotation to replenish nitrogen in the soil. It wasn't until the process of fermentation was discovered hundreds of years later that the beans were *eaten* as food.

Isoflavones are now known to be the chemical compounds in soy that block the TPO enzyme reactions needed to convert T4 to T3. Genistein and daidzein, two of the most publicized and studied of the isoflavone compounds, both inhibit these enzyme reactions in the thyroid that are involved in the iodine-adding ("iodination") step to convert T4 to T3. In fact, today it is recognized that a high-soy diet is one of the leading causes of *goiter* and subclinical hypothyroidism in Japan and other Asian countries where people eat a lot of these foods. Since the 1950s, the U.S. Food and Drug Administration (FDA) has also known that soy used in infant formulas contains antithyroid compounds, putting these soy-fed infants at particularly high risk for later thyroid disorders. Unfortunately, these studies in pediatrics don't get much publicity in midlife women's magazines or weight-loss books.

Since thyroid disorders are eight to twenty times more common in women, and since this incidence increases dramatically after age forty, you need to be aware that increasing your intake of soy supplements or soy foods may interfere with healthy function of the thyroid gland, thereby aggravating your weight problems and contributing to menstrual irregularities. The grain *millet* and red clover also have high concentrations of these compounds that interfere with thyroid function. One study from the United Kingdom in premenopausal women found that a daily intake of 60 grams of soy for one month (equivalent to about 1 to 1.5 cups of soy milk) continued to disrupt the menstrual cycle for a full three months after the soy supplement was stopped.

Isoflavones are also known to interfere with fertility, in humans and in other mammals. For example, cattle breeders have known for years that cows eating a diet high in red clover (high in isoflavones) have high rates of infertility and miscarriage, indicating disruption of ovarian function. Why don't you know some of this information? Soybeans are a major crop in the United States, both for use in this country and sold for export around the world. The food industry has a major financial incentive to find ways for you to eat soy in whatever form possible, including soy supplements. They have no financial gain from you having the medical information about adverse effects on the thyroid gland. You may read more about these issues in the references I provided in Appendix II.

If you are struggling with weight problems, clearly *any* interference with either the ovary or the thyroid hormone balance and function will make weight gain more of a problem and make it harder for you to lose weight. I recommend that midlife women who are overweight would be wise to avoid soy supplements and not change to a diet high in soy, since this is likely to make the T3 levels lower and less effective. In this respect, my recommendations differ from a number of current diet books that have jumped on the soy bandwagon for "menopause" diets for women. I think soy-caused thyroid disruption is a very significant, and underrecognized, saboteur of your weight-loss efforts.

THYROID INTERACTIONS WITH OTHER HORMONES

Thyroid hormones help to regulate reproductive function, and if there is a disturbance in the thyroid function, the ovaries are also affected. Your ovaries have receptors for the thyroid hormones and the thyroid gland has receptors for the ovarian hormones, so these glands are closely linked in their function. Early thyroid decline is one of the common causes of irregular menstrual cycles and lower ovarian hormone production leading to infertility . . . but also, you guessed it, more *middle spread* and *mental pause.* The loss of the optimal estradiol and testosterone from the ovaries means more loss of muscle, more sluggish metabolism, and . . . more fat gain. The higher incidence of thyroid disorders in women after menopause, compared to older men, may reflect unknown ways that ovarian decline also adversely affects brain centers that regulate the thyroid.

Higher-than-normal cortisol levels also interfere with normal thyroid function. Since cortisol rises as estradiol declines, this may be another mechanism for women to develop thyroid problems and then gain weight at midlife. High cortisol levels occur in Cushing's disease, prolonged severe stress states, use of high-progestin birth control pills, and use of corticosteroid medications (such as those for asthma or arthritis). When cortisol is too high, it pushes more thyroid hormone back into the bound, inactive portion. Less of the *free* T3 and T4 leads to more slowing down of your metabolism and more fat storage.

Thyroid hormones, in addition to estrogen, stimulate the production of GH, which, in turn, promotes the overall growth of bone and muscle. So if your thyroid hormones are lower than optimal, along with menopausal loss of estradiol, this means there will be a decrease in GH, too. Reduced GH in turn causes loss of muscle, which means . . . you guessed it, more fat. See how the pieces all intertwine and affect one another?

Thyroid hormones are also intricately related to the various neurotransmitters that regulate mood and pain pathways, and are known to cause problems with depression, anxiety, sleep, memory, and concentration when there is too much or too little thyroid activity. Remember, the thyroid hormones govern cell metabolism and energy pathways, and the brain is the biggest energy user in the body, as well as the most metabolically active. So if something goes wrong with the thyroid hormones, the first organ to be affected is usually the brain, leading to depressed moods. And if you feel sluggish and depressed, you don't exercise, and you typically don't eat very well, so you have more fat storage. Ultimately, whatever the cause of a biological depression, this disorder also typically causes high cortisol production, which is another stimulator of fat storage. See how quickly we can get trapped in a hormonal quagmire that overwhelms us?

THYROID EFFECTS ON MUSCLE TISSUE

Thyroid hormones have widespread effects on muscle metabolism. If you lose optimal thyroid effect, you don't build up more muscle, and then you have *less* of your active fat-burning tissue. In addition, too much or too little thyroid hormone can interfere with normal oxygen delivery to the skeletal muscle cells, which may help to explain the muscle pain, loss of strength, and increased fatigue that occur with thyroid disorders. The heart muscle is also very sensitive to the effects of thyroid hormone. Both hypothyroidism and hyperthyroidism may cause impaired oxygen delivery to the muscle, although the exact mechanisms may be different.

Excess thyroid hormone, such as in Graves' disease, or other causes of thyroid hormone excess—such as taking too much thyroid prescription medication or over-the-counter glandulars—can result in serious damage to the heart. Although the mechanism is not fully known, it appears that excess thyroid hormone disrupts normal blood flow to the heart, so there is diminished oxygen supply to the heart muscle. This can lead to a heart attack. Not enough thyroid hormone, on the other hand, may also contribute to damage to the heart muscle by decreasing oxygen delivery and causing more muscle damage, which can also lead to a heart attack. Optimal balance is key.

WILSON'S SYNDROME: DANGERS TO WATCH FOR

There has been a lot of attention on the Internet given to Wilson's syndrome, a condition Dr. Denis Wilson claims to have "discovered," in which T4 is not adequately converted to T3. Actually, this condition has been described in thyroid medical textbooks for a number of years and was not "discovered" by Dr. Wilson. It is one of many types of defects in the thyroid pathways that come under the larger heading of *thyroid resistance syndromes.* Failure to adequately convert T4 to T3 can have many causes, and I listed a few dietary ones earlier in this chapter. This condition clearly exists in some people, and may actually be even more critical to assess in women with weight problems since T3 is so critical to muscle and fat metabolism. As I said earlier, I think it is a *must* to check serum free T3 in such situations. The serum free T3 is highly accurate and specific for answering the question about whether the body converts T4 to T3.

As a way to see if you have low free T3, Wilson's syndrome materials recommend checking your morning basal body temperature under your arm (axillary temperature). Their directions tell you that blood tests are not reliable, and that you should increase the amount of T3 you take until your morning body temperature is back to normal at 98.6 degrees. They have ignored the advances in blood testing methods in the last fifteen to twenty years since these theories were first espoused. Current blood tests are highly reliable when used as I describe later in the chapter.

Proponents of the basal body temperature method have ignored basic female biology. They have completely overlooked women's *ovarian* hormones as important body temperature regulators. If low *estradiol* is the cause of body temperature problems, you won't be able to get your body temperature back to "normal" just by taking T3 hormone. The combination of low estradiol with excess T3 can cause lethal heart effects. In addition, there are still other endocrine factors that determine your basal body temperature. If something other than low T3 is the cause of your lower body temperature, you can become toxic on thyroid trying to get your temperature up by adding T3. *It can be very dangerous to follow Wilson's protocol.* Women have actually died from heart arrthymias due to excess thyroid following Wilson's guidelines.

I recently saw a fifty-two-year-old woman who had a free T3 level of over 750 following the "Wilson's protocol" and increasing Cytomel doses to reach desired basal body temperature. Her free T3 level should have been only about 300. When I saw her she was thyrotoxic as a result of many months of thyroid excess. She had high blood pressure, palpitations, shortness of breath, chronic insomnia, nervousness, anxiety symptoms, increased sweating, and her bone loss had gone from mild to severe osteoporosis. Her estradiol level was less than 30 pg/ml, and even though she was taking large amounts of T3, her morning body temperature was still 97.4 degrees and she was gaining middle-body fat.

This was a very dangerous situation for her. I was concerned that she was developing congestive heart failure from the thyroid excess and was at serious risk of a heart attack. Women who take increasing thyroid hormone trying to get their body temperature "back to normal" may end up not only having a heart attack, but they are also at high risk for rapid bone loss leading to hip or spine fracture. Excess thyroid is one of the leading *preventable* causes of osteoporosis in older women who are not taking estrogen.

Today, with the sensitivity of current test methods, we can get a reliable answer to the T3 issue. This is more reliable and safer than relying on body temperature. You also need reliable blood tests of estradiol and cortisol before you use body temperature to decide that you have a thyroid problem. Your physician needs to be careful in how thyroid medication is used and the measures relied upon to make dose decisions. And, *you* should not change your thyroid medication on your own, without specific guidance from your physician, based on reliable blood test information.

GETTING YOUR THYROID TESTED AND INTERPRETING THE RESULTS

Most standard thyroid panels only check the total hormones, but I find these standard profiles are inadequate to help us understand the thyroid factors in weight gain because it is really the amount present in the free form that determines how effectively your thyroid hormones are working. This is why I always check free T3 and free T4 in my patients, and you should ask your doctor to do the same. There is not a major difference in cost, and the information gained is far more helpful in sorting out what you may need in the way of fine-tuning your thyroid balance.

The following thyroid tests are the ones I think are important for women with weight problems, and they can be done on any day of your menstrual cycle if you are still menstruating:

◇ ultrasensitive TSH
◇ free T4 (levothyronine)
◇ free T3 (triiodothyronine)
◇ antimicrosomal antibody (also called antithyroid peroxi-dase antibody, or anti-TPO)
◇ antithyroglobulin antibody
◇ TRH stimulation test (I generally don't find that this is nec-essary if the ones above are done)

There is one type of *thyroid resistance,* however, that we don't yet have a good blood test to check, and that is tissue resistance to the effects of T3 even when adequate hormone level is present. Body temperature isn't reliable in this situation either since other hormone imbalances may cause lower body temperature. If your physician suspects resistance to T3 at the cellular level, but all the labs are "normal" *and* other hormones have been adequately restored to optimal, then it may make sense to have a trial of very low dose T3 (such as only 5 mcg of Cytomel or a compounded sustained release T3). If this is done, then it is important that you be checked regularly to be certain you aren't getting too much thyroid effect, which will increase bone loss and may trigger heart rhythm disturbances.

WHAT'S NORMAL VERSUS WHAT'S OPTIMAL

Keep in mind that if someone tells you that your thyroid tests are "normal," you still may have a subtle thyroid dysfunction contributing to your weight problems. It is a common occurance that women are told their thyroid is normal, without having the complete thyroid tests done. Of course, what most people, and many physicians, don't realize is that a "normal range" on a laboratory report is just that: a *range*. A person may require higher or lower levels to feel well and to function optimally. I think we must look at the lab results alongside the physical problems described by each individual. After all, we are treating people, not lab values. It is also possible that one or more lab measures may still fall in the normal range and yet other, more subtle, measures may be abnormal. This is when it is very important to listen to the woman, and her descriptions of what is wrong, with an open mind and with trust in what she says and knows about her body.

WHEN TO CONSIDER STARTING THYROID MEDICATION

On most laboratory scales, hypothyroidism is considered to begin at TSH values greater than about 5, although many physicians don't treat with thyroid medication until the TSH rises over 8. In my opinion, such a rigid view overlooks the point I made earlier: weight gain, menstrual irregularity, infertility, PMS, depression, and memory loss in women are occurring long before the TSH goes that high. Waiting until TSH is above 5 is waiting too long, in my view, and allows symptoms such as weight gain and insulin resistance to get worse unnecessarily. Since different labs have different units and reference ranges for free T3 and free T4, I can't give you specific guidelines here for those target values.

I prefer to take a "stitch-in-time-saves-nine" approach and begin treatment earlier, typically when the TSH is about 4, especially if thyroid antibodies are high, or if the free T3 or free T4 are lower than optimal and women are having symptoms of low thyroid. This fits with current studies that indicate women may not have normal fertility or optimal ovarian function if the TSH is much above 2. The earlier treatment is begun, the less likely you are to have other adverse effects of low thyroid such as high blood pressure, elevated cholesterol, and serious weight gain, and the easier it is to regain optimal health.

I do not advocate using thyroid hormone supplements solely for weight loss if all of the laboratory studies are completely normal, including thyroid antibodies. If women are given thyroid hormones when they don't have a thyroid problem, it can cause serious problems: impaired sleep, impaired immune function, rapid bone loss, heart rhythm disturbances, and damage to heart muscle fibers. Excess thyroid can also cause significant wasting of skeletal muscles throughout the body, leading to more weakness and more fatigue that makes you incorrectly think you need thyroid. If you also have low estradiol and testosterone, this is another cause of muscle loss. It is critical to check both ovarian and thyroid hormones carefully before making treatment decisions. I talk more about thyroid treatment options in chapter 14. Don't be tempted to take a "quick fix" approach to weight loss and ramp up your thyroid medication on your own, hoping to increase your metabolism. It is potentially dangerous.

Chapter 9

CORTISOL AND STRESS:

FAT-PROMOTERS FOR THE OVER-30 WOMAN

STRESS. For most of us, it conjures up awful images of body-wrecking effects: cancer, heart attacks, high blood pressure, infertility, allergies . . . the list goes on and on. But all of us live with stress, all of the time, both the stress of constant change going on within the body systems, and the stress of constant interaction with the outside world. But did you also know that stress can make you fat?

Stress sets off a series of hormonal changes that are more profound for women at midlife than for men, and these hormonal changes trigger the outpouring of additional hormones and chemical messengers that dictate how much fat we use or store. Not everyone *gains* weight when under stress, cortisol (the major stress hormone) is not the only contributor that makes us fatter. Other factors include: the balance of hormones, food choices we make (do we become ravenous, or are we unable to eat?), medications, our genes, our metabolic rate, adequacy of vitamins and other nutrients, and our attitudes.

Stress is always present until we die. We can't eliminate it completely. My goal is to help you be successful in eliminating the "stress traps" that make you fatter:

◇ **Stress Trap #1:** Eating at the wrong time of day, especially late at night, when you are stressed. This plays right into the waiting fat-storing hands of cortisol and insulin.

◇ **Stress Trap #2:** Eating more potatoes, pasta, breads, sweets for "comfort." Excesses of these foods also play into the fat-storing actions of cortisol and insulin.

◇ **Stress Trap #3:** Eating the wrong balance of foods, such as too *low* in fat or too restricted in carbs. The wrong balance of protein-carbs-fats adversely affects your thyroid and ovarian hormone activity.

◇ **Stress Trap #4:** Taking over-the-counter hormones to self-treat stress symptoms. Examples: using DHEA to boost energy, or melatonin to help you sleep. Both make you hungrier and store more fat.

◇ **Stress Trap #5:** Taking soy or herb supplements to relieve stress-induced hormonal imbalance symptoms (insomnia, hot flashes, etc.). Soy isoflavones and some herbs can block the proper action of both thyroid hormones and estradiol as I described in chapter 8.

◇ **Stress Trap #6:** Becoming a couch potato. Lack of physical activity and aerobic exercise further feeds the fat-storing actions of cortisol.

◇ **Stress Trap #7:** Drinking alcohol or smoking cigarettes, or pot, to relax. They block the effective actions of your key metabolic activators: estradiol, testosterone, T3 and T4.

Recognize yourself in any of these? Let's explore how stress aggravates our midlife "middle spread and mental pause"!

HOW OUR BRAINS PERCEIVE STRESS

Stressors are stimuli that trigger body responses to help us adapt to changes. These stressors may be *external* situations in our lives, or *internal* changes in our body. This is a good thing, essential to our survival. Stress of any form—positive or negative—elicits the same brain-body reactions. Our brain constantly perceives and processes information coming to it from the world around us and also from moment-to-moment changes inside the body. The brain uses this incoming information to tell the body how much food to eat and whether to release our fat stores for energy or store fat for future emergencies.

Stress-induced changes affect our weight-regulating neurotransmitters, how fast food moves through our gut, what kinds of food we want to eat, how efficiently our body processes foods, how well our nerve endings respond to food, and all aspects of metabolism. With prolonged stress of any kind—physical, environmental, situational, psychological, spiritual— the body's balance, or homeostasis, is disrupted and we see symptoms that are caused by two major factors: the "acute" stress response of increased activity of the "fight-or-flight" (adrenaline) pathways, and the "chronic" stress response of increased production of cortisol. Both of these sets of physical changes conspire to make you fatter by promoting abdominal fat *storage* instead of fat breakdown.

Your brain oversees all your thoughts, feelings, moods, and behaviors (including eating), and all of these are affected by both external situations and by internal body fluctuations. This means that all the biochemical changes throughout the body are affected by both physical causes and psychological ones. Eating is a brain-regulated behavior that is profoundly affected by the outpouring of cortisol when we are stressed. Cortisol and other stress hormones affect us both physically (e.g., release of hunger-promoting chemicals) and psychologically (e.g., habits, food preferences). For example, "anxiety" may be caused by falling blood sugar (internal physical change) *or* by worry (internal psychological feeling) *or* by a car pulling out in front of you (external physical event).

"Acute" stress symptoms may include feeling really hungry, craving sweets or alcohol, irritability, panic attacks, sweats, pounding heartbeat (palpitations), restless sleep, bad dreams, and others. "Chronic" persistent stress symptoms include overwhelming fatigue; low energy; feelings of sluggishness; bloating and mental fuzziness; comfort food cravings; insomnia; allergy attacks; infections (like colds, flu, and yeast); depression; low sex drive; and loss of your zip and zest. How do the stress hormones make you fatter? How does declining estradiol and testosterone make you more susceptible to cortisol's fat-promoting effects? How do the stress hormones affect your thyroid? Let's explore this.

CORTISOL, ITS DAILY RHYTHMS AND WHAT IT DOES

Cortisol is a member of the *glucocorticoid group* of hormones produced by the adrenal glands, and it prepares our body to deal with the effects of stress. Cortisol and its fellow glucocorticoids are major metabolic regulators, having several effects on your weight-regulating pathways in addition to their many other effects. Cortisol has a definite daily (diurnal) rhythm to its secretion, normally beginning to rise for the day about 4:00 to 5:00 A.M., and peaking about 8:00 to 9:00 A.M. We need the effects of rising cortisol to get our biological engines going to start our day. Levels should be gradually falling over the day and be lowest at night. When we are stressed, this normal daily rhythm may be blunted, shifted in time, or even completely reversed. For example, you may have low levels in the morning, rising (instead of falling) as the day unfolds so that you have unusually high levels in the afternoon or evening instead of in the morning. We often see this pattern in our midlife women patients who describe feeling like "I wake up tired, and I finally seem to get going in the evening and then I can't sleep."

Two brain centers, the hypothalamus and pituitary, govern cortisol output from the adrenal glands via three hormones. *Corticotropin-releasing hormone* (CRH) and ADH from the hypothalamus stimulate release of the pituitary hormone, ACTH, which, in turn, stimulates the adrenal gland to release cortisol. The normally rising blood levels of cortisol feed back to the brain, letting the pituitary and hypothalamus know the message was received and cortisol has been made. As a result, levels of ACTH, CRH, and ADH drop back down to baseline. But when we are stressed, levels of ACTH, CRH, and cortisol *all* rise, and these normal daily rhythms are interrupted, leading to excessively high cortisol levels over more of the day.

Cortisol levels higher than normal over time lead to high blood pressure, high cholesterol and triglycerides, high fasting glucose, excess insulin release and resistance to insulin effects, increased risk of diabetes, repeated infections (from cortisol's immune suppression), thin skin, easy bruising, muscle weakness, and increased rate of bone loss. Excess cortisol causes marked fat deposits around the middle of the body, breasts, upper back and arms, as well as a rounded puffy face that is called "moon facies." Together, these negative changes are called *Cushing's syndrome,* a medical name for cortisol excess, whether from too much cortisol being produced by the body, or from cortisol-type medications (glucocorticoids, such as prednisone) you may be taking for asthma, arthritis, and other medical problems. Whatever the cause, prolonged high cortisol leads to serious medical problems and a higher risk of early death, usually from heart disease, or infections that don't respond well to treatment.

If you have been under severe, unrelenting stress for long periods of time, such as many months to several years, the adrenal glands eventually may lose their ability to respond properly with increased cortisol, and you may enter a phase of adrenal insufficiency or "exhaustion." The hallmark of this condition is a *lower*-than-normal cortisol, along with sodium that is abnormally low and potassium that is abnormally high. Adrenal insufficiency may arise for unclear reasons not related to persistent severe stresses, a condition called *Addison's disease.* True Addison's disease (adrenal insufficiency, AI, or low cortisol) is uncommon. AI is almost always associated with severe weight *loss* (rather than weight gain seen with high cortisol), lower-than-normal blood pressure, significant fatigue, muscle weakness, and loss of pubic and axillary body hair.

HIGH CORTISOL AND HIGH STRESS

There is a two-way connection between ovarian hormones and stress. First, declining estradiol is itself a "stressor" to the body that causes increased cortisol output and loss of optimal function of norepinephrine, serotonin, dopamine, and acetylcholine. These chemical "communicators" are all involved in regulation of weight and body fat, appetite, muscle growth/repair, sleep, mood, memory, thirst, sex drive, and pain regulation. Second, stress leads to poor food and vitamin intake, low energy, and difficulty coping . . . which then adds further stress . . . which suppresses estrogen and thyroid function even more. These back-and-forth processes feed back on each other and make the stress effects even worse. See how you get caught in the traps?

Stress-induced decline in estradiol causing elevated cortisol and these adverse effects on brain chemical messengers is a significantly overlooked trigger for fat gain in midlife, and it is also a physical factor contributing to having difficulty coping. When my estradiol is too low; I certainly don't sleep well, feel my best, or think well, and that stresses me!

So here we have the downward spiral:

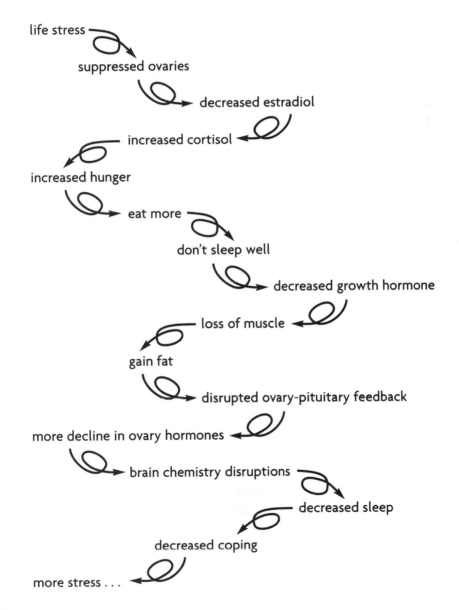

life stress

suppressed ovaries

decreased estradiol

increased cortisol

increased hunger

eat more

don't sleep well

decreased growth hormone

loss of muscle

gain fat

disrupted ovary-pituitary feedback

more decline in ovary hormones

brain chemistry disruptions

decreased sleep

decreased coping

more stress . . .

So we are back to the beginning of the list. When midlife hits, it seems we are caught in one after another of these quicksand pits. No wonder it is so difficult and frustrating to try and lose weight.

STRESS AND ILLNESS

Figure 9.1 shows some of the ways that *stressors* of all kinds require the body processes to change and adapt. Hormonal change is one of those stressors that means that the body systems must constantly be changing and adapting. These changes themselves may become additional stressors on the body and contribute to yet more stress overload. The interconnections and the ways in which hormonal production may in turn be altered by stress on the body are often overlooked when women seek medical care. The two-way nature of these pathways is a critical connection, throughout all facets of women's health, that has been the frequently overlooked "missing link."

HIGH CORTISOL FROM OTHER CAUSES

Life stress is the usual trigger that comes to mind as a cause of increased cortisol, but in addition to decline in your ovarian or thyroid hormones there are many other causes: taking steroid medications, infections, dieting, alcohol overuse, drug use, chronic exposure to pollutants or allergens, as well as the more usual psychological triggers such as fear, worry, anger, and other negative moods. When we are "stressed" by physical changes *or* by psychological states, and cortisol goes *up*, decreased ovarian hormone production, and altered thyroid function, leads to menstrual irregularity. Mother Nature built in a protective effect to prevent us from getting pregnant if our bodies are too "stressed" to be healthy enough to sustain a pregnancy and nurse the infant. Worldwide studies consistently show a correlation between high life stress and lower levels of ovarian estrogen, testosterone, and loss of the normal cyclic production of progesterone. If this high-stress state continues, it may lead to infertility in younger women or earlier menopause in older women. This is the reason I think it is important that we check all of these hormones together, particularly when you have been under a lot of stress.

Figure 9.1
STRESS EFFECTS

TYPES OF STRESSORS			
LIFE SITUATIONS	**PSYCHOLOGICAL**	**PHYSICAL**	**ENVIRONMENT**
finances	fears	hormone change	pollutants
work	worries	diet	allergens
relationships	body image	illness	weather
community	midlife angst	alcohol, drugs	toxins

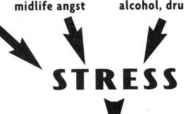

STRESS

**DISRUPTS BODY BALANCE (HOMEOSTASIS),
LEADING TO—**

PSYCHOLOGICAL SYMPTOMS
food binges
"panic attacks"
disrupted sleep
irritability, anxiousness
depression
angry outbursts
desire for alcohol, drugs

"FIGHT-OR-FLIGHT" SYMPTOMS
racing heartbeat, palpitations
sweatiness, clamminess
nausea/loss of appetite
increased hunger, sweet cravings
blood sugar swings
headaches
diarrhea, "irritable bowel"
allergy flares, skin rashes

PHYSICAL HEALTH PROBLEMS
weight gain
insulin resistance, diabetes
high blood pressure
heart disease
chronic fatigue
infections (viral, bacterial, yeast)
autoimmune disorders
malignancies

SPOTTING EARLY CLUES

Are there any clues that come early in the process of hormone change that alert you to problems before you gain a lot of weight? I think there are, but all too often these "early warning" symptoms are discounted by doctors, or explained away by patients as "I guess I'm just under a lot of stress." One clue, often missed by physicians, is that women who later developed weight problems had increasing food cravings—usually for sweets or rich, fatty foods (duh!)—and "anxiety" or "racing heart" episodes, usually right before their periods were due to begin. They tell me about having "blood sugar swings," "mood swings," or "horrendous palpitations" and pounding sensations "as if my heart were going to literally jump out of my chest." Often the heart-related symptoms are so pronounced that women don't notice the appetite changes or the connection with food cravings.

These clues often happen before they have serious weight gain, but many times doctors label these problems "anxiety" or "stress," so a woman who is experiencing this cluster of problems will often be told to relax more and reduce stress. But then it happens again, and again, and again . . . usually with the menstrual cycle, but doctors still don't seem to pay much attention to this connection. Oftentimes, they simply prescribe medication to relieve "anxiety." The "fight-or-flight" symptoms ease up, but food cravings and inexorable weight gain continue. If the underlying cause of such episodes is really the brain effects of diminished estradiol, along with beginning glucose intolerance and insulin resistance, then anxiety medications won't help very much.

Cortisol starts creeping up, estradiol declines some more without being addressed, and then you start having those torturous nights of restless, disrupted sleep. Sleep disruption adds to overstimulating cortisol and interrupting the normal daily cortisol pattern, so you wake up tired, hungry, foggy-brained, and with muscle aches . . . and the downward spiral toward persistent middle spread and mental pause has begun! I can hear you saying to yourself as you read this, "How does *estradiol* affect the *brain* to make me *fat*?" As I described in chapter 5, decreases in estradiol cause loss of many brain messengers, and that, in turn, further stimulates the cortisol release, which leads to more insulin release, which makes you store fat. See how the pieces connect? Take a look at the following sequence of events.

Figure 9.2
BRAIN-BODY EFFECTS OF ESTRADIOL DECREASE

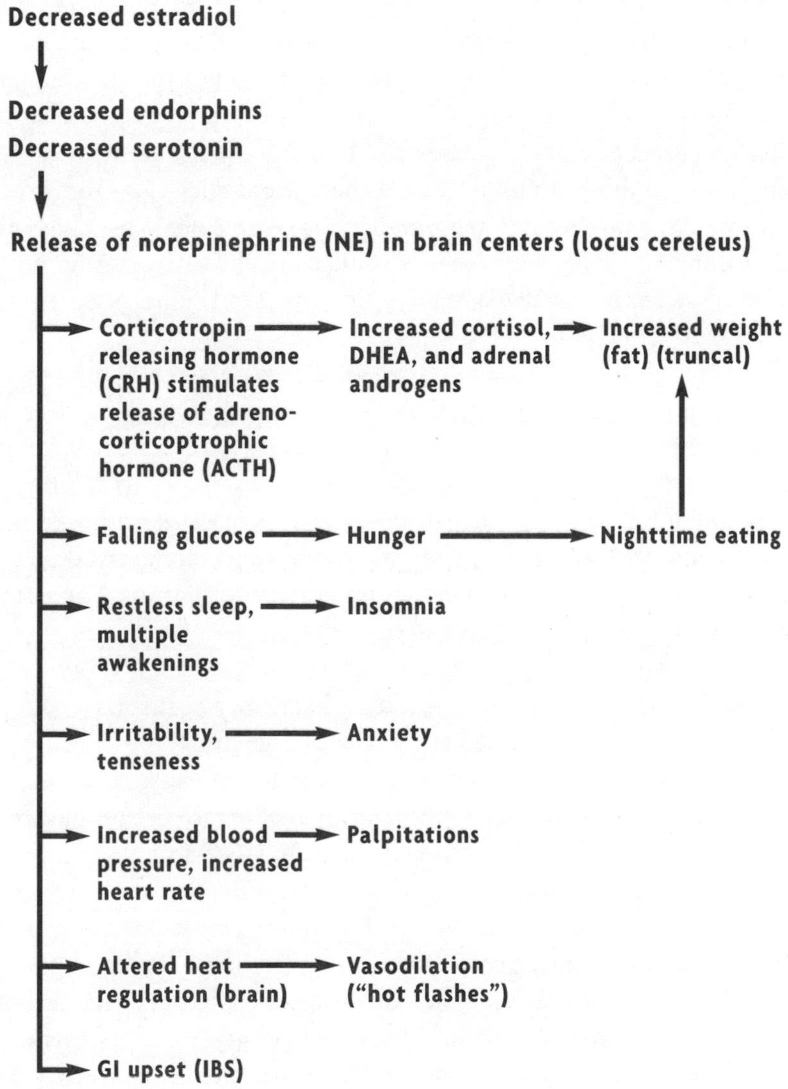

Decreased estradiol

↓

Decreased endorphins
Decreased serotonin

↓

Release of norepinephrine (NE) in brain centers (locus cereleus)

→ Corticotropin ⟶ Increased cortisol, → Increased weight
releasing hormone   DHEA, and adrenal   (fat) (truncal)
(CRH) stimulates   androgens
release of adreno-
corticoptrophic
hormone (ACTH)

→ Falling glucose ⟶ Hunger ⟶ Nighttime eating

→ Restless sleep, ⟶ Insomnia
multiple
awakenings

→ Irritability, ⟶ Anxiety
tenseness

→ Increased blood ⟶ Palpitations
pressure, increased
heart rate

→ Altered heat ⟶ Vasodilation
regulation (brain)   ("hot flashes")

→ GI upset (IBS)

© 1995, revised 2001 by Elizabeth Lee Vliet, M.D.

So there you are, falling estradiol triggers release of brain chemicals and leads to a whole cascade of events spreading *throughout* the body and making your fat-storing machinery pack on the pounds. The endorphins, your natural mood elevators and pain killers, are also involved in appetite regulation to either stimulate appetite or to make you feel full and satisfied. These physical events are so common, and start so gradually, that many women don't even notice them until the hormone drops become greater during perimenopause and you start having actual hot flashes. Suddenly, the hot flashes, or "power surges" hit, and we are *aware* of something new happening. Most doctors have not been taught these hormone-brain-body connections, so they don't realize that there are earlier clues to women's midlife weight gain. Women tell me they know "it's a physical, chemical kind of thing," but they have been told that it's "just stress," and no one checks the hormone levels. Women's intuitive (and more often correct) insights are overlooked.

Then there is the decrease in serotonin that occurs due to both persistent stress and to the loss of estradiol. Serotonin helps maintain sleep and decrease anxiety, so a drop in serotonin *adds* to the episodes of awakenings at night and aggravates the adrenaline-induced feelings of irritability, tension, palpitations, and . . . hunger! What you typically eat more of is the carbs, because that's a way the body makes more serotonin. And then, all that cortisol and insulin are lurking around that fat cell, waiting greedily to grab those carbs and make them into more fat.

Remember, too, that gaining excess body fat is itself a profound stressor on all of the body systems. Obesity makes your cortisol–weight gain problems worse by further interfering with ovarian function, including the way the hormones themselves govern the weight pathways. For example, the erratically falling estradiol levels prior to menopause fire off the brain's "alarm center" in the limbic system, causing a burst of norepinephrine that disrupts the appetite-regulating center in the hypothalamus. The hypothalamus responds to the "alarm" by sending out chemical messengers that make you want to eat more so you are prepared for the impending "emergency." Make sense? This sequence of physical changes is very real, and when it occurs day after day, it contributes to your getting fatter. I'll bet you didn't know that it takes only about fifty extra calories each day to add ten pounds of body fat in a year. Do this for a few years, and you see why you "suddenly" have an extra fifty pounds to lose.

GETTING TESTED FOR CORTISOL

If you've been under a great deal of stress and are gaining weight, ask your physician to check your cortisol levels.

An 8:00 A.M. *serum* cortisol level is the most reliable *first* step in checking for low or high cortisol. If this is *higher* than about 20 µg/dl, then other tests can be ordered to clarify the cause. The typical ones that are done include serum ACTH, twenty-four-hour urine for urinary free cortisol, and Dexamethasone Suppression Test (DST). A CRH stimulation test may be appropriate, and is usually done by endocrinologists. If these follow-up tests are abnormal, imaging studies (MRI, CAT scans, etc.) are usually ordered to check the adrenal glands and pituitary for possible tumors causing the excess cortisol production.

If the 8:00 A.M. cortisol is lower than 5 to 7 µg/dl, serum ACTH and ACTH (Cortrosyn) stimulation tests are generally done next to evaluate the cause of adrenal insufficiency (for example, adrenal destruction or pituitary dysfunction). If the 8:00 A.M. cortisol is greater than 10 µg/dl and your serum electrolytes (sodium, potassium) are normal, this makes it *very unlikely* that you have adrenal insufficiency. You should have other hormone systems tested, as I describe in chapter 11, to determine other causes of your symptoms such as fatigue, weakness, and low energy level. But remember, marked weight *loss* occurs in virtually *all* people who have adrenal insufficiency. If you are *gaining* weight, this usually occurs only in *excess* cortisol production syndromes, not adrenal insufficiency.

Stress and high cortisol have multiple adverse effects on the brain and body through many mechanisms beyond the ovary hormones, and more than just adding pounds to your middle The chart on page 148 lists some of the major ones, and in chapter 14, I will talk about steps for you to discuss with your physician to help you restore cortisol to normal if it is out of the healthy range.

For further information about the ways that prolonged stress and high cortisol can damage the body and lead to accelerated aging, I suggest you read *Why Zebras Don't Get Ulcers,* by Robert M. Sapolsky. This will help you better understand why stress management and *cortisol reduction* are crucial components of a sound *weight reduction* program.

ADVERSE HEALTH CONSEQUENCES OF EXCESS CORTISOL OR CORTICOSTEROID MEDICINES

◇ Abdominal fat gain

◇ Increased risk of heart disease by promoting plaque buildup in arteries

◇ Increased total cholesterol, LDL and triglyceride levels, lower HDL

◇ Increased risk of diabetes due to increased levels of blood glucose

◇ Aggravated insulin resistance

◇ Loss of normal collagen metabolism (the basis of healthy ligaments and tendons), leading to injuries, joint and back pain

◇ Disruption in the sleep cycle, leading to less restorative sleep, diminished GH, and decreased muscle repair at night, which add to the damaging effects of declining estradiol on the same pathways

◇ Interference with normal thyroid function, leading to *less* of the available T3 that is so important for cellular metabolism throughout the body

◇ Immune suppression, leading to more infections and illnesses

◇ Increased need for antioxidants, vitamins, minerals as well as proper balance of macronutrients, yet when we are stressed and don't feel well, we often don't get the nutritional balance we most need

◇ Hair loss, thinning skin, easy bruising

MELATONIN: THE "NATURAL" SLEEP AID THAT BUILDS FAT

People often take "natural" supplements when under stress. Lately, melatonin has become one that people reach for as a sleep aid. But in addition to being the "night" hormone secreted during darkness, melatonin has a different kind of "dark" side when it comes to its effects on body fat. It helps to think of melatonin as the hormone of hibernation—it triggers the body changes that help Mama Bear slow down her metabolism, store fat for the long winter, and remain sleepy and slowed down. Researchers have found this effect in studies of melatonin injected into other animals that don't typically hibernate: they overeat, oversleep, are lethargic, and have a slowed activity level. No wonder then that I regularly hear from our women patients that they began having an increase in fatigue, food cravings, and drowsiness (not to mention headaches and depressed mood) after starting melatonin supplements. Ask yourself, is this how you want to feel each day?

In studies of SAD, researchers gave melatonin to women who had been successfully treated with bright light therapy. Melatonin administration did not fully blunt the success of bright light as an antidepressant, but the women who received melatonin did have a significant increase in other symptoms characteristic of SAD: fatigue, increased appetite, carbohydrate craving, weight gain, and social withdrawal. The increase in these symptoms was not seen in women receiving placebo.

The interaction between melatonin and serotonin may help to explain some of these observations. Melatonin is made in the brain from serotonin, and the same area of the brain that regulates melatonin release also regulates serotonin production. Since serotonin is used to make melatonin, it stands to reason that when melatonin levels go *up*, serotonin levels go down. This may help to explain the symptoms of increased carbohydrate cravings experienced by SAD sufferers, since carbs shift amino acid balance in a way that allows the brain to make more serotonin. High-carbohydrate meals enhance all the other amino acids moving into body tissues from the bloodstream, which leaves more tryptophan, serotonin's building block, in the blood so it can be taken up into brain cells to make serotonin.

But what if you are *taking* melatonin supplements? The supplements contain much higher levels of melatonin than the brain normally makes. It appears that these high levels of melatonin end up suppressing serotonin production, which in turn triggers the intense carbohydrate cravings, headaches, and depressed mood that women describe.

Recent studies have shown an alarming connection in *women* taking melatonin supplements: they had much higher serum levels of cortisol than did women taking placebo. Melatonin's effect on cortisol was not seen in the men. So when women take melatonin at night to help improve sleep, they are hit really hard: The melatonin itself makes you hungrier, makes you more efficient at storing fat, and stimulates cortisol production (which makes another way you unwittingly increase your fat storage). Most of the studies quoted in popular books touting melatonin as a powerful "anti-aging" hormone with sleep-promoting effects were done in men or male animals. All of this just goes to show that studies done in men cannot be applied to women with the assumption that there will be the same effects. Women's bodies respond differently than men's to hormones. If you are struggling with weight gain, I urge you not to take melatonin on a regular basis.

THE BOTTOM LINE

Cortisol, corticosteroid medicines, and melatonin all promote fat storage. The higher your cortisol stays, and the longer it is elevated, the more you store pounds around the middle of the body. As I showed you in the chart on page 148, elevated cortisol has a host of negative effects on your health. Not only do you have the physical consequences of excess fat, you have the resulting psychological stress and emotional pain of being fat in a culture that idolizes thinness. Then, when you feel lousy about yourself, you eat more to ease the pain. I know, I have done that, too. All of these changes together push us inexorably toward more weight gain and a higher risk of diabetes, high blood pressure, heart disease, and stroke. My professional and personal experiences have taught me that, to break out of the trap and regain your healthy, fit body, it takes *all* of the integrated approaches I describe in Part Three, *Your Hormone Power Plan.*

Chapter 10

YOUR SUGAR-REGULATING HORMONES

AND HOW THEY CAN MAKE YOU FAT

How many of you have experienced food cravings with your menstrual cycle? I'll bet most of you nodded yes as you read that question. Have you ever had chocolate cravings the week before your period? Yup, I know that one well! I can remember times when I was in the top ten for Chocolate Queen. And then there were the late night runs to the 7-Eleven for a "chocolate fix" to help me survive studying for exams in medical school . . . but only if I happened to be studying intensely and stressed at the same time as the week before my period! So what is happening with our ovary hormones that makes us feel like we are out of control with these cravings in the second half of our cycle . . . and it seems to get worse, not better, as perimenopause hits?

A QUICK REVIEW: METABOLISM BASICS

Food is our metabolic fuel to stay alive and grow. Digestion breaks food down into smaller, simpler molecules (glucose, amino acids, fatty acids) so that it can be absorbed into the bloodstream and delivered throughout the body to the trillions of cells that make up our organs and tissues. Ultimately, amino acids (from proteins) and fatty acids (from fats) are metabolized to glucose, which is combined with oxygen and "burned" to provide energy to run the cells, much like your car burns gasoline to power its engine. *Metabolism* is the name for this entire process of breaking down foods into smaller molecules, and "burning" (oxidizing) them to make energy for our body's growth and repair.

WHAT ARE YOUR SUGAR "FUELS" AND HOW ARE THEY REGULATED?

Glucose is one of those simple molecules that is both made in the body and created by digestion of food we eat. For example, glucose and *fructose* molecules hooked together make a compound called *sucrose,* one you know as *table sugar,* that is very easily and rapidly converted to glucose. A larger "storage" form of glucose is a compound called *glycogen*, which is made up of hundreds of glucose units, like a long train composed of a line of individual boxcars. Glycogen provides a compact form for the liver and muscles to store as ready energy that can be quickly released if your blood glucose drops too low or you have a sudden need for more energy, such as starting to run.

Although there are other sugars, such as fructose, that are made in the body or obtained from the foods we eat, glucose is the easiest and most plentiful fuel for all of our cells to use. Glucose is carried in the bloodstream and is the one that is usually meant when you hear the term *blood sugar.* When I use *blood sugar* in this book, I am referring to glucose. Inside the cells, glucose is oxidized in the presence of oxygen to create energy, and it is the primary fuel that the brain uses to survive. Other cells in the body, such as in the muscles, can use all of the simple molecules listed above, but the brain needs a steady supply of glucose for it to work properly. When glucose levels are too low, it causes unpleasant, and sometimes frightening, symptoms we describe as hypoglycemia; when glucose is too high over a long period of time it causes the disease diabetes mellitus (hyperglycemia).

What are some of these symptoms? For example, if glucose levels are either *too low* or if they *fall rapidly* after you eat, you may experience anxiousness, heart palpitations, pounding heartbeat, sweating, nausea, fuzzy thinking, irritability, difficulty concentrating, memory loss, or crying for no reason. Symptoms are caused by the brain's lack of its glucose fuel (called neuroglycopenia), and by the brain's "alarm" response to the stress of a potentially dangerous shortage of glucose. The central alarm center sends out a surge of "norepinephrine," one of the "fight-or-flight" hormones, that triggers the adrenal glands to release their stress hormones. The surge of "fight-or-flight" chemicals makes you feel overstimulated, anxious, nervous, sweaty, nauseous, and so forth. These reactions are part of the response to prepare you to deal with having to fight or flee, and they cause a *rise* in blood sugar to give you the energy you need for an impending emergency.

On the other hand, if your glucose levels are too high for long periods of time or if there's too rapid a rise after you eat, the high levels befuddle the brain, making you feel extremely sleepy, unable to keep your eyes open, and lethargic, and causing fuzzy thinking, problems remembering things, and difficulty concentrating. You may also feel nervous and anxious due to the rise in glucose causing an abrupt rise in brain serotonin. If glucose gets seriously out of control, and levels remain critically low (hypoglycemic coma) *or* extremely high (diabetic *hyperglycemic* coma), brain damage or even death can occur if not treated promptly.

HOW GLUCOSE IS REGULATED: THE ROLE OF INSULIN AND GLUCAGON

Since glucose and oxygen are the critical fuels the brain needs for survival, there are fairly narrow ranges of each that are optimal for the brain to work properly in all its complex functions. Since there are such severe consequences of glucose changes, the body has ways of keeping glucose from "swinging" to dangerous extremes. Insulin and glucagon are the two major regulators of the amount of glucose in your bloodstream at any given time. They act in opposite ways, so they are called the counterregulatory hormones. When these two hormones are working normally, insulin keeps blood glucose levels from getting too high, and glucagons prevents blood glucose from getting too low. Insulin serves to lower glucose levels by moving glucose from the blood into muscle cells where it can burned to provide immediate energy, or by moving it into fat cells where it is stored as fat for future energy needs. Glucagon has the opposite effect: it stimulates the liver and muscle cells to break down the stored glycogen and sends the glucose molecules rushing out of the cell into the bloodstream to raise blood sugar when levels drop too low. In addition to actual high or low blood glucose levels, the *rate* of rise and fall in glucose is a crucial factor that can also lead to the symptoms I mentioned above, and triggers insulin and glucagon release.

However, as we get fatter, insulin and glucagon don't work as well, so our body has more difficulty keeping blood sugar in the healthy range. That's when problems like hypoglycemia (low blood sugar), glucose intolerance (rapid rises and abrupt falls), insulin resistance, and diabetes mellitus develop. Let's look at each of these and how it relates to weight gain, middle spread, and "mental pause" for women in midlife. Think of each of these "conditions" as being part of a continuum of changes along the path from being completely normal to becoming diabetic. Although it may not occur *first* in the process, I will talk about *insulin resistance* first because it is the most serious of the early stages before diabetes develops.

INSULIN RESISTANCE AND SYNDROME X

Insulin is a major *anabolic* (tissue-building) hormone of metabolism, governing many aspects of glucose regulation, body-fat storage, and a host of other functions. Without enough insulin, you will die because you need insulin to help get the glucose from the bloodstream to the cells that must have it for fuel to live, and into the fat cells for glucose to be stored as triglycerides for later energy needs. But unlike the anabolic effects of testosterone to build muscle and bone, insulin is an anabolic hormone that *builds fat*. Insulin is a very potent promoter of fat storage (*lipogenesis*), and it is a potent inhibitor of fat breakdown (*lipolysis*). Insulin actually works to increase the ratio of fat to muscle, so the more insulin stimulation you have, the less of the fat-burning muscle cells you have. Excess insulin is a signficant nemesis if you are female, and having trouble losing fat.

Triggers of excess insulin that hit you at midlife include:

◇ constant dieting with the wrong kinds of foods, eating excessive high-carbohydrate foods
◇ increased stress with high cortisol
◇ loss of estradiol
◇ high free testosterone relative to estradiol
◇ disrupted sleep
◇ high levels of DHEA
◇ declining thyroid function
◇ less physical activity

Normally, when glucose is rising, insulin is produced in order to move the glucose out of the bloodstream to be used by muscle or stored as fat. The insulin level is supposed to then quickly drop back down to baseline after the insulin has done its job. But as we get older and have more body fat, the insulin receptors don't seem to work as well. The cells become distorted in shape and size and this makes the "lock," or receptor site for insulin, get all "warped" out of proper alignment. As a result, the insulin molecule "key" no longer fits easily into the receptor, leading to impaired insulin responsiveness. When this happens, glucose levels remain high after you eat because the insulin, even though present, isn't working as well as it is supposed to. This causes your brain sensors to detect continuing high glucose levels, and the brain signals the pancreas to release even *more* insulin to bring the glucose down. Your bloodstream and cells are flooded with insulin. Then suddenly, when all this insulin starts working, the glucose rushes into the cells, and your blood glucose level plummets.

We call this response "reactive hypoglycemia" (low blood sugar), and when it happens you feel ravenously hungry and also tend to feel shaky, sweaty, nauseous, lightheaded, fuzzy thinking, and have heart palpitations along with a racing pulse. You can see how this drop in blood sugar would create intense food cravings, especially for sweets. As soon as you give in to them, however, the whole cycle starts over. You have a rapid rise in glucose that makes you feel lethargic and sleepy, and have trouble concentrating. Then when the glucose falls too fast from the excess insulin, you feel sweaty, anxious, irritable, or weepy. For perimenopausal women, this pattern is accentuated by the menstrual cycle hormone changes. If you pay attention to the timing of how you feel relative to when and what you eat, as well as where you are in your cycle, you may begin to pick up clues that your normal insulin sensitivity isn't working, which means you are becoming insulin resistant. A waist measure greater than thirty-three inches is another clue that insulin resistance is creeping up on you.

Insulin resistance refers to this entire pattern—high levels of both insulin and glucose in the bloodstream and excess insulin causing glucose to be stored as fat instead of being used up for immediate energy. Since the insulin isn't working properly to deliver a steady supply of glucose to working muscle cells, the effect is the same as if you weren't getting enough food. The cells are not getting the fuel they need, so you get hunger signals continually and eat more, even though there is plenty of fuel (glucose) circulating in the bloodstream. It's like you have a leak in a gas line. Even though you keep filling the tank (eating), the fuel never gets to the engine so it can work. What's worse is that your fat cells are also screaming for more food to store. The excess insulin is making your body better at storing excess fat, and less effective at allowing your fat stores to break down for energy for the muscles and rest of the body. Over and over each day this pattern repeats, and you get fatter and fatter and fatter while you eat less and less and less.

Insulin resistance also causes:

- ◇ impaired immune function, making you more susceptible to infections
- ◇ increased buildup of the smooth muscle in artery walls, leading to reduced blood flow to critical organs
- ◇ plaque buildup in the arteries, leading to strokes and heart attacks
- ◇ more platelet stickiness, leading to increased risk of clots

It is not a pretty picture. With all these damaging effects on the blood vessels, you can see why excess insulin, particularly when our estradiol is too low, is now considered to be a risk factor for developing heart disease and early heart attacks.

This process leads to the development of Syndrome X, a serious metabolic syndrome more common in women, which dramatically increases your risk of early heart disease, diabetes, and death. The "deadly quartet" that makes up Syndrome X includes excess insulin/insulin resistance, middle-body obesity (high waist-to-hip ratio), high blood pressure, and high cholesterol and/or high triglycerides. Syndrome W is another name you may read about in the news that is given to this same cluster of problems more common in women. Syndrome W stands for:

◇ Women
◇ Weight (gain)
◇ Waist (over 33 inches)
◇ White-coat hypertension (i.e., high blood pressure at the doctor's office)
◇ Worry (stress/high cortisol)

When we have our optimal levels of estradiol, we are less likely to have problems with insulin resistance because the estradiol helps improve insulin response in the cells. But loss of estradiol is not the only way that our ovaries are involved in this insulin pathway. Researchers have found insulin receptors in the ovary. Insulin acts at these ovarian receptors to change the enzymes in the ovary so that they make more androgens rather than the normal estradiol-estrone balance. Higher androgens then feed back on the glucose-regulating hormones and cause more insulin production; the higher insulin levels stimulate more androgens being made by the ovary. It is an insidious cycle that makes a woman grow fatter and fatter and fatter. This is a major cause of the marked weight gain in young women with PCOS.

A milder form of this imbalance occurs in perimenopausal woman who are losing estradiol and "unmasking" the effects of their androgens, DHEA and testosterone. As you develop a shift toward more androgen effects instead of the normal estradiol balance, you have more body fat around your waist and deep inside the abdomen (visceral fat), similar to males. Low-fat, high-carbohydrate diets make this problem worse by stimulating more insulin production by the pancreas. More insulin pushes the body to store more abdominal fat. More abdominal fat then makes for more insulin resistance. Around and around we go, fatter and fatter we grow.

Some of you may see yourself and your own struggles in this description. I know I have certainly been caught in this trap and, at first, didn't realize what was happening. So what do you do about this problem of excess insulin? There are four major areas to be balanced in order to help keep you from overproducing insulin, getting fatter, and progressing toward greater risk of diabetes as you get older. You will read more about this in later chapters. Here are a few key ideas to get you started thinking now about how all this fits together. These are the key components of *Your Hormone Power Life Plan:*

◇ **The balance and timing of foods you eat each day.** Skipping meals and eating large amounts in the evening lead to more insulin and more fat storage. High-carbohydrate foods increase insulin production.

◇ **How much you exercise.** Exercise acts like an "invisible insulin" to facilitate delivery of glucose to the muscles, lowering high blood glucose. Exercise decreases the problem of insulin resistance, helps you burn fat for fuel, and helps you build more muscle, which then increases your metabolic rate.

◇ **Your hormone balance.** This helps oversee how much body fat you have and where it is stored on your body. Restoring optimal levels of estradiol, testosterone, and thyroid all help reduce insulin resistance, increase your metabolic rate, and build healthy muscle. (Then you have the energy to go out and exercise!)

◇ **Getting control of stress to lower cortisol.**

See how it all fits together? Each of these components plays an important role in controlling hypoglycemia, glucose intolerance, insulin resistance, or diabetes. *Your Hormone Power Life Plan* will show you a better balance of protein, carbohydrates and *healthy* types of fat to break out of the insulin trap, as you will see in chapters 15 and 16.

HYPOGLYCEMIA AND GLUCOSE INTOLERANCE

Hypoglycemia, low blood sugar, usually goes hand in hand with having difficulty handling glucose normally, a situation we call *glucose intolerance.* Both of these imbalances are common early phases in a progression toward developing diabetes. Hypoglycemia is defined as a blood glucose level below 50 mg/dl, but you may have *symptoms* of hypoglycemia at levels above that if the glucose is *falling* rapidly. It's similar to a smoke detector in your home that doesn't distinguish between the serious smoke of a fire and the expected smoke that occurs when you broil a steak in the oven. It sends out an alarm for both.

Because glucose is a critical fuel for our brain cells to survive, brain sensors are set to warn us at the slightest indication that glucose supplies are not adequate, whether from *falling* glucose or *an actual low* level. This is why diabetics sometimes check blood sugar when they have symptoms of hypoglycemia, but find that the level is high. They have likely experienced a high glucose falling to a lower level that sets off the brain alarm, even though the actual level is still above normal. This is also the same way that you can experience symptoms of hypoglycemia only a short while after eating. An overshoot of insulin production, triggered by too much refined carbohydrate food, causes your glucose levels to fall too fast, even though glucose may not drop below the magic number of 50 to qualify for a "diagnosis" of hypoglycemia. Your brain and body haven't read our textbook definitions, they just know what they need to function!

Glucose intolerance simply means that you have a tendency to "swing" between higher-than-desirable blood sugar levels after you eat and rapidly falling or lower-than-desirable levels two to four hours later. It is an early warning that you are having problems regulating glucose to keep it steady. This situation should be a clue that you have to change your eating habits. Sometimes it is hard for you to realize that the same trigger—rapidly falling glucose levels—may cause all your food cravings and anxious, panicky feelings.

If you ask your doctor what's wrong, you typically get told that you have an anxiety disorder or are overeating from depression and need an antidepressant or antianxiety medication. I find that many physicians don't realize that a rapidly falling glucose level can trigger a hypoglycemic "fight-or-flight" reaction even though the glucose level doesn't drop below 50. So, in case you have been told you can't be having these problems because your glucose is "normal," that may not be correct. You may have the hypoglycemia symptoms when your glucose falls quickly, even if your blood glucose is in the "normal" range. This problem is common in glucose intolerance and insulin resistance and can be resolved by changing the way you eat and improving your hormone balance, as we will explore later.

DIABETES MELLITUS

Diabetes is a deadly disease. *It kills twice as many women every year as breast cancer does.* Most women don't know this, and are far more fearful of breast cancer. Diabetes is becomingly alarmingly more common as Americans get fatter and fatter, and it is a woefully underrecognized medical problem, especially in midlife women. It is a devastating, killer disease. If diabetes is not treated early and aggressively, it leads to high blood pressure, kidney damage, nerve damage, severe pain of the hands and feet, visual loss, memory damage, depression, dementia, as well as early heart attacks, strokes and premature death in both women and men. Diabetes attacks the tiny end arteries throughout the body that provide blood to all our cells. This is why the complications of diabetes are so diverse and hit so many different organs.

Diabetes is a much greater problem for women than for men for two reasons: more women *get* diabetes, and women tend to have more severe and more frequent diabetic complications. Women have smaller arteries than men, so they get into trouble faster as diabetes damages arteries throughout the body. Type 2 diabetes is the form caused by excess body fat, and this type of diabetes is far more common in women. Depression is also more common in women, and in women with diabetes, depression occurs with a threefold greater frequency. Then women get yet another hit: Certain antidepressants, such as tricyclics, may cause even higher blood sugar, memory loss, a marked increase in carbohydrate craving, and more weight gain—all of which make the diabetes worse.

The *wrong* choice of birth control pill (e.g., high-progestin pills) or the wrong type of hormone therapy can aggravate weight gain, make glucose control worse, and cause more yeast infections, which are already more prevalent due to the diabetes. And then you have an additional burden: osteopenia and osteoporosis are also more common in women with diabetes than in nondiabetic women. This happens as high levels of glucose lead to decreased bone building, decreased response to the parathyroid hormone, and decreased response to a type of vitamin D needed to build healthy bone. So it is clear that diabetes needs to be diagnosed early so that you have the best chance of preventing these catastrophic health consequences.

Loss of optimal estradiol as you reach perimenopause is one more factor that pushes you toward increased risk of developing diabetes. Estradiol actually helps to *improve* our sensitivity to insulin, and makes us *less likely* to become glucose intolerant and insulin resistant. Estradiol also helps keep our SHBG levels in the healthy range, which helps prevent the excess free androgens that aggravate insulin resistance. Excess glucose in diabetes generates more of the cell-damaging free radicals, so we need more antioxidants (such as vitamin E and vitamin C) to prevent this damage. Estradiol is also an antioxidant, and when this hormone is declining, you are even more sensitive to the cell-damaging effects of glucose-triggered free radicals.

Excess glucose makes platelets more sticky and more likely to clot. Prior to menopause, our estradiol helps prevent excess platelet "stickiness," and we have a lower risk of serious blood clots. When you have lost your healthy level of estradiol and also have elevated glucose, you now have two factors making for more platelet "stickiness" and clumping, which leads to clots and stroke. Eating a high-carbohydrate diet makes this problem even worse: One Harvard study found that women aged thirty-eight to sixty-three who ate a diet high in refined carbohydrates had a 40 percent greater risk of having a heart attack or stroke than did women who ate a diet lower in refined carbohydrates. Diabetes complications can begin *years* before the disease is diagnosed, so that's why I keep emphasizing that you need to watch out for the early signs of glucose intolerance and get tested.

GETTING TESTED TO FIND OUT IF YOU ARE INSULIN RESISTANT

There are some helpful ways to detect insulin resistance. One is the Insulin Response to Glucose Test. It involves drinking a measured amount of glucose, then measuring glucose and insulin at regular intervals over six hours to see the pattern of rise and fall in both of these, correlated with any symptoms you experience with these changes in glucose and insulin. If this test is done without insulin levels, it is called a glucose tolerance test (GTT). The GTT tells how your body handles glucose, but does not identify insulin resistance.

Other doctors have said to my patients, "You don't need to do glucose or insulin tolerance tests, we don't do those to diagnose diabetes," or "It doesn't matter when in your cycle you do a glucose tolerance test, it's all the same," or "A three-hour test is fine, you don't need the full six hours." I disagree on all those points. I am not simply looking for diabetes, I am looking for the early change of insulin resistance and for objective laboratory data that help to explain patients' descriptions of uncontrollable food cravings, difficulty losing weight, mood swings and other physical symptoms. Also, it is clear from the women's descriptions that there is a definite *cycle-specific* characteristic to these cravings, so we *must* do the testing at the time when women experience these symptoms and cravings or we won't discover the physical changes that trigger them. If we do only a three-hour measure of glucose-insulin response, we miss the last two or three hours when the most significant abnormal changes tend to occur, both in the glucose and insulin values as well as in the symptoms.

We typically do these tests in my offices, so that our staff can observe directly when a woman is having symptoms, and how she is being affected. Most physicians just look at the numbers for each hour of the test, and if the numbers fall into the "normal" range, the patient is told "everything's normal," without asking *you* how you *felt* during the test. Most patients are never asked if they had any symptoms during the GTT. It seems to me that this overlooks the most crucial information: what *you* have to say about what you were experiencing as the glucose and insulin levels rose and fell. I also have our patients keep a timed symptom log of everything experienced throughout the test, and my staff makes written observations as well. We frequently also do a short cognitive assessment (to check memory, attention, concentration, etc.) at each hourly blood draw. These combined observations are discussed in detail when we go over the test results at a follow-up appointment.

This integrated information from you, from our staff observations, and from the lab results then allows us to correlate your symptoms with actual fluctuations in blood glucose and insulin levels. What has emerged from this approach has been remarkable in properly identifying overlooked problems, and in helping each woman learn how her body responds, what's contributing to the sensations she experiences, and what will be needed in order to create eating plans designed to constructively help her lose weight and relieve symptoms. It helps us decide the best spacing of meals as well as the most optimal *balance* of carbohydrate, fat, and protein.

This approach also helps me to see whether you may need an adjustment to your particular HRT or birth control pills or any other medications to improve your glucose tolerance and help minimize insulin resistance. Nine times out of ten, this process leads us to the insights, and data, we need to help you turn things around and finally be successful with your weight-loss efforts.

MENSTRUAL CYCLE CONNECTIONS

Since the 1930s, and perhaps earlier, doctors have observed that women have more abnormal changes in their glucose regulation during the second half of the menstrual cycle when progesterone is the dominant hormone. In twenty years of work with PMS and menopausal hormone changes, I have been studying the connections between cyclic changes in estrogen and progesterone and how these hormones affect blood glucose, glucose tolerance, insulin resistance, food cravings, binges, and weight gain.

I have found a strikingly consistent abnormal pattern of glucose and insulin response in women who have been experiencing middle-spread weight gain, bloating, food cravings (especially for sweets), and worsening PMS. If you are still menstruating, I recommend that you do the Insulin Response to Glucose Test on Days 20–24 of the menstrual cycle, or about a week before your period is due. This timing allows us to check how the rise in progesterone affects your symptoms and the insulin-glucose response. As estradiol declines at midlife, this abnormal glucose tolerance and increased insulin resistance gets worse. This is especially true if you are still having high progesterone rises with ovulatory cycles at the same time your estradiol is decreasing and your androgens are being "unmasked" as they move into the free, active state. The women I have evaluated with this integrated approach typically show a pattern with the following characteristics:

⋄ Rapid early rise in glucose in the first half hour
⋄ Higher than expected 1-hour peaks of glucose and insulin
⋄ Rapid fall off in glucose (sometimes as early as hour 2), triggering symptoms of the adrenaline "fight-or-flight" response (panicky feelings, nausea, dizziness, fuzzy thinking, rapid heartbeat, among others)
⋄ Insulin levels that are too high, for too long, especially since the glucose levels have already started falling too low and causing symptoms
⋄ Glucose levels at the fourth and fifth hour of the test that are lower than normal and associated with symptoms of adverse brain effects: impaired memory, concentration, dizziness, drowsiness, low energy, increased pain, tearfulness for no reason, etc.

Figure 10.1
NORMAL PATTERN OF GLUCOSE REGULATION

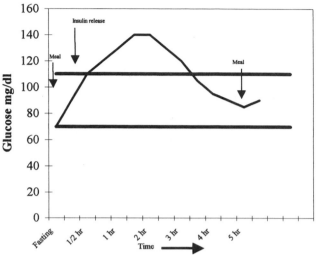

Chart shows the rise and fall in glucose following a meal. The "normal" steady state range for glucose of about 65 to 110 mg/dl is shown by the heavy horizontal black lines above.

INSULIN

Insulin serves to move glucose from bloodstream into cells; the effect of insulin release is to lower blood glucose back into the normal, steady state range.

"Insulin resistance" means that insulin levels rise too high, or remain high too long, causing a rapid fall in blood glucose that leads to low blood glucose (*hypoglycemia*). Higher than normal insulin levels also causes more fat storage, especially around your waist and upper body.

WHEN GLUCOSE LEVELS ARE TOO HIGH

Glucose levels that are too high, or rising too fast, produce brain symptoms such as anxiousness, sleepiness, headaches, fuzzy thinking, low energy or fatigue, and difficulty concentrating. Other symptoms of high blood glucose include increased thirst, increased urination, blurred vision, slowed stomach emptying (leads to burning "reflux" pain), sluggish bowels, etc.

When glucose levels remain above 200, it is called *hyperglycemia* (high blood glucose). Over time, hyperglycemia results in *diabetes mellitus*.

© 2001 by Elizabeth Lee Vliet, M.D.

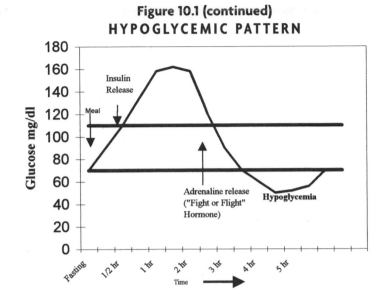

Figure 10.1 (continued)
HYPOGLYCEMIC PATTERN

WHEN GLUCOSE LEVELS ARE TOO LOW OR FALLING

Symptoms are produced two ways:

1. Activation of the "Fight-or-flight" Pathways
⋄ Palpitations (heart pounding or skipping)
⋄ Racing heart beat (tachycardia)
⋄ Anxiety, panic attacks, fearful thoughts
⋄ Dizziness, "woozy" feelings
⋄ Nausea, "butterflies" in the stomach
⋄ GI upset, possibly diarrhea
⋄ Shortness of breath
⋄ Numbness around mouth/nose
⋄ Numbness of hands or fingers

2. Brain symptoms from low glucose (neuroglycopenia)
⋄ Fuzzy or scattered thinking
⋄ Difficulty concentrating
⋄ Difficulty thinking clearly on complex tasks
⋄ Headaches, usually dull, diffuse aching; may also be pounding or throbbing; low glucose may trigger migraines in susceptible people
⋄ Mood "swings", labile (changeable) mood
⋄ Irritability, anxiety, tenseness
⋄ Feeling blue, sad; crying easily for no reason

© 2001 by Elizabeth Lee Vliet, M.D.

TOXIC EFFECTS OF EXCESS GLUCOSE

EXAMPLES OF COMMON SYMPTOMS

Weight gain

Fatigue, low energy

Excessive sleepiness after eating

Lethargy

Food cravings

Memory and concentration problems

Excessive thirst

Increased urination

Blurred vision

Mood changes, depression

Increased frequency of yeast infections

Headaches

DAMAGES

Formation of AGEs (advanced glycosylation end products)

Arterial smooth muscle overgrowth

Increased platelet stickiness, leading to clots

Increased "leakiness" (permeability) of blood vessels

Loss of blood vessel elasticity

Reduced clearance of lipoprotein particles

Buildup of plaque in arteries

Increased formation of free radicals that damage cells

Loss of myelin around nerve cells, death of axons

Impaired nerve impulse conduction

Impaired immune cell function

Impaired enzyme function

Depleted antioxidant vitamins *(vitamin C especially)*

Depleted magnesium, potassium

Increased bone loss

TOXIC EFFECTS OF EXCESS INSULIN

EXAMPLES OF COMMON SYMPTOMS

Waist measure greater than 33 inches
Eating less and still gaining abdominal fat
Overall weight gain
High blood pressure
Food cravings, especially sweets and simple carbs
Frequent episodes of reactive hypoglycemia
Memory and concentration problems
Mood swings

DAMAGES

Promotes fat formation (lipogenesis)
Inhibits fat breakdown (lipolysis)
Increases cell division, leading to aging of cells
Vascular damage (see also glucose), especially endothelial cells
Enhances adverse androgen effects on lipids (elevated cholesterol,
    increased LDL, lower HDL, increased triglycerides)
Increases blood pressure
Decreases levels of antioxidants such as vitamin E
Death of nerve cells, leading to cognitive damage, etc.
Increases risk of dementia (Alzheimer's form and others)
Impaired immune function
Plays key role in growth of cancer cells
Increases risk of breast, endometrial, colon, liver, and pancreatic
    cancers, especially in women

PROGRESSION

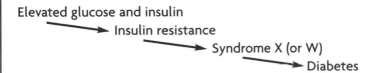

Elevated glucose and insulin
　　　　　　　Insulin resistance
　　　　　　　　　　　　Syndrome X (or W)
　　　　　　　　　　　　　　　　Diabetes

© 2001 Elizabeth Lee Vliet, M.D.

OTHER TESTS FOR GLUCOSE AND INSULIN LEVELS

In addition to the Insulin Response to Glucose Test that I have described earlier, *fasting glucose and insulin* measurements are helpful. These levels should be measured after fasting in the morning, at least twelve hours after your last meal. A healthy fasting glucose should be in the range of 65 to 100 mg/dl. Although some labs show that a "normal" fasting glucose goes up to 110 to 115 mg/dl, newer diabetes research suggests that if your fasting glucose is above 100, this is suspicious for beginning glucose intolerance that could mean you are at higher risk for developing diabetes. The criteria to diagnose diabetes mellitus have been revised recently to reflect our awareness that even mild elevations in fasting glucose levels may lead to increased risk for damage throughout the body and earlier development of diabetic complications. These new cutoffs are a fasting glucose greater than 126 mg/dl, a casual (random) glucose greater than 200 mg/dl along with symptoms, and a two-hour postprandial glucose greater than 200 mg/dl.

It is difficult to give you specific insulin values to look for because there are so many different assays used by laboratories throughout the country, and the insulin values are not as well standardized as are glucose values. Generally, *a normal fasting insulin is 6 to 25 micro-international units per milliliter (mIU/ml),* and a typical two-hour postprandial range is 6 to 35 mIU/ml.

Another way to check for early stages of glucose intolerance, insulin resistance, or diabetes is to measure your glucose and insulin at two hours after you eat a typical meal. This test is called a *two-hour postprandial glucose and insulin,* and it tells you how high your glucose and insulin rise in response to eating. If the two-hour postprandial glucose is at least 140 mg/dl but less than 200 mg/dl, you are glucose intolerant and at higher risk of becoming diabetic. If your two-hour postprandial glucose is over 200, you are considered to be diabetic and need a really thorough evaluation by your physician.

You have to check and see if this is the same reference scale used by the lab where you have your test done. If your lab appears to have a different reference range, and your two-hour postprandial insulin is at the high end or above the top of their normal range, then you are likely insulin resistant and at higher risk of becoming diabetic. High fasting and postprandial insulin levels are also seen in women with PCOS, and in perimenopausal women who are gaining middle-body fat. These high insulin levels make it even harder for you to lose those unwanted fat pounds, so it is important to "know your numbers."

Hemoglobin A1C is a measure of the amount of glucose that has been incorporated into hemoglobin, which is the oxygen-carrying molecule in your red blood cells. If you are developing problems in your body's ability to handle glucose, this test is a sensitive marker that can pick up these problems earlier and give us a way of seeing whether or not you have had high blood glucose levels over the past three months. If you already have diabetes, Hemoglobin A1C is used to monitor how well your diet and medications are improving your glucose control. Hemoglobin A1C will be *less than 6* if your glucose control is in a healthy normal range.

SUMMARY

There are many complex metabolic effects of the shifts in ovarian hormones during perimenopause and their interactions with insulin, cortisol, thyroid hormones, and the various brain "hormones" that serve as neuroendocrine "regulator messengers" to control body weight, fluid balance, appetite, food cravings, and other functions. Higher-than-normal insulin levels during the early stages of "insulin resistance" are just as damaging, if not more so, than high glucose levels. Since the complications of insulin resistance and diabetes mellitus are directly related to how long your glucose and insulin levels have been out of control, and how high they have been, you need to get on top of this problem early.

The American Diabetes Association (ADA) states that we currently have more people in the United States with *undiagnosed diabetes* than people who have been diagnosed. Part of the reason is that in the United States, we don't do the most sensitive tests I have described, and we wait too long to do those we do! Recommendations from the Centers for Disease Control (CDC) in 1998 said that with the rise in diabetes, every person should be tested by age twenty-five. The World Health Organization (WHO) recommends a return to the oral glucose tolerance test as one way of identifying people with insulin resistance sooner so that we can help prevent them from becoming diabetic. The ADA is still focusing on abnormal *fasting* glucose test results before doing more extensive testing. Especially for women, waiting until fasting glucose is abnormal means we are too late. The disease has already developed and has been doing its dirty work on your body. If these problems are diagnosed earlier and treated aggressively, it is possible to prevent or at least delay the onset of serious consequences such as nerve damage, kidney damage, blindness, strokes, heart attacks, and premature death.

Even if you don't develop diabetes, you will have much more difficulty losing excess body fat if you remain glucose intolerant and insulin resistant. You need to know these glucose and insulin numbers to plan how best to design your weight-loss program. If any of these results is abnormal, it is even more critical that you follow the meal plans I have outlined in chapters 15 and 16 to help prevent diabetes and higher risk of cardiovascular disease.

Part Three

Your Action Plan:

IMPLEMENTING

DR. VLIET'S

*YOUR
HORMONE
POWER
LIFE
PLAN*

Okay, so you suspect your hormones may not be functioning optimally. You have some of the symptoms of low thyroid but these same symptoms may also be due to low estradiol or too much testosterone. How do you know? What's the next step? Part Three is designed to help you get started, teach you how to get the right tests, how to get answers, what these answers mean, and how to take all this information and put it together to create your total plan for regaining your zest, vitality, and healthy body. Part Three has chapters that show you how to balance your hormones, how to eat a food balance that works *with*, not *against*, your hormones; and how to stimulate the fat-burning power of exercise, as well as capture your *mind* power to put all this to work for you.

One word of caution though: I suggest you follow these chapters in order and not try to tackle everything at once. This is not a quick fix. It is a solution designed to last a lifetime. This is *Your Hormone Power Plan* for *life* we are talking about now. I have found that it is important for my patients to get their hormones in balance before tackling too many of the lifestyle changes. Why is this? Because until you do so—you simply will not feel energetic enough to make the other necessary changes and stick with them. If you don't have enough estradiol or testosterone to run your body engines, how will you have the energy to exercise or prepare healthy meals? If you tackle this program "piecemeal," you're likely to feel frustrated and discouraged when it doesn't work the way you expect. Then, falling back into feelings of failure and disappointment generally leads you to experience more weight gain.

So to avoid having your hormone imbalance sabotage your efforts, I want you to first focus on getting your hormones tested using reliable blood tests, working with a knowledgeable physician. Find out where you *are* and then you will know where you have to *go*. This action plan is designed to help you identify what you may need to improve so that your weight-regulating systems will work properly. Once you have objective, reliable data about your hormones and other body measures, you can then implement the other steps of *Your Hormone Power Life Plan*. You will be amazed at the difference. You will now have the solid foundation of healthy hormone levels, and from this, you will be able to launch your lifestyle changes, increase your physical activity, and have the mental focus to stick with a nutritious eating plan.

This section may seem like a lot to accomplish, but there is no time limit. This is your life, remember. *Life* is not a dress rehearsal! YOU are all you've got. Don't compromise yourself. Do it right. Take it one step at a time and it won't feel so overwhelming. After all, as the old saying goes, How do you eat an elephant? . . . one bite at a time!

| Chapter 11 |

GET TESTED—

KNOW YOUR NUMBERS

Why bother with tests before you start on your weight-loss program? Why not just go ahead and begin a new meal plan? Wouldn't that be easier, cheaper, and faster? Perhaps. But then, how many "diets" have you tried in the past? Have they been successful? If not, do you know why not? Wouldn't it be nice to have some clues about *why* your weight-loss efforts may have failed in the past? I believe that getting a good comprehensive baseline medical evaluation, including the specific hormone tests I describe, gives you critical information to help you better design an integrated plan for long-term success. The following chart is an overview of my recommendations to put *Your Hormone Power Life Plan* into action.

DR. VLIET'S STARTING STEPS:
YOUR HORMONE POWER LIFE PLAN

1. **Examine your own health risks.** Look for symptom patterns, diagnosed diseases (e.g., high cholesterol, high blood pressure, diabetes, osteoporosis, and others).

2. **Check your family history.** Look for first-degree relatives (parents, siblings) with common problems that may affect metabolism and weight gain, such as diabetes, PCOS, elevated cholesterol, heart disease, high blood pressure, thyroid or adrenal disorders, hypoglycemia, history of obesity. Check for other hereditary problems such as autoimmune disorders, depression, osteoporosis, dementias, or cancers that play a role in your own risks, and provide clues to how important it may be for you to have optimal hormone balance as you get older.

3. **Work with a physician who will do objective tests.** Look for one who uses standardized laboratory procedures and blood (serum) measures. To start out, I recommend the following (described in more detail later in the chapter):

   ◇ *Serum levels of all of your ovary hormones.* This should include at a minimum FSH, estradiol, progesterone, testosterone, DHEA, DHEA-S.
   ◇ *Serum cortisol, TSH, free T3, free T4, thyroid antibodies.*
   ◇ *Fasting lipid profile* (cholesterol, HDL, LDL, triglycerides).

   ◇ *Metabolic profile* to check electrolytes, liver function, calcium, etc.
   ◇ *Fasting glucose and insulin, plus HgbA1C (glycosylated hemoglobin)* and a *2-hour post prandial glucose and insulin* (if waist is more than 33 inches).
   ◇ *Bone density of the hip and spine.* DEXA is the most reliable test to measure your "bone bank account." Heel and arm tests aren't well correlated with degree of loss at hip and spine, and these last two sites are ones where fractures are more critical.
   ◇ *Urine or serum test of N-telopeptide,* a measure of the rate of bone building vs. bone breakdown.

4. **Evaluate your lifestyle.** Look at the types of foods you eat, how much you exercise, your intake of calcium-zinc-magnesium and the antioxidants; habits such as smoking, alcohol use, drug use; make a list of all the OTC herbs or supplements and any prescription medications you are taking. Make a list of the things you are doing *right*, and a list of the unhealthy habits you want to change.

5. **Take stock of your stressors.** Make a list of the ones you can change and *want* to change, as well as the ones you can't change right now. Begin thinking about ways to relieve excess stress in your life.

YOUR HORMONE TESTS
AND WHAT THEY MEAN

Ovarian Hormones

Ideally, a baseline estradiol, progesterone, testosterone, DHEA, and DHEA-S should be done in your twenties or thirties when you are feeling really well. Having your healthy baseline gives you a target range to aim for with any later hormone replacement. Unfortunately, this is rarely done. These same tests are even more important as we get older and start having symptoms, including weight gain. If you are still menstruating, you need to check levels at the low point of the cycle (Days 1–3) and also check the ratio of estradiol to progesterone in the luteal phase (about Days 19–22). If you have stopped menstruating, or have had a hysterectomy, checking all of the ovarian hormones once for your baseline will usually do. Recheck these levels as symptoms develop, or intensify, after a tubal ligation, after hysterectomy, or when you start or change your hormone Rx. Checking levels after starting hormone therapy helps you be certain that you are above the currently accepted thresholds for preserving bone, brain, and heart and for other benefits of estradiol.

I have explained in earlier chapters (see Testing sections) what to look for in optimal ranges for each of the ovarian hormones. Please refer to these chapters for more details, but here is a summary of my clinical guidelines to refresh your memory.

Estradiol

In my clinical experience, women typically experience their usual energy level, mood, sleep, and memory when serum (blood) levels of estradiol are *above* 90 to 100 pg/ml, which is the lower end of the range for healthy menstrual cycle levels. Levels up to about 200 or so are the normal estradiol levels reached in the first half of the menstrual cycle before women reach menopause. At ovulation, estradiol levels are typically in the range of 300 to 500 pg/ml, and then in the luteal phase of the cycle (when progesterone is produced), a healthy level of estradiol is generally in the range of 200 to 300 pg/ml.

For restoring hormone function and health benefits after menopause, estradiol levels below about 90 pg/ml are generally too low to provide adequate relief of symptoms from hot flashes to muscle/joint pain and disrupted sleep and memory, not to mention maintaining a normal feeling of well-being. International research has found that estradiol levels below about 80 to 90 pg/ml result in increased bone loss after menopause. Cardiovascular benefits of estradiol have been found to occur at levels above about 80 pg/ml as a starting point. Therefore, I suggest you look for a level of about 90 or better and then correlate this with your symptoms.

Testosterone

In my experience, women typically experience their optimal normal energy level and libido when serum (blood) levels of total testosterone are between 40 and 60 ng/dl (which is 400 to 600 pg/ml using the same units for estradiol), with the percent of free testosterone at about 1 to 2 percent of the total. Levels below 30 ng/dl (300 pg/ml) are generally too low to maintain your usual libido, intensity of orgasm, energy level, and bone mass. The majority of menopausal women I have evaluated, particularly those who have had surgical removal of the ovaries in their thirties and forties, have had testosterone levels of less than 10 . . . with barely detectable amounts of free testosterone. No wonder they don't have any sexual desire left! Such low testosterone levels are also a significant factor in fatigue and low energy. As I described in chapter 7, I usually measure the total, free, and weakly bound forms of testosterone circulating in the bloodstream.

Levels of progesterone and DHEA are discussed in chapters 6 and 7, if you want to go back and read this material again. Be sure that you have the blood serum tests done to give a picture of both total and free hormones. Urine and saliva tests do not give as complete a picture of the hormone reserve that is available for action in the body, and I don't recommend them.

FSH

The follicle ("egg") stimulating hormone is produced by the pituitary gland in the brain. Its main function is to stimulate the ovary to "ready" new follicles each month, for release at ovulation. When the ovary stops making optimal estradiol (for whatever reason), the FSH *rises* as the brain tries to stimulate the ovary to keep up estrogen production. *High* FSH levels (above 20 mIU/ml) indicate that estradiol levels are too low, even if you are on hormone therapy. *If your hormone therapy dose is right for you* (and your brain), FSH comes back down to the lower level seen prior to menopause (less than 20). In my opinion, FSH is *not* the most sensitive marker of estradiol decline, so that's why I check both the FSH (brain) and ovary hormones (estradiol, testosterone, and progesterone).

Thyroid

I recommend the following tests be done: TSH, free T4, free T3, and thyroid antibodies (antithyroglobulin, antimicrosomal) for women, since these are more sensitive indicators of subtle (subclinical) thyroid disorders that may be affecting weight gain. I have described these tests, and some optimal ranges, in chapter 8.

Cortisol

This is the "stress" hormone produced by the adrenal glands. I recommend the 8:00 A.M. cortisol as a first step. If this is abnormal, I describe in chapters 9 and 14 some additional tests to consider. Levels that are too high may indicate a stress response to physical factors like sleep loss, hormone imbalances, medication side effects, drug use, and also to situational life "stresses." High cortisol (greater than 20 mg/dl) may also be a sign of an underlying more serious disease, such as Cushing's syndrome. Extremely low morning cortisol levels (less than 7 to 9 µg/dl range) may indicate chronic stress effects (sometimes called adrenal "exhaustion" or adrenal insufficiency) or a more serious disease, adrenal insufficiency. Check chapter 9 for more details and additional tests that may be needed if your cortisol is out of the desired healthy range.

Prolactin

This hormone is produced by the pituitary and can be measured in a simple, reliable blood test that is best done between 7:00 and 8:00 A.M. Elevated prolactin can be an indication of a pituitary hormone-producing tumor. These are usually benign, but may cause problems because the tumor is large enough (macroadenoma) to cause pressure on the optic nerve, resulting in visual changes, or the hormone production from a small tumor (microadenoma) is enough to disrupt ovarian cycles, cause loss of menstrual periods, and add to weight gain problems. If you are gaining weight and have symptoms (see chapter 3) that suggest elevated prolactin, I think your prolactin should be checked.

If the levels are too high and there are visual changes, generally an MRI of the pituitary is done to see whether the best treatment is medication to bring down the prolactin, or whether surgical removal may be needed to prevent permanent damage to the optic nerve. Dopamine boosters (*agonists*), such as bromocriptine (Parlodel), cabergoline (Dostinex), and pergolide (Permax) are the most common medications used to treat elevated prolactin. High prolactin levels respond very well to these medications, so this problem is treatable—it doesn't need to continue to sabotage your weight-loss efforts.

SHBG

This is a carrier protein in the bloodstream that binds the sex hormones, holding them in reserve to release as needed to activate hormone target cells throughout the body. Measuring this protein in the blood helps us determine whether a hormone imbalance has also affected the production of this protein, which in turn will determine the relative amount of estrogen and testosterone in the free, active fraction in your blood. Too much free testosterone and too little free estradiol, for example, can adversely affect your appetite as well as determine the areas on your body where fat is stored. SHBG is often abnormal in women with PCOS and returns to desirable ranges with appropriate treatment of the underlying hormone imbalance.

YOUR METABOLIC TESTS
AND WHAT THEY MEAN

Generally, for the following tests, I suggest you follow the reference ranges on your laboratory report to see if you fall into the desirable target ranges. If you are at the high or low end of the range, talk with your physician to see if it indicates a significant concern or "early warning" of possible future problems.

Fasting Blood Glucose (sugar)

The healthy range is 70 to 100 mg/dl. Low blood glucose, or *hypoglycemia,* is a fasting glucose less than 60. Fasting glucose between 100 and 110 mg/dl should be a warning that your body is changing in a negative direction and you need to do something about it (see chapter 10). *Glucose intolerance* is indicated by a fasting glucose of 111 to 125 mg/dl. Fasting glucose above 126 mg/dl is the new cut-off to indicate diabetes. Fasting glucose should be checked every two to three years after age twenty, if within normal limits. *It should be checked at least annually if you have high risk for diabetes* based on the following:

- ◇ family history of diabetes
- ◇ overweight
- ◇ have gained more than 20 pounds in the last year
- ◇ have gained weight around the middle of your body, waist is larger than 33 inches
- ◇ new onset sweet cravings, increased thirst, increased urination

Fasting Insulin

Insulin resistance is increasingly common in midlife women and is a significant factor that makes it harder for you to lose excess fat. It also greatly increases your risk of diabetes. I think this is important to check if you are seriously overweight, or if you have any of the risks I listed under glucose (see above). It is difficult to give you specific insulin values to look for because there are so many different assays used by laboratories throughout the country and the insulin values are not as well standardized as are glucose values. Generally a normal fasting insulin is 6 to 25 micro-international units per milliliter (mIU/ml), and a two-hour postprandial insulin range about 6 to 35 mIU/ml. You have to check and see if this is the same reference scale used by the lab where your test is done.

Hemoglobin A1C

This is a measure of the amount of glucose that has been incorporated into hemoglobin, the oxygen-carrying molecule in your red blood cells. I use this test to see whether or not you have had high blood glucose levels over the past three months. Hemoglobin A1C will be *less than 6* if your glucose levels have been in the healthy ranges. This test is a sensitive marker that can pick up glucose intolerance problems early. If you already have diabetes, Hemoglobin A1C is used to monitor how well your diet and medications are improving your glucose control.

Cholesterol

This test must be done fasting for reliable results, and must include HDL cholesterol to be useful in assessing risk of heart disease. Women also need to include fasting triglycerides with the fasting cholesterol profile. A cholesterol and triglyceride profile should be done at least every two to three years, beginning in early teen years, if you have no particular risk factors. After age thirty-five, or when the following situations exist, I recommend checking it more frequently, usually at least twice a year:

- ◇ if you have experienced extreme changes in weight
- ◇ if marked changes in the level of your activity have occurred
- ◇ if you have been ill or begin new medications that may affect cholesterol
- ◇ if you become menopausal (after surgery or naturally) and do not take estrogen; once a year if taking estrogen
- ◇ if you have high blood pressure or diabetes mellitus
- ◇ if you suspect or have been diagnosed with a thyroid disorder

- ◇ if you had previously been found to have high cholesterol or triglycerides
- ◇ if you smoke cigarettes or use other tobacco products
- ◇ if you drink more than 2 glasses of wine (or equivalent) daily
- ◇ if you take corticosteroids over a long period of time
- ◇ if you have experienced life changes or chronic diseases that affect cholesterol

Insulin Response to Glucose Test

This is an important test for insulin resistance and early clues to developing diabetes. It is particularly important in women who are struggling with relentless midlife weight gain or problems losing weight in spite of appropriate diet and exercise strategies. I have described this test, as well as the postprandial tests of glucose and insulin, in chapter 10, and I also describe how they should be done relative to the menstrual cycle if you still have periods and are experiencing food cravings at certain times of the cycle.

Electrolytes: Sodium, Potassium, Chloride

These three tests measure the concentration of salts in the bloodstream and tell us whether your kidneys and adrenals are working properly. The normal range is relatively narrow, but minor variations such as a sodium down to 133 to 134 (mEq/L) or potassium up to 5.5 (mEq/L) may be perfectly normal. If you take in too much sodium in food and beverages, your body holds on to extra water to dilute the sodium to a normal concentration. The extra water then raises the fluid volume in your arteries, which may lead to high blood pressure, so this is why the first treatment for hypertension is salt restriction. If you decrease salt intake, you lose excess water through increased urination, and blood pressure drops.

Levels of potassium that remain *too high* or *too low* can cause heart rhythm disturbances that are potentially serious. A potassium level that is *slightly above* the normal range is usually the result of laboratory variation or may occur if you are getting too much potassium from supplements or in your diet. If you take potassium supplements of any kind, your levels should be checked regularly to avoid high potassium that could be dangerous. A *low* potassium level may occur from taking medication (diuretics, cortisone, and others) that lowers your potassium, or it could indicate the possibility of an adrenal disorder.

Calcium, Magnesium, and Inorganic Phosphate

These are other important minerals that help regulate many body functions. The body very carefully regulates calcium, magnesium, and phosphates in the bloodstream to maintain a normal level because they are needed for normal nerve and muscle function, normal blood pressure and heart rhythm regulation, to make brain chemical messengers, to build bone, and to metabolize our foods. The serum (blood) calcium level is *not* a test for osteoporosis; it measures the amount of calcium only in the blood, not bone. If you are not taking in enough calcium or are losing it too quickly, such as with estrogen decline, your body will "raid" the calcium supply in the bones to maintain a normal blood level so your brain, heart, nerves, muscles, and other key body parts all work properly. When menopause occurs and estradiol is low, the body loses more calcium in the urine, even if you take calcium supplements, because estradiol is needed to properly absorb calcium from the intestinal tract and deposit it into bone. Low estradiol and increased urinary calcium is a cause of kidney stones in midlife women.

High serum calcium levels can indicate excess vitamin D intake, use of lithium or thiazide diuretics, as well as more serious problems such as severe osteoporosis, hyperthyroidism, myeloma, leukemia, hyperparathyroidism, metastatic cancers, and others. If your serum calcium level is high, your physician should check this further. *Low serum calcium* levels are often seen with too little intake of calcium and vitamin D, but may also be caused by various malabsorption syndromes, kidney and liver disorders, low function of the parathyroid gland, and others. If the calcium is low, check with your physician about further tests.

Low serum magnesium may occur from low dietary intake (common in American women) and also in GI disorders, alcoholism, hyperthyroidism, parathyroid disorders, use of some diuretics, kidney disease, and prolonged breastfeeding. *High serum magnesium* may occur if you take excess magnesium supplements or have hypothyroidism or adrenal or kidney disease. Magnesium imbalances affect many critical metabolic pathways, so this is an important mineral to check if you are having problems losing weight.

Low levels of phosphates occur with alcoholism, diabetes, gout, excess aspirin use, use of anabolic steroids, high DHEA and/or testosterone levels, overuse of diuretics, vitamin D deficiency, overuse of phosphate-binding antacids, severe vomiting or diarrhea, hyperparathyroidism, and other disorders. *High blood phosphates* may occur if you are taking too much vitamin D or have hypoparathyroidism or some types of bone diseases and other uncommon problems.

Liver Function Tests

Alkaline phosphatase, AST, ALT, GGT, and bilirubin are liver enzymes, and they are indicators of how well your liver functions. Many factors can cause high levels of liver enzymes, including use of some herbs, alcohol overuse, some medications, hepatitis, acute heart attacks, and other diseases. Mild elevations of these tests may be perfectly normal, for example, a GGT of 70 to 80. Slight increases in bilirubin may occur in prolonged fasting or Gilbert's syndrome, which is usually a benign problem.

Albumin and blobulin are proteins that are produced in the liver and carried in the bloodstream. They have important functions to make up antibodies and other immune messengers. Albumin is also the basic protein that helps build muscles and other organs. These proteins may be low due to poor dietary habits, chronic dieting, eating disorders, liver disease, and other more serious illness. If your results are significantly abnormal, your physician will suggest other tests to determine the cause. These blood tests are very reliable measures of liver function, and I recommend they be done as a baseline before you start a weight-loss program or a new medication.

Kidney Function Tests

Blood urea nitrogen (BUN), uric acid, and creatinine are breakdown products of protein that are excreted in the urine. These tests indicate how well your kidneys function. Most commonly, a low BUN is seen when you are overhydrated (drinking excess fluid) or when your diet is low in protein and high in carbohydrates. A low BUN could also be a sign of disease, so your physician should decide whether further tests are needed. If your creatinine is above 1.5, it may be a sign of kidney problems that need to be evaluated further. A very high BUN can also be an indication of kidney problems, but levels in the high 20s more commonly mean that you are simply dehydrated and not drinking enough water each day. Uric acid levels may also be low if you are eating a low-protein diet, and will improve if your diet balance is corrected. Uric acid levels may be too high due to excess alcohol intake, high triglycerides, too much dietary protein, and dehydration. High uric acid can cause gout, an inflammatory arthritis that typically causes severe pain in the feet or toes. There are simple, helpful diet changes that will usually reduce the pain, such as eliminating alcohol.

YOUR BONE MARKERS AND BLOOD COUNTS: WHAT THEY MEAN

N-telopeptide (collagen cross-linked NTx)

This is a breakdown product of bone that can be measured in blood or urine. If the urine test is used, it must be the *second* morning urine specimen to be accurate. If the body is breaking down bone faster than it is making new bone, NTx will be high (greater than 35). If you are "in balance" and the body is making new bone and breaking down old bone at about the same rates, this number will be *low*, or less than 35. If the NTx is too high, even if your bone density is still good, it indicates that you are already beginning the process of excessive bone breakdown and are at higher risk for later-life fractures. You should be taking more aggressive steps now to preserve bone, since just taking calcium and exercising regularly will usually not be enough to reverse this process. If you are taking hormone therapy to preserve bone, or taking medications such as Actonel, Fosamax, Miacalcin, or Evista, the goal is to have an NTx of about 35 or less.

Complete Blood Count (CBC)

This test measures a number of different cells in the bloodstream, and checks for various types of anemia, as well as more serious problems such as leukemia. I recommend that you have a CBC done as part of your annual checkup.

Hemoglobin and Hematocrit

Red blood cells (RBCs), hemoglobin, hematocrit, MCV, MCH, MCHC, and RDW are measurements of cell numbers and size, and help show whether you have anemia as well as define the type. The normal levels for hematocrit and hemoglobin differ for men and women, but generally a hematocrit level below 38 is considered anemic. It is not something to be greatly concerned about if you are only slightly below or above the average range.

White Blood Cell Count (WBC)

Your white cells fight infection and help immunity. They include granulo-cytes, lymphocytes, and mononuclear cells (monocytes). The percentages of each type vary, and the safe range is generally quite wide. It is a concern only if any *one* cell type shows up as a very high percentage such as 80 or 90. Neutrophils routinely can go up to 80 or 90 percent or more during infections. Lymphocytes and monocytes may also get high in viral infec-tions. It is usually not a serious problem if they are slightly elevated or slightly low. The normal range for the white blood count is 4.5 to 10.6×10^3; levels above 10.6×10^3 usually indicate that an infection is present.

Platelet Count

Platelets are the clotting factors that are the first line of defense in bleeding. A platelet count below 100,000 is a significant abnormality and should be evaluated by your physician. A slightly elevated count is not of great con-cern, but if it is much above 500,000 your physician should evaluate it.

YOUR OTHER TESTS AND WHAT THEY MEAN

CA 125

This is a cancer antigen that may be elevated in both ovarian cancer and several benign conditions such as fibroids, ovarian cysts, endometriosis, adenomyosis, and early pregnancy. I find this a useful component in evalu-ating women with weight problems because it is a useful clue to the pres-ence of the unrecognized benign conditions I listed above that have to be addressed in planning appropriate treatment. CA 125 is currently the only available blood test that could alert us to an ovarian malignancy and is the best "early warning" test we have at this time, even though it is not diag-nostic for ovarian cancer. I think it is important to have done if you have a family history of ovarian cancer, or if you have vague abdominal symp-toms (gas, bloating, distension, change in bowel movements, pain, etc.) that are not responding to other measures.

Ferritin

This is a measure of the body's iron stores. Optimal levels for women are about 50 to 90 ng/ml. The concern about iron and heart disease is that *high* ferritin levels indicate excess iron that may increase your risk of heart disease. If your serum ferritin is in the normal range, it is fine to continue multivitamins that contain iron. High ferritin levels (over 150), may cause damage to liver, kidneys, and brain as well as cause a whole host of other problems such as fatigue, weakness, muscle and joint pain, diabetes, and, in men, impotence. If your ferritin is over 125, I suggest you stop taking multivitamins that contain iron and consider donating blood at the Red Cross to decrease your iron stores. *Hemochromatosis* is a hereditary disorder leading to iron overload. You should ask your physician about having further tests to determine whether you have hemochromatosis if your ferritin is over 200 and *not* related to taking iron supplements. You may request information from the American Hemochromatosis Society (see Appendix II).

Low ferritin (less than about 40) is associated with insomnia, "restless legs," fatigue, muscle pain and twitches, poor exercise tolerance, hair loss, and other problems. If your levels are low (even without anemia yet showing on your hemoglobin and hematocrit), I suggest taking a multivitamin that contains iron. You may also want to discuss with your physician whether to add an additional iron supplement for about six to nine months until ferritin reaches 50 to 90.

What about Saliva, Hair, and Urine Tests?

You may have seen ads for testing your hormones by saliva, hair analysis, or urine. There has been quite a consumer marketing campaign for these tests over the Internet, through newsletters, and by direct mail. Based on reputable medical studies, these tests are not reliable enough to properly decide your treatment, particularly with something as critical to your health as your hormones. I believe in offering options to my patients, so I have tried these methods and have been greatly disappointed in the lack of accuracy of these tests. I stopped using saliva tests over seven years ago because of these problems. Current international research has actually compared the saliva and serum results in the same person, at the same time of day, and found the saliva tests vary so much as to be totally unreliable. A medical reference on this issue is included in the resources for the progesterone chapter.

In addition, the values from these have not correlated well with the descriptions of the women themselves, whereas serum tests correlate *very* well with my patients' self-descriptions. I have continued to use the "gold standard" serum tests that are used in worldwide hormone research and are much more reliable and clinically useful in helping women design appropriate hormone strategies.

FINDING "OPTIMAL" LEVELS VERSUS "NORMAL" REFERENCE RANGES

Getting your hormones and other labs checked can often be confusing when the results come in and your physician says everything is "normal" because the tests are within the lab's "normal" range. This may be quite misleading. First of all, the reference ranges for women's ovarian hormones in particular are often too broad to be meaningful. Second, you have to consider that a given number is not necessarily the "optimal" number for you to feel your best. If your estradiol or testosterone or thyroid is at the bottom of the normal range, that may not be enough to give your brain and body the "hormone power" fuel it needs for optimal performance. On the other hand, sometimes your hormone levels may be slightly higher that the "normal" range, but this may be where you feel the best. Ultimately, my medical approach is to listen to what you say about how you are feeling, and not just treat lab numbers. My desire is to carefully integrate the lab results with what you describe so *together* we can make the best decisions about appropriate treatment approaches for you.

BENEFITS OF COMPREHENSIVE HORMONE TESTING

Other physicians have often been critical of the test recommendations I have just discussed, saying that it is "too expensive" to check women's hormones. I think it is too expensive *not to* know what is happening with these crucial metabolic regulators in your body. Besides, it is difficult to put a price tag on improving someone's quality of life. I think in the long run it is less expensive to check hormone blood levels than to do all the myriad tests, evaluations, and multiple medicines that I see being given to women because hormone problems are not recognized. It also does not make sense to me (in time or economics) for women to undergo a series of psychotherapy sessions thinking that their weight gain is just due to stress or an "empty nest" or a bad relationship. Clearly, having reliable information about hormone levels has made an enormous difference to the women who had been told their symptoms were "all in their head" and who now have a hormone regimen that is right for them. Many of my patients have been able to stop expensive medications to lower blood pressure and cholesterol, as well as eliminate a variety of pain or antidepressant or sleeping medications when their estradiol levels were again in the optimal ranges.

In my opinion, the hormone blood tests are efficient, reliable, cost-effective, and psychologically helpful in identifying a physical cause of excess weight gain at midlife and around menopause. There are too many "hidden" medical, psychological, and relationship costs if you don't know your physiological measures. You may find that it is too costly to your quality of life *not* to have this information as you plan how to best achieve your health goals.

KNOW YOUR BODY NUMBERS: WHY YOU NEED TO THROW AWAY THE SCALES

Weight (on the scale) is misleading for women in midlife, so *throw away your scale*. (Yes, that means get up and do it *now*.) You don't need it, because it will only make you depressed and discouraged. The scale does not show progress with fat loss and muscle gain because muscle *weighs* six times as much as fat tissue.

These following measures give you a more reliable indication of the "fatness" of your body and your progress toward losing excess body fat as you use *Your Hormone Power Life Plan*. I will describe each one below. I urge you to get these done now, keep a record of your starting point for each one, and then track your progress at monthly intervals using these measurements as your guide to healthy body changes:

◇ Body composition . . . . .Goal: 22 to 30 percent fat
◇ Waist-to-hip ratio (WHR) . . . .Goal: less than 0.8
◇ Waist circumference . . . . . . .Goal: less than 33 inches
◇ Body mass index (BMI) . . . . .Goal: less than 25 to 27

BODY COMPOSITION

This term refers to the amount of body fat you have relative to the amount of lean body mass (muscle, bone, and connective tissues). We all need a certain amount of body fat for stored energy, heat insulation, shock absorption, and, in women, to provide a source of estrogen (estrone) that helps preserve bone as we get older. Generally, healthy women have a higher percentage of body fat than do men as a reflection of our biological role to sustain pregnancies. From a medical, health-risk standpoint, we generally define obesity as being more than 33 percent body fat for women and more than 25 percent body fat for men. You know the saying, "You can never be too rich or too thin"? Well, for good health, you *can* be too thin if you are a woman over thirty. As we get older, women lose bone more rapidly if their body fat percent drops much below 24 to 25 percent. So, if you are over thirty, I don't recommend that you push to get below about 25 percent body fat.

How do you determine your percent body fat? Scales that measure body fat are now available to consumers, but they are not as reliable as the more accepted measures of body composition such as body calipers, electrical impedance, DEXA, and hydrostatic weighing (see Appendix I for definitions of these terms).

Muscle and bone *weigh* far more than fat tissue, so if you are exercising or taking hormones, which both build muscle, you will not see as much change in pounds on the scale as you will see in body composition changes and with the way your clothes fit. Gaining more muscle and losing fat tends to make your body leaner, more compact, leading to a loss of inches. At the same time, however, you could see an *increase* in pounds as you build heavier muscle and bone. For general purposes of tracking your progress, skinfold measures with calipers by an experienced person at your health club or the electrical impedance method is fine. You don't really need the more expensive DEXA or hydrostatic weighing.

WHR: ARE YOU A PEAR OR AN APPLE?

Your health risk from excess body fat is determined by both how much fat you have and where the fat is located. I talked in earlier chapters about women's normal "pear" shape with hip-and-buttock fat patterns, and men's pattern of fat buildup around their bellies, giving them more of an "apple" shape. Women, however, undergo an undesirable midlife transformation: We become apple shaped during the hormone changes of perimenopause. The pounds of perimenopause are more dangerous to our health than pounds we put on around hips and buttocks earlier in life. As an interesting switch, overweight men become pear shaped.

If your fat is concentrated mostly in the abdomen, like an apple, you are much more likely to develop the serious health problems associated with obesity, such as diabetes. We have a simple way to measure whether someone is an apple or a pear. The measurement is called a waist-to-hip ratio (WHR).

Calculating Waist-to-Hip Ratio

To find out your WHR, measure your waist at its narrowest point, then measure your hips at the widest point. Divide the waist measurement by the hip measurement. Example: A woman with a 35-inch waist and 46-inch hips would do the following calculation: $35 \div 46 = 0.76$. Your health goal is a WHR of less than 0.8.

WHRs of more than 0.8 for women or 1.0 for men mean you have become an "apple." You are at increased health risk because of the middle-body fat distribution.

Checking your waist measure is an even simpler way of telling whether you are becoming an apple. As a general guideline, your goal for a healthy body should be a waist measure of less than 33 inches.

BMI

BMI, or body mass index, is a term new to many women, but it is the measurement of choice for many physicians and researchers studying obesity. BMI uses a mathematical formula that includes both your height and weight. BMI is calculated by taking your weight in kilograms divided by height in meters squared (BMI = kg/m2). BMI tables are available that have already done the math and metric conversions. To use the table, find the appropriate height in the left-hand column. Move across the row to the given weight. The number at the top of the column is the BMI for that height and weight.

In general, if you are age thirty-five or older, you are obese if your BMI is 27 or more. If you are younger than thirty-four years old, you are considered obese with a BMI of greater than 25. *A BMI of more than 30* usually is considered a sign of moderate to severe obesity with increased health risks for developing diabetes, heart disease, and other problems. The BMI measurement poses some of the same problems as the weight-for-height tables. Many times, doctors don't agree on the cutoff points for "healthy" versus "unhealthy" BMI ranges. BMI also does not provide information on your percentage of body fat. However, like the weight-for-height table, BMI is another useful number to help you track your progress.

WEIGHT-FOR-HEIGHT TABLES

Most people are familiar with weight-for-height tables. We have used them in medical offices for decades to determine whether a person is overweight. They usually have a range of acceptable weights for a person of a given height.

Many versions are available, all with different weight ranges. Some tables take a person's frame size, age, and sex into account; others do not. A limitation of all weight-for-height tables is that they do not distinguish excess fat from muscle. A very muscular person may appear obese, according to the tables, when he or she is not. I find that these are generally not as helpful for women, particularly if you are building muscle and bone with exercise and hormone therapy. Still, these tables can be used as general guidelines, if you keep in mind that taking estrogen and testosterone build more lean body mass, so the higher end of the weight range for a given height may be more appropriate for you.

BEYOND THE BLOOD TESTS: PUTTING IT ALL TOGETHER

Hormonal imbalance is commonly not recognized or is misdiagnosed, so it is important for you to seek a thorough evaluation in addition to the hormone assays. There are many other, often incorrect, diagnoses given to women who, in fact, have declining estradiol, insulin resistance, PCOS, PMS, or menopause: some of these are mental disorder, manic-depressive illness, major depressive disorder, atypical depression, chronic fatigue, chronic candidiasis, panic disorder, anxiety disorder, stress reaction, and others. The goal of a comprehensive evaluation is also to make certain that you do not have another medical problem causing similar symptoms, and to ensure that any previously unrecognized secondary disorders, which may be contributing to your symptoms, are diagnosed and properly treated.

Once you have the results of your various tests, you and your physician should review this information together, and explore in the next chapter ways to boost your hormone levels to the optimal ranges I have described to help you restore a healthy metabolic balance so that all the other strategies will work more effectively. If you are having difficulty getting your hormone concerns to be taken seriously, however, it may be helpful to locate a specialty clinic to focus on these issues and give you more helpful resources and suggestions.

I have designed the *HER Place* programs in Tucson, Arizona, and Dallas–Ft.Worth, Texas, to help women get hormone levels properly tested and to identify dietary, lifestyle, hormone, and alternative therapies to help hormonally related weight gain. We feel that a comprehensive evaluation of all these factors is important to get you started on the right track, with objective information that guides you in making the right choices to improve your health. For those of you who are not able to visit us for a consult at *HER Place*, these are the recommendations that I think are important for you to pursue in your local health care settings to provide the best possibility of identifying the factors that may be interfering with your progress.

TAKE CHARGE!
DR. VLIET'S GUIDE TO PERIODIC
PERSONAL HEALTH SCREENINGS

1. **Start your personal medical records notebook.** Keep an up-to-date list of diseases present in your family and copies of all your laboratory tests, mammograms, Pap reports, and other important health information.

2. **Perform self-exams.**
      Breast: monthly, just after menses
      Skin: a nurse practitioner colleague calls this "your mole patrol," giving yourself a good look to see if any moles or skin "bumps" exhibit changes in size, shape, or color over time; every six months from adolescence through age 35, monthly along with your breast exam after age 35. Report any suspicious changes to your physician or nurse practitioner.

3. **Undergo a physical examination by your physician.**
      Height and weight: annually
      Blood pressure: Every year ages l4 to 40; two or more times per year after age 40; two or more times a year before age 40 if you

      ◇ have elevated or borderline blood pressure
      ◇ take oral contraceptives
      ◇ have had a hysterectomy (with or without ovaries removed)
      ◇ have a history of heart disease
      ◇ smoke cigarettes or use other tobacco products
      ◇ are more than 10 percent overweight
      ◇ have chronic diseases that require periodic blood pressure screening
      ◇ take corticosteroids
      ◇ have kidney disease.
      ◇ have thyroid disease
      ◇ drink alcohol on a daily basis

      Breast: Every 1 to 3 years, ages l6 to 39; *annually after age 40.*
      Pelvic Exam: Every 1 to 2 years beginning when you become sexu-ally active; *every year after age 40; every 3 three years if you have had a complete hysterectomy (removal of uterus, cervix and ovaries) for noncancerous reasons (ACOG guidelines).*
      Pap smear: Begin when you become sexually active. Every l to 3 years after two negative results, ages 18 to 39. Every year after age 40; every 3 three years if you had a complete hysterectomy (removal of uterus, cervix, and ovaries) for noncancerous reasons (ACOG guidelines).
      Hormone Levels and Other Lab Tests: As indicated and described above.

© 1995, revised 2001 by Elizabeth Lee Vliet, M.D.

Endometrial (uterine) tissue biopsy: American College of Obstetrics and Gynecology recommends an *annual* biopsy in women who are intolerant to progestin or progesterone and are taking estrogen alone. American Cancer Society recommends *one screening test* for the following situations (frequency of additional tests based on physician recommendations):

⋄ if you have anovulatory cycles
⋄ if you have a history of infertility
⋄ if you have abnormal uterine bleeding
⋄ if you are postmenopausal and considering estrogen replacement therapy (ERT) or HRT
⋄ if you develop bleeding a year or more after menopause and are not on any hormone therapy
⋄ if you are taking tamoxifen

Bone density measurement: I recommend this be done for a baseline by age 40, or earlier if multiple risk factors for bone loss are present. Waiting until after menopause is too late in my opinion. I recommend Dual Energy X-Ray Absorptiometry (DEXA) as the safest and most useful procedure. DEXA uses far less radiation and is much less expensive than CT scans. Heel and wrist scans are not as reliable as DEXA scans of hip and spine: the former are often normal even when significant bone loss is present in the hip or spine.

Mammogram, alone or with breast ultrasound: Baseline exam at age 35 if no family history of breast cancer. If there is a positive family history of breast cancer in mother or sister(s), the baseline should be done *before age 35*. Normal risk: every 1 to 2 years from age 40 to 50. High risk (positive family history): annually from age 35 onward. Normal risk: Every year after age 50.

Rectal exam for occult blood (digital): Once a year after age 40.

Proctosigmoidoscopy or colonoscopy: for polyps, tumors, bleeding, etc. Every 3 to 4 years after age 50; annually if at high risk for cancer.

Electrocardiogram: Baseline at age 40, then every 3 to 5 years. There is controversy about the value of screening exercise (treadmill) "stress" EKG in women. I recommend that this be done if you are beginning a new exercise program and are overweight or have existing medical problems. Such testing may also be recommended by your physician if you develop chest pain or shortness of breath with mild exertion.

Chest X ray: Annually if you are a smoker or have a significant family history of lung cancer. Every 3 to 5 years if symptoms warrant.

Sexually transmitted diseases: Annually or more often if high risk based on having multiple sexual partners *or if you have failed to use a condom.*

Tuberculosis: Annually if in healthcare profession or high risk.

© 1995, revised 2001 by Elizabeth Lee Vliet, M.D.

Chapter 12

EXPLORING HORMONE MYTHS
AND MISUNDERSTANDINGS

"Hormones." Myths abound. Misunderstandings permeate media stories. *Estrogen equates with Premarin. Estrogen causes cancer. Estrogen prevents heart disease. No it doesn't. Estrogen makes you fat; progesterone makes you lose fat. Estrogen is good. No, it's bad. Estrogen is "lethal." Testosterone makes you grow a beard. Progesterone is a "wonder hormone" that cures all your problems. DHEA is the "antiaging" hormone* (ever wonder how you "stop aging" and still manage to be alive?).

No wonder women are confused. Every women's health book says something different. News headlines and articles only get part of the story—usually the most alarming part. Scary headlines sell newspapers. No one seems to care whether they give you *all* the crucial information—we live in an age of sound bites, not in-depth reporting.

If you are really going to understand *why* you gain weight at midlife, you need the comprehensive testing I just outlined in chapter 11. To break out of the vicious cycle of inexorably getting fatter and fatter, a critical component of your success will be to correct any hormonal imbalances. Healthy diet and exercise alone are not enough if you have any of these hormone problems. Balancing your hormones is your next step. If you are overweight, insulin resistant, or actually have diabetes, getting all these hormones (estradiol, progesterone, testosterone, DHEA, cortisol, insulin, and thyroid) back into a healthy, optimal balance is what's going to help you get "unstuck" and achieve long-term success.

While you may be accepting what I have written so far, you may also be saying to yourself, "But, are hormones safe? Are they *really* helpful? Won't I *gain* weight from taking hormones? Everybody I talk to is doing something different. What's the difference with all the types of hormones I hear about? How do I know what is right for me? How do I make *sense* of all this."

I want to answer your questions with some key points to clarify these common myths and misunderstandings about hormones. I base my information on the extensive worldwide research over the last fifty years. I have read thousands of medical articles on these subjects, and I have attended national and international conferences where leading researchers in the world have presented their work. I can't cite all of these studies in the limited space of the Resources section; I have, however, listed key review articles and journals you may want to peruse. I also refer you to my first book, *Screaming to Be Heard*, in which I provide hard-hitting, in-depth background information on these issues.

HORMONE MYTHS:
LET'S SET THE RECORD STRAIGHT

Hormone Myth #1: "Hormones make you fat."

Fact: Taking hormones does not cause weight gain. Loss of our premenopausal hormonal balance does.

Whether it is too little estradiol, too little thyroid, too little testosterone, or too much insulin, too much cortisol, or an excess of androgens, it is the *imbalance* that leads to gaining fat around the middle of your body. The most important issue is *balance*. The right hormones, in the right balance for you, actually help you lose excess body fat more readily.

The Post-menopausal Estrogen-Progestin Intervention (PEPI) trial tested several hormone combinations, compared to placebo, in menopausal

American women. The study lasted several years, so it could show longer-term changes and effects on weight, metabolism, blood pressure, cholesterol, triglycerides, clotting factors, and other variables. Even though women were given the types of hormones most likely to cause weight gain (Premarin and Provera), *none* of the hormone therapy groups showed a gain in weight. The only group that gained weight was the placebo group taking no hormones. Recent studies from other countries, with various hormone combinations, show the same thing: Postmenopausal women *not taking* hormones consistently have higher percent body fat and more middle-body obesity than women who *are taking* hormones after menopause.

Hormone Myth #2: "Estrogen makes you gain weight; progesterone makes you lose weight."

Fact: The reverse is true: Progesterone is the fat-promoting hormone that helps you store fat for pregnancy.

Take a look back at all the mechanisms for this that I summarized in chapters 5 and 6. Think about your own experience as well. When in your menstrual cycle do you get the hungriest and have food cravings? Isn't it usually the week before your period? This is when *progesterone* is the dominant hormone. Estradiol is highest the first half of the cycle, before ovulation. Your body gives you the answer.

Hormone Myth #3: "Hormones cause cancer."

Fact: Hormones don't *cause* cancer.

If that were really true, young women with the highest hormone levels would have the highest cancer rates. This is not the case. The highest cancer rates are found in postmenopausal women. In particular, postmenopausal women who are obese have the highest rates of breast, endometrial, colon, and pancreatic cancers. Estrogen and progesterone may facilitate the growth of an existing cancer, but there is *no data* that show either hormone *causes* cancers.

The flip side of the coin is that there is even better news about the *protective* effects of birth control pills on two cancers: they reduce your risk of ovarian cancer by more than 50 percent, and your risk of endometrial cancer by more than 75 percent if you have been taking them five years or longer.

Hormone Myth #4: "All estrogens are the same."

Fact: No, they are not. The three estrogens made by your body have important chemical differences and actions in the body, including different effects on your metabolism.

This is even more true for the plant estrogenic compounds (phytoestrogens), synthetic estrogens, and the mixed, animal-derived estrogens such as Premarin. Even though doctors prescribe these products, they are different molecular "keys" and don't quite fit the "locks" of the estrogen receptors in our body to cause the same responses that our own 17-beta estradiol does.

Hormone Myth #5: "All progestins are the same."

Fact: No they are not. Progesterone is the hormone made by your ovaries. Progestins are man-made ("synthetic") molecules that are chemically different from your body's progesterone.

Some progestins are derived from progesterone (e.g., Provera or medroxyprogesterone acetate, MPA) and some are derived from testosterone (e.g., Micronor or norethindrone), called "androgenic" progestins. This important difference affects their properties and the way they act in your body. For example, Provera is more likely to cause increased appetite, weight gain, bloating, breast tenderness, loss of libido, and depressed mood compared to the androgenic progestins like Micronor, which have less of these effects, but in some women may cause more acne or irritability.

Hormone Myth #6: "All birth control pills are the same."

Fact: No they are not. Different pills contain different ratios of estrogen and progestin, as well as different chemical types of progestins.

The higher the progestin (P) relative to the estrogen (E), the more likely you are to have increased appetite, weight gain, low sex drive, fatigue, headaches, and negative moods (irritability, depression). The better the E:P ratio, the less likely you are to gain weight or have trouble with "blood sugar swings." If you are gaining weight on your current birth control pill, talk with your physician about trying a brand with more estrogen and less progestin. I list these in chapter 13.

Hormone Myth #7: "Hormones aren't your problem, you just need to eat less and exercise more."

Fact: Doctors have really missed the boat here. Even if you cut your calories drastically and exercise more, your body will thwart you and hold on to fat if your overall hormone balance isn't optimal.

Go back and review what I have explained in chapters 5 through 10 to see all the ways our metabolism slows down and stores more fat when our hormones are out of whack. Even subtle imbalances can wreck havoc with your efforts to lose excess fat.

Hormone Myth #8: "You are too young to need hormones."

Fact: Not true. Women of any age can have hormone imbalances that cause weight gain.

The youngest patient I saw was an eight-year-old girl who suddenly "ballooned up" thirty pounds with no significant changes in her diet or activity and no growth in her height. Her DHEA was seriously elevated (in fact, she was probably on the way to having PCOS when she got older), and she also had elevated thyroid antibodies even though her TSH was normal. As you read earlier, both of these hormone problems can cause rapid weight gain. I see many teenagers and young women in their twenties who have gained thirty to sixty pounds in just a few months with the serious hormone imbalances of PCOS.

Hormone Myth #9: "You couldn't have hormone problems, your FSH is normal."

Fact: A high FSH (greater than 20) is a late stage in the transition to menopause.

Your levels of estradiol have been declining for several years before the FSH goes up, and if we check only FSH, we miss these earlier changes in estradiol. Again, the loss of estradiol is a key factor in our tendency to have more trouble with insulin resistance as we get older.

Hormone Myth #10: "You can't be having hormone problems, you are still having periods."

Fact: Women can have lower-than-optimal estradiol and thyroid hormones and still menstruate.

Loss of occasional menstrual periods is also a late stage in the transition from our reproductive years to menopause. What you will notice, and what doctors often ignore, is that your periods are *changing* as your estradiol declines or your thyroid isn't optimal. When your estradiol declines, your flow is lighter, darker, and shorter in duration than when your estradiol is optimal. Periods stop altogether when the hormone decline or thyroid disease becomes more severe.

Hormone Myth #11: "You can't be having hormone problems, your vagina shows good estrogen effects."

Fact: Women can have normal estrogen effect for vaginal lubrication and not have optimal estradiol levels to effectively run our metabolic pathways.

Estrogen-sensitive pathways in the brain, such as those that govern metabolism, appear to require higher levels to maintain normal function than do the estrogen receptors in the vagina.

Hormone Myth #12: "I am too old to start hormones."

Fact: You are never too old to feel better and have improved "hormonal health."

There are a number of benefits from estradiol and testosterone, in particular, that can help you maintain healthy body composition, regardless of age. Some major ones are gain in lean body mass (muscle and bone), improved metabolic rate, better memory, improved sleep (which lowers cortisol, improves GH, allows muscle repair at night, etc.), and improved insulin sensitivity, to name a few.

Hormone Myth #13: "There is no need to check hormone levels because they vary too much."

Fact: Not true. There is no greater variance in the lab tests we use for ovarian hormones than for the other standard lab tests we use, such as for cholesterol.

Besides, telling women we don't need to check hormone levels because they vary has to rank as one of the dumbest statements I hear physicians make to women! That's like saying we shouldn't measure blood pressure because it varies all day, or we don't need to check glucose in a diabetic because it varies. How do you know where you need to *be* if you don't know where you *are*? A 1998 study found that as many as 45 percent of the women on estrogen actually had serum estradiol levels below the thresholds for protective effects on brain, bone, and other target organs, even though they reported their symptoms were relieved. The authors concluded that monitoring symptoms alone is not enough; assessment of serum hormone levels is crucial to ensure adequate estradiol levels to provide the desired benefits.

HORMONE MISUNDERSTANDINGS: LET'S GO BEHIND THE HEADLINES

The "myths" I have discussed above are statements that are factually incorrect, and I have presented the medically correct information. But there are a number of hormone "misunderstandings" that arise when news headlines present only part of the story. For these, I have given you additional background to help address concerns you may have.

Hormone Misunderstanding #1: "Taking estrogen after menopause increases your risk of breast cancer."

Clarification: The studies showing this increased risk have been ones in which women were using Premarin.

Premarin is the horse-derived mixture of estrogens that is chemically very different from the human 17-beta estradiol. Two studies that media articles commonly cite, which showed an increased risk of breast cancer in women on estrogen, are the U.S. Nurses Health study—in which Premarin was the estrogen used by most of the women being followed—and a Swedish study using *estradiol valerate,* a synthetic estrogen more potent than our natural 17-beta estradiol. The authors of the Swedish study published an update in 1992 and the revised data did *not* show any increase in breast cancer risk as they had initially reported in 1989.

Even with the U.S. Nurses Health study, which showed increased breast cancer risk, the increase in breast cancer was found *only* in those estrogen (Premarin) users *who also drank alcohol,* not in *all* of the estrogen users. We know that alcohol increases the level of the estrone form of estrogen, and daily alcohol use is a separate risk factor for breast cancer.

Premarin gives high blood levels of horse-derived (equine) estrogens that are more potent than the human estradiol in their attachments to the estrogen receptors. These horse estrogens are not easily metabolized by our body's enzyme systems and therefore have the potential to build up in the breast tissue the longer you take them. I think this is potentially a mechanism for increased risk of breast cancer, so I do not prescribe the equine estrogens. There are many studies showing no increased risk in women taking estrogen after menopause. I have not found any studies in the medical literature that have shown an increased risk of breast cancer in women who are taking only *the native human 17-beta estradiol* after menopause.

Hormone Misunderstanding #2: "Combined estrogen-progestin therapy increases the risk of breast cancer."

Clarification: This is also based on one study in which Premarin and Provera were the hormones being used.

In addition, this effect was seen only in *lean* women, not heavier women, for reasons that are still unclear. As I have said elsewhere, Premarin and Provera are chemically quite different from the natural forms produced by the human ovary. If you are concerned about breast cancer risk, this is another reason I think it is wise to avoid these particular forms of hormones.

Hormone Misunderstanding #3: "I don't have any symptoms, so I don't need hormones."

Clarification: Both symptoms and health risks should be included in your decision making.

Don't focus on just whether you have symptoms. The crucial issue is whether you are missing silent, subtle changes that may be significantly affecting your health, such as abdominal fat gain, insulin resistance, glucose intolerance, bone loss, brain effects (memory loss, sleep disruption), and adverse cholesterol changes. You need to assess these other factors with the testing that I outlined in chapter 11. Then consider: Which hormones will help which of my health risks? Which health risks may be made worse by the wrong type of hormones? Which type and route of taking hormones is best suited to my needs and preferences?

Hormone Misunderstanding #4: "I went through menopause smoothly, I don't have hot flashes anymore, so I don't need hormones."

Clarification: This is similar to the comments I made in #3. You may not have hot flashes any longer, but are you gaining weight? Is your waist more than 33 inches?

Then you may have some of the *metabolic* effects of low estradiol. Take a look at the results of your lab tests and see if there are any imbalances that could be helped with proper hormone balance. This may be a reason to start hormone therapy, regardless of whether you have hot flashes.

Hormone Misunderstanding #5: "I'm 65, so I don't need hormones anymore."

Clarification: For the same reasons I described in #3 and #4, reaching a particular age is no reason to stop hormones if you have been taking them and feeling well.

Remember, our loss of muscle and memory, along with gain in body fat, gets worse the older we get unless we address the hormone imbalances that perpetuate these problems. As a result, older women may be in *greater* need of the benefits of hormone therapy than younger women.

Hormone Misunderstanding #6: "Testosterone causes liver damage."

Clarification: This is based on use of the synthetic methyl testosterone in oral form, and at significantly higher doses than we use today for women.

These problems have not been seen with proper physiologic replacement with bioidentical testosterone in micronized form, especially using nonoral forms such as creams or patches (available in other countries, not yet in the United States).

Hormone Misunderstanding #7: "My libido is still low; I need more testosterone."

Clarification: Not necessarily. More testosterone may not produce any improvement in sexual desire, and may actually interfere with normal sleep and mood and pain regulation as well as cause more middle-body weight gain.

There are some interesting findings from recent research on sexuality in women. First, women need optimal levels of estradiol in order for the brain testosterone receptors to work properly in stimulating the sexual desire–arousal circuits, so it doesn't always follow that *more* testosterone is better. Second, women, more so than men, are sexually aroused by the quality of the relationship to an even greater degree than being aroused as a result of their hormone levels. Male sexual response is more purely "biologic" than women's; female sexual desire clearly has biological components with estradiol and testosterone, but for women, the emotional-intimacy connections are also a major part of becoming sexually aroused.

Hormone Misunderstanding #8: "Estrogen and the birth control pill cause blood clots."

Clarification: The estrogen data on this issue were based on oral estrogen, primarily Premarin.

Newer data on the patch (transdermal) form of estradiol, our bioidentical premenopausal estrogen, shows that estradiol actually *decreases* the risk of thrombophlebitis (blood clots) through a number of mechanisms that I described in detail in *Screaming to Be Heard.*

Old data on birth control pills causing blood clots were based on use of the pills by cigarette smokers. Cigarette smoking is a separate risk for blood clots and strokes. Reanalysis of the old data, separating women into smokers and nonsmokers, showed that *nonsmokers* did not show this higher risk of blood clots and strokes. The older studies were based on the older, very high dose (over 100 mcg of ethinyl estradiol and 1 to 2 mg of progestin) formulations used in the 1960s. None of those high-dose pills are even available today. Today's formulas contain a fraction of the hormone content used when the pills first came out. About 1990, birth control pills were FDA-approved for use in nonsmoking women over age forty because the potential benefits far outweighed the risks.

Hormone Misunderstanding #9: "My friend is taking PremPro. Why should I take something different?"

Clarification: Every woman's needs are different.

Your body, your genes, your metabolism, and your health issues are different, as is your lifestyle. If hormone therapy is truly individualized, you would not expect to take exactly the same amount and type as your friend takes. It's crazy for so many doctors to continue this "cookbook," "one-prescription-fits-all" approach to women's hormone needs that has been the standard approach in the United States for decades. It's equally nonsensical for you to buy into faulty logic when your health is at stake.

Hormone Misunderstanding #10: "HRT doesn't prevent heart disease."

Clarification: This headline is based on the Heart, Estrogen-Progestin Replacement Study (HERS), and doesn't take into account serious shortcomings of the study itself.

These shortcomings include the fact that the women already had heart disease with blockage of the coronary arteries when the hormones were started; and that the hormone product being used was PremPro, a product combining horse-derived estrogens and a potent synthetic progestin (MPA). None of the women were given estrogen alone, or a bioidentical form of estrogen, to compare a natural estradiol with estradiol plus synthetic progestin.

To everyone's surprise, including the researchers, women taking the combined hormones had 50 percent *more* heart attacks than women taking placebo, and 3 percent more clotting problems in the first year of the study. This is what the news articles focus on, leading to the "misunderstanding" above. There are several critical points the news articles "overlooked" that would put this information in better perspective.

⋄ During the *last* two years of the study, women on the combined HRT had 40 percent *fewer* heart attacks, more consistent with many studies that show hormone therapy reduces heart disease risk.

⋄ HERS participants taking combined HRT had an 11 percent reduction in LDL ("bad") cholesterol and a 10 percent increase in HDL ("good") cholesterol. These were positive changes, though not as good as the improvements in cholesterol measures seen when estrogen (particularly 17-beta estradiol) is used alone, or is used with *natural* progesterone instead of the synthetic progestin MPA.

⋄ It takes, on average, about one and a half to two years before a reduction in cholesterol will show a decrease in heart disease risk. The women in the HERS trial were not in the study long enough to see the full benefit of hormone therapy.

But there are other serious problems with the HERS design. In the 1970s and early 1980s, British researchers Dr. Campbell and Dr. Whitehead showed that the horse-derived estrogens had the potential to have much worse effects on heart disease risk measures than our own natural 17-beta estradiol. Even though the negative effects of Premarin and Provera (combined to make PremPro) have been known for over twenty-five years, the HERS researchers still chose to use the horse-derived estrogen and the synthetic progestin.

Progestins like MPA reduce the beneficial effects of estrogen on a number of heart disease risk factors, such as the good cholesterol levels, blood vessel wall "elasticity," fibrinogen levels, and others. The PEPI trials, published in 1995, showed that natural progesterone did not have the same negative effects on cardiovascular measures as MPA. But the HERS researchers *still* chose to use only the synthetic progestin in the study. As a consumer, you should be aware that this study was funded by a grant from the company who makes PremPro. To those of us who have long advocated use of more natural forms of hormones for women, it was actually encouraging news to see our concerns demonstrated so clearly in the HERS results.

What's the "take-home" message as you consider hormone therapy? If you already have heart disease, or its risk factors, I suggest you avoid using a continuous combined horse-derived estrogen and synthetic progestin product like PremPro. If you are already on PremPro and have problems with weight gain, high blood pressure, high triglycerides, glucose intolerance or diabetes, insulin resistance, high cholesterol, or a history of heart problems, I suggest you to talk with your physician about changing to the bioidentical human forms of estradiol and progesterone. Transdermal 17-beta estradiol, alone or with natural progesterone (for women with a uterus), has better benefits on these metabolic pathways.

A FINAL "MISUNDERSTANDING": DEALING WITH YOUR INSURANCE PLAN

Insurance companies in the United States express concern about the growing health care costs of obesity as a factor in increased risk of diabetes, high cholesterol, high blood pressure, heart disease, and breast and endometrial cancers. They have extensive databases showing that obesity is a far greater problem among women than among men, and that this gender discrepancy commonly begins following a woman's first pregnancy. You would think that your insurance company would want to *help* women in their weight-loss efforts. Facts suggest otherwise.

We get letters from "managed" care insurance plans on an almost daily basis in both of our medical offices asking us to change our prescriptions to one of their "preferred formulary" prescriptions such as Premarin. Preferred formulary medications are typically older, cheaper, and often generic versions of medications that may be similar, but not necessarily identical to, the product that you and your doctor have decided you should take. Your insurance carrier is doing this to save money. Insurance carriers pressure doctors into changing your prescription medication to one that costs them less, regardless of whether it is as effective or may cause more side effects.

Let's look at an example from my practice. A thirty-nine-year-old woman requested my help to identify causes of her weight gain and to improve her hormonally triggered migraines. Her PMS had become severe as she got older, and her gynecologist started her on Demulen birth control pills. Her migraine headaches began soon after, and her weight began ballooning upward. Her doctor tried another brand of pills without success. Then her prescription plan said she had to change to a "preferred formulary brand" (Nordette or LoOvral) if she wanted reimbursement. She tried both.

All of the birth control pills she tried made her headaches and weight gain worse. The headaches became so severe she required care in the emergency room to break the migraine cycle. By the time I saw her, she was pretty desperate for relief. She was understandably fed up with the whole idea of birth control pills, and said, "I guess I'll have to try and put up with the PMS, because if I don't find a way to lose this weight and get my headaches under control so I don't miss work, I will lose my husband and my job."

I explained how the estrogen and progestin ratios in these brands had worked against her. These brands are all *higher* in either dose or potency of the progestin. High-progestin pills aggravate headaches and also trigger more weight gain than we see with low-progestin pills that have a better balance of estrogen (ones like Ovcon 35, Yasmin 35, Modicon, or Orthocyclen). Her own health insurance plan had made her problems worse by insisting she use these high-progestin pills. The health plan's required formulary products also resulted in increased *cost* for her medical care—she now needed more prescription medications for her headaches, she now needed medicine to control high blood pressure caused by the high-progestin pills, and she had numerous ER visits to treat acute, severe headaches. So, did the insurance company really save money? And this list doesn't include the cost to the woman herself of buying new clothes as her weight escalated out of control, or the pain and anguish she suffered as she watched her body shape change and her self-image plummet.

It is true that all these brands had similar safety profiles and similar effectiveness at preventing pregnancy, but they have profound differences in side effects and effects on appetite, metabolism, weight gain, and headaches. Pharmacists often say to us, "They are the same; it is only a 5 (or 10) microgram difference in the estrogen," or "It is only a half milligram difference in the progestin." If you are experiencing weight gain or headache problems, these small changes in progestin may lead to major differences in how the pills affect you.

You deserve better, so speak up when someone is trying to get you to change to a "preferred formulary" product. You can insist on being given more information about what the differences may be and how this could affect other problems you may have. If you try a formulary product and it causes more problems for you, and your plan doesn't allow you to use a product "off formulary," then file an appeal (using the process outlined by your health plan) and push to be allowed to use safer and more effective products that work for you.

GETTING STARTED ON
YOUR HORMONE POWER LIFE PLAN

The pounds of perimenopause—the ubiquitous plague of the baby boomers. Hormone imbalance at midlife has important implications for your health and well-being. Big contributors to this progressive middle spread are lower-than-optimal estradiol and imbalance of your androgens, insulin, cortisol, and possibly thyroid as well. These imbalances respond to a variety of hormonal therapies and other medications that will serve as a foundation to help you use the mind-body approaches and healthy-living lifestyle choices.

I've taken you through the facts behind the myths and misunderstandings. It's now time for you to make the decision that you feel is right for you. If you are fed up with being fatter than you want, check your baseline hormone levels as I outlined in chapter 11 before you just start "taking something." Then go step-by-step through the options I describe in chapter 13 to help you make sound decisions about getting your hormones balanced for an effective fat-loss plan. To win the weight and wellness game, take charge! Tap into *your* hormone power.

Chapter 13

BALANCING YOUR OVARIAN HORMONES

FOR WEIGHT LOSS

D *ear Dr. Vliet,*

You may share my story in your book. I suffered many years, so I want my story told to help other women. For two months after my hysterectomy I felt fine, but then began the frustrating journey through seven doctors, eleven different hormones, six antidepressants, and three NSAIDs [nonsteroidal anti-inflammatory drugs] trying to find a way to stop the sadness, the tears, the joint pain, the fatigue, the hopelessness: wondering if I was going crazy, gaining weight with many of the medications, developing high blood pressure, searching for a doctor who could tell me what was going on in my body.

Why seven doctors? One female doctor told me I was afraid of getting old, sad that I could no longer bear a child. Another female doctor told me there was absolutely no connection between hormones and the way I was feeling. Yet another female doctor thought I was depressed. So much for the theory that only male doctors often misunderstand, dismiss, and devalue women.

They gave me so many different hormones . . . I felt like a clinical trial.

Not one of them helped me. And since I was crying, sad, lethargic, I must have depression; let's try amitriptyline, Prozac, Paxil, Serzone, Zoloft, Wellbutrin SR. Only the last one helped somewhat: the rest made me jumpy or zoned out; most increased my appetite and weight but destroyed my sexual response.

Self-help books told me to control my thoughts: I'm tough, I thought; I'll get through this. When I feel like crying I'll count backwards, I'll recite Bible verses, I'll pray, I'll plan my goals for the week. The tears and sadness were always stronger than my resolve. One popular book by a physician touted progesterone as the *menopausal answer; another physician's bestseller warned women against using any hormones because they are dangerous and women don't need them for a natural passage like menopause. I thought to myself, birth is a natural passage as well, but most women and most doctors welcome assistance to ease the symptoms that last at most twenty-four hours. Menopause is soooo much longer!*

One day I just stopped the hormones and the antidepressants because I felt so defeated and frustrated. I thought I was out of options. I was tired of contradictory advice. I didn't feel important enough to continue my search for a way to feel better. One night on the Internet, I discovered information on your book, Screaming to Be Heard. *Within three weeks after devouring the book, I called to set up an evaluation. After you started me on thyroid, testosterone, and estradiol, I felt better physiologically, psychologically, and emotionally. After six years of searching I had found answers. I am now losing weight more easily, back on my road to regaining my healthy body. But what about those millions of women who just give up and follow their doctors' ill-advised ideas?*

Thank you, Dr. Vliet, for your knowledge. Without it I could not have resumed my life as a business owner and university teacher, nor could I have cared for my mother, who eleven months after I first saw you was diagnosed with a brain tumor. She, and my CEO Mary Kay Ash, have always championed women: "You can do it!" was their motto, and with your medical wisdom, I did!

—Lynne

Lynne's initial evaluation showed many problems to address: significant weight gain (BMI greater than 29), very low estradiol and testosterone, high cortisol, excess insulin, elevated glucose, high cholesterol and triglycerides, and an early phase thyroiditis. These medical problems were quite serious. She and I had a lot of complex "fine-tuning" to do to get all her metabolic "hormone power" back. As you see from her comments, her patience for the journey and her willingness to implement all the suggestions we made empowered her to reach her goals: improved energy, safe and effective fat loss, and improved long-term health risks.

Now, take a look at "Mara's" story. Even a woman who was "doing everything right" and didn't have major medical problems as Lynne did, was still gaining weight and losing stamina. Optimal balance helped her, too.

"Mara" at forty-eight is a serious triathlete and Ironman competitor, but she was having problems losing strength and getting fatter around her waist in spite of intense workout regimens in preparation for the Hawaii Ironman competition. She had been competing in the triathalon for over a decade and this change in her ability was really bothering her. She talked with several doctors, who didn't seem to understand how important this was for her, and just said, "What do you expect? You're getting older!" (How many times have you heard that one?)

Mara had not yet stopped menstruating, but she did have occasional hot flashes and had noticed that she no longer slept as soundly as she used to. She was also frustrated with her middle-spread fat and its stubborn refusal to budge, in spite of heroic exercise and diet efforts. Granted, she clearly wasn't obese, but her extra pounds were affecting her competition readiness, her stamina, and her sense of self-esteem. She was beginning to feel angry and betrayed by her body, when strategies she had used successfully in the past no longer worked. Even her trainer had noticed that her workouts weren't building muscle the way they should, and he was puzzled by these changes in her condition. She was convinced this was somehow related to her hormone balance, but no one would check her levels. When she had her consult with me, her testosterone was 26 ng/dl, and her estradiol was also extremely low at 21 pg/ml. This would be like trying to run your car on gasoline *vapors* instead of a full tank! She just didn't have the hormone "metabolic fuel" to run her body and build muscles. Even though she was still having light periods, her FSH at 99 was well over the menopausal "threshold" level of 20. In order for her to improve muscle mass, regain her strength and energy for competitions, as well as sleep normally, she needed to have her healthy hormone levels restored! Once we did this, she competed successfully in the year 2000 Hawaii Ironman Triathlon and her body is once again one she recognizes.

INTRODUCTION

Balancing your hormones is an intricate process involving all the various hormones, the *types* of hormones you need, and the best *route* of delivery (pills, patches, creams, injections, vaginal applications, etc.) to give you the most stable levels. In this chapter you'll learn more about what's involved to get your ovarian "hormone power" back so you will be able to lose excess fat more easily and regain your energy and health.

Here's a "road map" to show how I organized the discussion for each hormone, estrogens, progesterone, progestins, testosterone, and birth control pills:

- ◇ "Natural" or bioidentical products
- ◇ Synthetic or "mixed" products
- ◇ Background information on pros and cons of each
- ◇ Products to avoid if you are gaining weight
- ◇ Delivery systems: advantages and disadvantages for various health problems
- ◇ Dose comparisons by type

NATURAL VERSUS SYNTHETIC: WHAT DOES THIS MEAN?

I hear a lot of women talking about wanting to take only natural hormones, and use of the words *natural* and *synthetic* can be very confusing, to patients and doctors alike. This seems a good time to explain these terms.

Whether a compound is biologically "natural" (to plants or horses or whatever), is not the issue. The crucial point is whether the molecule shape, makeup, and structure is *exactly identical* to what is made in the human body, to provide the perfect "key" to unlock the body's receptor sites. A compound that meets these requirements is called "bioidentical." It's like getting a spare key for your car from the locksmith. The manufacturer (the ovary) stops making your own hormone at menopause so a "locksmith" (the laboratory) makes an exact duplicate hormone molecule for you to have to use if you choose to.

In common usage today, "synthetic" has come to mean "artificial," but that is not always correct. Synthetic simply means "produced by synthesis," or "to make." Synthroid and Estrace are "synthetic" in that they have been made in the laboratory rather than within a biological organism, but they are "natural" in being the exact molecules made by the thyroid and ovary, respectively. Other examples of exact copies of our bodies' hormones synthesized in the laboratory are Humulin (insulin) and cortisone (cortisol).

"Natural" or bioidentical hormones are made in the laboratory; the process is called "synthesizing." The sources for most of these "natural" human forms of ovarian hormones are actually building blocks found in wild yams and soybeans. The laboratory steps then convert these plant compounds into chemical molecules identical to those made in the human body for 17-beta estradiol, progesterone, or testosterone, which can then be made into standardized tablets, patches, creams, gels, and injectables for our prescriptions. Since the hormone quantity in each tablet is known, specific tailoring to each woman can be accomplished easily. So, we are able to synthesize a natural, bioidentical compound to replace what our body no longer makes.

The flip side of this coin is that something "natural" may be foreign or "supernatural" for the human body. Consider Premarin again. It is a "natural" mixture of estrogens because it is made by a biological organism, the pregnant mare. But it contains types of estrogen that were never found in the human body, ones that are more potent, and more long-lasting in the body, than our human 17-beta estradiol. In effect, it is a "*super*natural" estrogen for women that has some very undesirable consequences, as I explain later.

Another example is the "natural" estrogen-type compounds (genistein and others) found in soy and red clover and many other plants. These are "natural" substances since they come from biological plant sources. These compounds are "*un*natural" for our bodies, however, since we don't make these same compounds and don't have the enzymes to change the genistein or clover isoflavones into 17-beta estradiol. These molecules act very differently at our body's estrogen receptors, and don't have the full protective effects on heart, brain, and bone that 17-beta estradiol does. Furthermore, If you try to get enough active hormone from plant/herbal sources alone, you really are not able to determine how much you are taking and whether the amount is right for you because they aren't standardized.

Don't be misled by clever wording in advertising. While "natural" bears the mystique of being "better for you," it isn't always the case. If you aren't sure about whether you are taking, or considering taking, natural or synthetic hormones, check the chart I've created to guide you.

DIFFERENT ESTROGENS, DIFFERENT EFFECTS

All estrogens are not the same, and Premarin is not the only estrogen, as I explained in chapter 12. Premarin is only one brand of estrogen among many brands available. It is natural for the horse, but is not "natural" for your body, nor does it even provide very good levels of the 17-beta estradiol that your body made before menopause. If you have a weight problem, Premarin (and the Provera prescribed with it) often aggravates it, for a variety of reasons I will explain later.

WHAT ARE THE NATURAL HUMAN ESTROGENS?

17-Beta Estradiol (E2)

This estrogen, often called just "estradiol," is our primary, biologically active, premenopausal estrogen that is the optimal "key" to activate our estrogen receptors and provide all the benefits we associate with "estrogen therapy." There are several brands of 17-beta estradiol commercially available in this country, and all of these brands use a form of estradiol that is derived from soybean or wild yam precursor molecules purified in the laboratory to make the *identical molecule* made by our ovary before menopause. The comparative studies that have been done, as well as my clinical experience, show that the bioidentical human form of 17-beta estradiol is more easily tolerated, with fewer side effects and better positive effects on glucose regulation, insulin sensitivity, muscle and connective tissue, brain function, pain regulation, and bone markers.

FDA-Approved 17-Beta Estradiol Brands in the United States

- ◇ Estrace tablets and vaginal cream (FDA approved in 1976)
- ◇ Gynodiol tablets; generic estradiol tablets
- ◇ Alora, Climara, Vivelle, Vivelle DOT, Estraderm, Esclim transdermal patches, in multiple strengths
- ◇ Vagifem vaginal tablets
- ◇ Estring vaginal ring
- ◇ Combination products (estradiol with progestin): Activella, Combi-patch, Ortho Prefest

In addition to these FDA-approved products, *estradiol USP* is available for various generic products (not all are as reliable as the brands, so be aware of this problem), as well as for compounding pharmacists to use in making tablets, creams, gels, and injections in other dose strengths than are available in the FDA-approved products. Keep in mind that 17-beta estradiol is what your ovary made before menopause, and what keeps your body's cellular machinery working at optimal effectiveness. When you think about hormone replenishment for the optimal metabolism, energy, and well-being, think about restoring the "key" that your body always had and now needs!

Estrone (E1)

This is the estrogen that, after menopause, is still made in fat tissue from the androgen, androstenedione; it is the one that is associated with higher risks of breast and uterine cancers. It is metabolically less active than E2, but serves as an estrogen reservoir for our bodies.

There are a number of products that primarily deliver estrone, and I don't recommend these if you are having difficulty losing weight. The estrogen products that give high levels of estrone and relatively little of the 17-beta estradiol are Premarin, Prem Pro, Prem Phase, Estratab, Estratest, Cenestin, Menest, Ogen, Ortho-Est. Overweight women already have higher estrone relative to estradiol, so using an estrone product just makes this imbalance worse and makes your metabolism even more sluggish. In addition, high estrone is associated with a greater risk of breast and endometrial cancers.

Estriol (E3)

Estriol is the weakest estrogen, made in the placenta during pregnancy, not normally found in high levels in a nonpregnant woman. Many studies have shown it does not preserve bone, heart, or brain benefits seen with E2.

Estriol has been studied extensively in Europe over several decades. It really isn't the "forgotten estrogen" as some books claim; it just isn't used much because studies have clearly shown that it doesn't provide the degree of protective effects on bone, heart, brain, and nerves as does 17-beta estradiol. If someone tells you that your estriol level is low, that's a normal finding if you are not pregnant. Since menopause is not a time you are planning to be pregnant, estriol doesn't really make much sense for hormone therapy.

Some authors claim estriol prevents breast cancer, but no protective effect of E3 has been found in reputable medical studies, other than the known effect of full-term pregnancy prior to age thirty in reducing breast cancer risk. Whatever role estriol plays in reducing breast cancer risk is not an independent effect of estriol, but rather is thought to occur along with other breast changes that happen with a full-term pregnancy before age thirty.

There are no FDA-approved estriol products in the United States because it has not been found effective to preserve bone and the other benefits of estradiol. Women who use estriol have it made by compounding pharmacists in a variety of forms. For some women, estriol relieves milder symptoms (vaginal dryness, mild hot flashes, for example). Many studies have demonstrated that estriol does not improve sleep, in contrast to what has been shown with 17-beta estradiol. Estriol also does not have significant beneficial effects for improving pain, memory, mood, and the "brain fog" symptoms that are so common in midlife. I have treated a lot of women who had been put on estriol and suffered from "brain crash" when it didn't work as well as estradiol on these crucial brain pathways.

Another emerging concern as more "natural hormone" practitioners use estriol is the studies from England over the past twenty years that showed higher doses of estriol (needed to give symptom relief) will also stimulate the endometrium of the uterus to thicken just as other estrogens do. Thus, if you take *enough* estriol to really help your symptoms, you still have to watch for endometrial hyperplasia just as you would if you took any of the estradiol products.

Plant Estrogens (Phytoestrogens)

These are estrogenic compounds found in several hundred different plants, including soybeans, red clover, grains, and many others. The phytoestrogens are biologically weaker than the native human estrogens and don't have the same effects at the human estrogen receptors as our own estradiol. Some of the phytoestrogens are "activators" (agonists) and some are "blockers" (antagonists), and some have mixed agonist-antagonist effects. These different actions are dose and concentration related, and occur due to small chemical changes in molecular arrangements. All of the phytoestrogen precursors require chemical conversion in the laboratory to make the bioidentical human form of 17-beta estradiol. Since the human body does not have the enzymes needed for these changes, taking phytoestrogen supplements does not provide the critically necessary 17-beta estradiol.

These differences help explain an apparent discrepancy: In China and Japan, where diets are high in phytoestrogens, women do not typically describe hot flashes, but they do continue to have bone loss after menopause. There is currently a serious problem with osteoporosis in Japan; their research indicates that phytoestrogens alone do not provide enough estrogen effect to protect against osteoporosis and decline in cognitive function, even though the plant sources may be helpful for mild symptoms. Ginseng is another plant recommended by herbalists as a "natural" source of estrogen. Ginseng gives little measurable estrogenic effect, and can cause high blood pressure, insomnia, anxiety, and agitation if taken in large amounts.

Double-blind, placebo-controlled, prospective studies from the international menopause literature have found that phytoestrogen products were no more effective than placebo, even for controlling hot flashes. Phytoestrogens are less potent than 17-beta estradiol, but because the blood concentrations are so much higher when today's isoflavone supplements are used, it is quite easy to "overwhelm" the tiny concentration of estradiol. By competing with your body estradiol at cellular receptors, these high concentrations of isoflavone phytoestrogens can interfere with action or production of your own body estradiol.

Synthetic Estrogens

All of these estrogens have slightly different chemical structures from the three human forms, and are more potent than human estrogens. They have somewhat different effects and side effects as a result of these chemical changes.

Ethinyl estradiol (EE). This is the most common form of estrogen found in the birth control pills that are widely used in perimenopausal women who may need better control of irregular cycles, symptoms, and erratic bleeding. Birth control pills are not widely used in the United States for postmenopausal HRT because they provide more estrogen effect than is generally needed after a woman reaches menopause. EE is found in a new menopause product, *Femhrt,* in a much lower dose than in birth control pills. The problem with Femhrt is that it has as much progestin as many birth control pills (1 mg norethindrone), but so little estrogen that women in our practice who tried it didn't like the way they felt. Plus, they gained more weight because the high progestin content made them so hungry! Ethinyl estradiol is available alone as the brand Estinyl, used in some countries for hormone therapy, but it is not a birth control pill since it contains only the estrogen.

Estradiol valerate. A chemically different estrogen, more potent than 17-beta estradiol, and rarely used in the United States for hormone therapy. It is used commonly overseas for postmenopausal ERT in oral and intramuscular injectable forms.

Ogen (piperazine estrone sulfate). A synthetic estrone that is chemically similar to, but not exactly the same as, human estrone. If you are using this product, you may still have some residual symptoms due to the lower amount of estradiol and the piperazine chemical ring part of the molecule. I don't recommend Ogen for women with any kind of muscle or bladder pain syndromes because I have found that this chemical difference makes it more likely to aggravate the pain problems. I also do not recommend Ogen for overweight women due to the additional estrone load it delivers.

Figure 13.1
TYPES OF ESTROGEN PRESENT
IN POPULAR PRODUCTS

Cenestin* (synthetic plant-derived conjugated estrogens)	Premarin[†] (conjugated horse-derived estrogens)	Estratab[‡] (esterified estrogens)	Estrace tablets[†] Patches: Alora, Vivelle DOT, Climara, Esclim (17-beta-estradiol soy/yam derived)
estrone 58%	estrone 49.9%	estrone 88.8%	
equilin 28%	equilin 22.8%	equilin 5.9%	
17-α-dihydro equilin 15%	17-α-dihydro equilin 13.5%	17-α-dihydro equilin 2.6%	
	17-α-estradiol 3.6%	17-α-estradiol 1.2%	
	δ-8,9-dihydro estrone 3.7%		
	equilenin 2.8%	equilenin 1.1%	
	17-β dihydro equilin 1.4%		
	17-β estradiol 0.5%		17-β-estradiol 100%
	17-α-dihydro equilenin 1.4%		
	17-β-dihydro equilenin 0.4%		

*Cenestin product information from manufacturer's prescribing information
[†]Premarin advertisement, Journal of the American Medical Association, February 8, 1995, and manufacturer's prescribing information
[‡]From manufacturer's prescribing information

© 2001 Elizabeth Lee Vliet, M.D.

Nonhuman, Mixed Estrogens

Cenestin. A plant-derived estrogen product formulated to have the mixed estrogens found in Premarin; delivers predominately estrone.

Premarin. Conjugated equine estrogens derived from pregnant mares' urine; delivers high levels of estrogens not found in the human body, plus higher levels of estrone and very little 17-beta estradiol. Prempro and Premphase contain the horse estrogens plus synthetic MPA.

Estratab. Esterified estrogens, similar to Premarin, plant-derived; delivers primarily estrone.

Estratest. Esterified estrogens plus methyl testosterone. Delivers primarily estrone, so I don't recommend it.

Refer to figure 13.1 for the list of all the different types of estrogens contained in the above products. *Estrace (17-beta estradiol)* contains none of the other compounds shown above, thereby reducing the overall estrogen amount delivered per dose when compared to the above types. For women who are struggling with weight gain, I suggest that you avoid the mixed estrogen products, and use one of the 17-beta estradiol products I have listed in this chapter.

PROBLEMS WITH PREMARIN

Three decades ago (late 1970s, early 1980s), two leading British menopause researchers, Dr. Whitehead and Dr. Campbell, did studies of the potencies of the different types of estrogens and the effects of the various estrogens on different organs in the body. Their work raised some serious issues about adverse effects of horse-derived estrogens for women, but most of their questions and concerns have been ignored in the United States where over 80 percent of the estrogen prescriptions are for Premarin.

Conjugated equine estrogens in Premarin are about three times more potent in stimulating the liver production of renin substrate, which is used to make angiotensin in the body, a factor that causes increased blood pressure. Estrace and Ogen, two other estrogens used in Campbell and Whitehead's work study, did not show this elevation of renin substrate, and did not have the tendency to cause high blood pressure that was seen with Premarin. If you are overweight and already have high blood pressure, this is an important difference.

Premarin was more likely to lead to elevated triglycerides than the human estradiol, particularly when estradiol was used in patch form and bypassed the liver "first-pass" metabolism. This is also important for women with weight problems, since they also tend to already have high triglycerides.

Other important differences, particularly relevant for overweight women, emerged from the Nurses Health Study. This study reported an increased risk of breast cancer in women on long duration estrogen. But what the news articles failed to tell you was that these women were primarily taking Premarin, and the Premarin users who also drank alcohol regularly were the ones who had the increase in breast cancer risk. What do obesity, alcohol, and Premarin have in common related to breast cancer? They all cause higher-than-normal levels of estrone.

We know several important things about the horse-derived estrogens: equine estrogens stay in the human body much longer than our natural estradiol, anywhere from eight to fourteen weeks after the last dose; equine estrogens have stronger "attachment strength" (affinity) for our estradiol receptors (especially the breasts, where estrogens may concentrate in the fat tissue), and equine estrogens give much higher total blood level of estrogens following an oral dose of Premarin than is seen with a comparable dose of Estrace. All of these problems are made worse when women have high estrone due to excess body fat.

ADVANTAGES AND DISADVANTAGES OF VARIOUS DELIVERY SYSTEMS

Oral Estrogens

All of the various products for 17-beta estradiol deliver the identical estrogen made in our body. The primary difference between pill form and transdermal patch form is that oral estrogens all have to be metabolized (changed) first in the liver, called the first-pass effect. This has some pluses and some minuses. A plus is that if you have a very low level of HDL, you may want the boost of having the oral estrogen stimulate the liver to make more HDL. This is a pharmacologic, or druglike, effect of estrogen first going through the liver.

Patches, creams, and gels of estradiol still give you the beneficial physiological (natural) effect of estradiol to maintain the normal level of HDL cholesterol, they just don't give you that rapid, extra liver stimulation to make more HDL. For women who have high total cholesterol and low HDL, however, an oral form of estradiol provides more decrease in total cholesterol and a more significant increase in HDL for cardiovascular protective effects. The patch may be all that is needed for women who have a normal cholesterol profile.

Some minuses of the oral estrogens are that they may lead to higher blood pressure, higher triglycerides, higher estrone, and more likelihood of gallstones if you have a predisposition to those problems. Otherwise, which form you use—pills or patches—becomes a matter of personal preference.

The Transdermal Estradiol Patch

Transdermal estrogen patches deliver the human 17-beta estradiol in a way that is the most "natural" of all. The estradiol is absorbed through the skin, directly into the bloodstream, similar to the ovarian process before menopause. Direct delivery to the bloodstream bypasses the first-pass metabolism in the liver that breaks down some of the hormone, making it unavailable for its normal functions.

The estradiol patches stick to the skin and stay in place for several days for the hormones to be slowly absorbed. Each brand of patch lasts for a slightly different period of time, and women metabolize the hormones at different rates, so it may take a little experimenting to find the patch change schedule that is right for you.

There really are only two drawbacks to this form of estradiol: the skin irritation from the adhesive may bother some women, although adhesives vary by manufacturer, so experiment with different brands; and some women don't like the cosmetic appearance of having a patch on their body.

Advantages of the Estradiol Patch
(especially if you have weight problems)

- ⬦ Patches keep blood levels of estradiol fairly steady, similar to the hormone production by the ovary (helpful for women with blood pressure or "hormonal" headache problems).
- ⬦ Estradiol by patch gives better improvement in glucose control and insulin sensitivity than oral estrogens.
- ⬦ Patches do not lead to further elevation of estrone (as seen with oral forms) since the estradiol bypasses the liver first pass.
- ⬦ Estradiol in a patch is less likely to be adversely affected by other medications, since the estradiol is not metabolized first in the liver.
- ⬦ Transdermal delivery of estradiol does not elevate triglycerides as occurs in some women taking oral estrogens.
- ⬦ Estradiol by patch is less likely to cause gallstones.
- ⬦ Patches maintain benefits of estradiol on HDL to LDL cholesterol even though this form of estradiol delivery doesn't raise HDL as rapidly or quite as high as oral estrogens.

Creams, Gels, Injections, and Implants (Pellets)

All of these delivery methods bypass the liver first pass, so they will have similar results and benefits as I outlined for the patch. Their main drawback, as a group, is that the stability in estradiol level is not as good as with the pills and patches. Creams and gels, in particular, often rise too fast and wear off too quickly for many women, leading to a pretty bumpy road and more symptoms from the fluctuations in estradiol blood levels. Injections and implants, in the usual way they are used, tend to cause excessively high levels at the outset and then wear off unpredictably, leaving you again feeling like you are on a roller coaster ride. While I have used all of these approaches, they are a little more tricky to stabilize and keep estradiol even and consistent each day. Sometimes, what I find works best is a combination of the above options. The key is finding what gives the best results for each individual women and not being locked in to any one approach.

PROGESTERONE AND PROGESTINS

It will help you understand this section if you go back and review the terms I defined in chapter 6 for progesterone and progestins. This is a list of some examples of the types of natural micronized progesterone and common progestins available in menopausal products and birth control pills:

◇ Micronized (natural) progesterone: Prometrium, Crinone
◇ Androgenic progestins:
    Norethindrone: Micronor, Aygestin; Birth control pills: Ovcon, Modicon, Necon, and several other pills; also in HRT products Activella, Femhrt, CombiPatch
    Levonorgestrel: Alesse, Levlite, Levlen, Levora, Nordette, Norplant
◇ Progestational progestins:
    Medroxyprogesterone acetate: Provera, Cycrin, Amen, Depo-Provera
    Norgestimate: Ortho-Cyclen, Ortho-Prefest
    Desorgestrel: Desogen, Ortho-Cept, Mircette

Earlier you read about progesterone's role in storing fat for pregnancy and nursing, so you may wonder why you should take this hormone at all.

If you are menopausal and still have your uterus and want to take estrogen, then you take progesterone (or a progestin) in some form to oppose the estrogen effect on the lining of the uterus and prevent excess buildup that could later become hyperplasia or cancer. If you are premenopausal and using birth control pills, the progestin prevents pregnancy by suppressing ovulation, keeping the uterine lining thin, and changing cervical mucus to be "inhospitable" to sperm.

There are several good ways now that you can use progesterone, or a low-dose synthetic progestin, to prevent hyperplasia and yet not have an overly adverse impact on your appetite and weight. The difference is determined by which type you take, in what form, and for how long, as well as the balance with estradiol.

If you have a weight problem, and have already had your uterus removed, then I would strongly encourage you *not* to add progesterone (pills, patches, creams, or gels—either prescription or over the counter) to your therapy. It clearly does make you hungrier, it makes you more likely to remain insulin resistant, and it diminishes GH production—to name a few of the points I made in chapter 6. There is also evidence now that estrogen alone is safer than estrogen plus progesterone/progestin in terms of breast cancer risk, so if you do not have a uterus, there are many reasons to avoid taking this hormone. Why complicate your weight-loss efforts if you no longer need to protect the uterine lining from developing hyperplasia or cancer?

Side Effects of Progestins

Synthetic progestins, whether in birth control pills or given in post-menopause, are the most common cause of unpleasant side effects associated with hormone therapy: increased ("ravenous") appetite, weight gain, fluid retention, irritable mood, depressed mood, headaches, decreased energy, bloating, breast tenderness, loss of libido, among others.

To minimize the negative effects, it is important to check: the relative balance of progestational and androgenic activity, and the balance of progestin relative to estrogen in the preparation. Newer progestins like norgestimate and desogestrel are the *most progestational* and *least androgenic* of the synthetic progestins. This means they are less likely to cause acne, but may be more likely to cause weight gain, loss of libido, or depressed mood. Progestin-only products, like Norplant and Depo-Provera, as well as pills such as Micronor that contain no estrogen, typically have the worst side-effect profile of all, because you get all the negative effects of the progestin without any compensating benefits of the estrogen *unless estrogen is added as a separate pill or patch.*

Route of Delivery

How you take progestin is another factor that will influence side effects. Oral progestins or progesterone are more likely to have more unwanted mood and appetite side effects because of the compounds that are made by the liver in the first-pass metabolism. With transdermal delivery, either by suppositories, vaginal gels, prescription cream, or patch, the hormone isn't metabolized by the liver before it is absorbed into the bloodstream. You may have to try different methods to see what works for you.

MY SUGGESTIONS FOR FINDING WHAT'S RIGHT FOR YOU

My approach of individualizing hormone therapy for each woman rather than using the cookbook approach of doling out Premarin-Provera has met with great success. One of my patients, a woman judge, called me and practically shouted over the phone in a jubilant voice about my changing her to natural progesterone: "It was 10 million times better than Provera. I can live with this, I don't feel crazy and bloated anymore."

Another fifty-three-year-old woman, who had been having very bothersome side effects of depression, weight gain, lethargy, and "all that PMS feeling again" with the Provera phase of her HRT, was also pleased with a changeover to natural progesterone with the Estrace: *I'm feeling great! I can't believe the difference in how I feel taking the natural progesterone. I don't feel so depressed and slowed down like I did. I used to hate those fourteen days on Provera, and sometimes I didn't even take it. I didn't want to tell my doctor, but I just didn't like how I felt on the Provera.*"

Another new combination product that has worked well for many of our patients is Activella, which contains 1 mg 17-beta estradiol and 0.5 mg norethindrone. This estrogen-progestin ratio is better than most of the other combination products on the market, and it is the natural human form of estradiol. We have seen less of the bleeding and spotting with this product compared to Prempro, CombiPatch, and Femhrt. Women also tell us that they don't have as much bloating, breast tenderness, and weight gain with Activella as they do with the other combination products.

Birth control pills using less than 1 mg of norethindrone (or equivalent) with 30 to 35 mcg of ethinyl estradiol are the ones I have found less likely to overstimulate your appetite and contribute to weight gain. Examples of these are Ovcon 35, Modicon, Necon, Ortho-Cept, and Ortho-Cyclen. Higher progestin pills such as Alesse, Mircette, Loestrin, and others are *more likely* to cause weight gain.

Ortho Prefest (1.0 mg 17-beta estradiol and 0.09 mg norgestimate, alternating with plain estradiol tablets) uses a different approach: steady estradiol and intermittent progestin delivery. There are three days of estradiol alone followed by three days of combination estradiol and norgestimate in a continuously repeated regimen. This dosing regimen is proposed to capitalize on our emerging understanding of hormone-receptor dynamics:

delivery of estradiol alone stimulates new hormone-receptor growth, thought to maximize estrogenic benefits, and the combined delivery of progestin with estrogen then down-regulates hormone receptors. It may be a good option for some women who don't have many side effects with progestins and who don't like having monthly bleeding.

I see some potential problems with this regimen for you to consider before asking your doctor about trying it. If you have been struggling with excess weight, insulin resistance or diabetes, migraines, tension headaches, depression, bladder pain, or fibromyalgia, even the intermittent progestin may still be more than you can tolerate. The fluctuating progestin levels from starting and stopping the norgestimate every three days may be a particular problem for migraine sufferers and increase the frequency of headaches. If you don't have any of these problems, and don't like having monthly bleeding, you may want to ask your doctor about trying Ortho-Prefest and see how you do.

Progestasert and *Mirena* are two intrauterine progestin-delivery systems. These are options to explore if you have gained a lot of weight and have trouble with increased appetite when you take the progestin or progesterone. These products are used primarily for contraception rather than for progestin therapy in menopausal women, but they may be a good alternative if you are overly sensitive to other forms of progestins.

Progestasert and Mirena release a small amount of daily progestin directly to the lining of the uterus, and there is very little progestin absorbed into the total body circulation. The dose of progestin is smaller because it is delivered directly to the uterine lining. These two reasons are why the intrauterine systems do not have the usual unwanted side effects of progestin or progesterone taken orally or transdermally. A number of studies have shown that these products delivers enough progestin to effectively suppress the buildup of the uterine lining. If you have a uterus and want to continue estrogen but nothing else has worked to give you a progestin you could take, you may want to ask your doctor about trying Progestasert or Mirena.

Even with natural progesterone, there are still some women who simply aren't able to tolerate any progestogen, synthetic or natural. Women who are markedly sensitive to progesterone or progestins may experience intolerable degrees of depression, loss of libido, pain flares, headaches, lethargy, bloating, breast tenderness, and weight gain. For these women, the American College of Obstetricians and Gynecologists (ACOG) published the ACOG Progestin Consensus Statement in 1988 (still valid today) that says: If a woman is intolerant to the progestin, it is acceptable to use unopposed estrogen as long as she is willing to have an annual endometrial biopsy and report immediately any abnormal bleeding.

Many physicians are reluctant to use this approach because of the endometrial cancer issue, and because of the erratic and potentially serious bleeding problems that can occur with long use of estrogen only. Going without progestin and having an annual biopsy is an avenue you may explore with your doctor if you have not been able to find any progestin that you can use and natural progesterone doesn't work for you, and if you don't tend to have bleeding problems that could be made worse with this approach.

The use of estrogen alone tends to be a greater concern in women who are not getting adequate health care and who have bleeding over a long period of time that is not being properly evaluated. But, for women who have a lot of side effects with the progesterone or progestin, and have severe cardiovascular risks or other problems precluding use of progestogens, then the ACOG position does provide an option for you as long as you take responsibility to see that you are appropriately monitored. There are really not any hard-and-fast rules in this situation, so it once again comes down to an individualized approach.

TO BLEED OR NOT TO BLEED WITH PROGESTINS

If you are on a *cyclic* progesterone or progestin regimen, when you stop the progestin each month, you will have some degree of menstrual-type "withdrawal" bleeding. This is what you want to have happen in order to reduce the endometrial cancer risk by getting rid of the lining of the uterus.

On the other hand, many women don't like having menstrual-type flow after menopause and may choose to take a progestin every day. The use of any progestin every day suppresses the lining and stops all bleeding in about 80 percent of women after about six months of continuous progestin use. The other 20 percent of women taking progestin daily tend to continue to have annoying, erratic bleeding and spotting. If you fall in this last group, you may want to talk with your doctor about going back to a cycling regimen so that you have more predictable bleeding patterns. Current research has shown that it is medically safe in terms of reducing endometrial cancer risk if you cycle the progesterone or progestin every other month or even every third month. Whether the progestin is given cyclically or daily, the goal is to minimize the amount to the least possible dose that protects the endometrium in order to reduce the likelihood of unpleasant side effects.

Recent research has shown, whether the progestogen is given monthly or every two or three months, it is the duration of the progestogen phase that is needed to protect the endometrium from hyperplasia. One study of 398 women found that in those who took the progestogen for only seven days, 3.5 percent (14 women) developed cystic hyperplasia after several years. When the duration of progestogen was increased to ten days or more, not a single woman developed cystic hyperplasia. If you are supposed to be taking a progestogen, make certain you take it for the full time your physician has recommended, even if you should start bleeding earlier, before you have finished your progestin/progesterone cycle. If you continue to start bleeding early each time, talk with your doctor about changing the dose or type of progestin.

There is some good news in all this: The longer you are on hormone therapy, what characteristically happens is that the uterine lining does not build up as much as it did earlier in your life so the actual flow is shorter and lighter.

For women who feel strongly that they do not want any more monthly bleeding, another combination or regimen being used is the continuous regimen of giving estrogen and progestin together every day, called continuous-combined therapy. This can be done with various tablet options for estradiol plus progesterone or low-dose progestin. Activella is a good option for this. It is a new combination tablet without as much adverse effect on weight as those products with higher progestin dose such as Combi-Patch and Femhrt. Activella uses the bioidentical 17-beta estradiol with 0.5 mg norethindrone (less appetite stimulation than Provera or MPA).

A caution for women with weight problems: I have a concern that taking the progestin every day may make weight loss more difficult, unless you use just a low dose of norethindrone that doesn't have as much appetite-stimulating effects as we see with progesterone and Provera. For some women, the daily progesterone or progestin may interfere with optimal estrogen effects on the brain and lead to more irritability, depressed mood or insomnia. In addition, if you have abnormal cholesterol or triglycerides, taking progestins daily may make this problem worse. Daily use of the progestin may also contribute to difficulties regulating blood sugar in women with diabetes or insulin resistance. If you are considering the option of daily progestin, you may want to review these pros and cons with your physician to decide what is best for you.

WHAT ABOUT WILD YAM
AND PROGESTERONE
OVER-THE-COUNTER CREAMS?

Disogenin (and others) is a plant precursor molecule found in wild yams, soybeans, and a variety of other foods that has some very mild effects similar to both progesterone and estrogen. This is used in many over-the-counter nonprescription creams. These plant precursors are not the same chemical molecule as either progesterone or estradiol, and do not have the exact same effects in the body—even though the marketing claims try to make you think they do. This compound will not prevent endometrial cancer, so you can't depend on these over-the-counter creams for this purpose. These *phytosterols* (phytoestrogens, phytoprogestins, etc.) can be synthesized into progesterone or estradiol in a laboratory, but not in your body.

A lot of women have been misled about these over-the-counter creams sold in health food stores, on the Internet, and in health catalogs. Women are treating themselves using these products in the mistaken idea that they are "safe," have "no side effects," and can even help weight *loss*. These claims are *not* substantiated by reputable medical research. In fact, as I have explained, progesterone promotes fat *storage*. Be aware that many of these products have significant progesterone effects, even though they are sold as "natural" and/or as "wild yam extract."

Many have very high doses of USP progesterone added to them, sometimes shown on the label and sometimes not. The standardized FDA-approved prescription progesterone vaginal cream, Crinone 4 percent, delivers 40 mg per application, and the recommended amount is one applicator every other night for only six doses a month. Using Crinone 4 percent cream would deliver an average of 20 mg a day over twelve days. This is the amount that research to date has shown is sufficient for preventing endometrial hyperplasia.

Many of the over-the-counter progesterone creams deliver amounts of progesterone far in excess of the amount delivered by FDA-approved Crinone 4 percent cream. The excess amount of progesterone in many of the over-the-counter creams accounts for such side effects as weight gain, bloating, breast tenderness, headaches, low libido, acne, sweet cravings, depressed mood, lack of energy, fatigue, backaches, and other effects of high levels of progesterone. Just think about the last trimester of pregnancy when progesterone is highest and you have an idea of what may occur with large amounts of progesterone in skin creams.

If you are using one of these products, you need to let your doctor know. Read the label carefully to see if it says "progesterone" in addition to wild yam extract. If you have been having any of the symptoms I mentioned above since starting one of these products, I suggest you stop the product and observe what happens with your appetite, fluid retention and sweet cravings. It is important that you also keep in mind that too much progesterone relative to estrogen can cause heavy bleeding and painful cramps with menstruation. This is a point many women don't know, and the makers of these creams don't tell you. Women, and many doctors, tend to focus only on bleeding problems that occur when there is excess estrogen relative to progesterone, but it is also true that constant use of progestins or progesterone without the right estrogen balance can cause erratic, heavy bleeding. Your gynecologist needs to know what over-the-counter "hormonally active" creams or herbs you may be using.

CAPTURING THE POWER OF TESTOSTERONE

You've read about the powerful role of testosterone in building lean body mass: muscle and bone. This is what you want to maintain as one of the best ways to help tackle the midlife middle spread. Testosterone also helps improve your flagging libido and energy level and improves your sense of well-being, so there are a number of reasons to consider adding this hormone to replenish what you have lost as the ovary declines. Just don't go overboard! Too much testosterone will add those pounds to your waist, as I explained in chapter 7.

Types of Testosterone—Natural and Synthetic

We don't yet have in the United States an *optimal* FDA-approved commercial product to deliver just natural, micronized testosterone in steady levels for women, although there are several good ones for men. Let me explain what *is* available, and what issues you need to consider as you work with balancing this hormone.

Methyl testosterone (MT). This was the first FDA-approved testosterone product available. MT is a synthetic, more potent form of testosterone, chemically different from the form made by the human ovary or testicle. The addition of the methyl group to testosterone made it possible for the hormone to be taken orally without being broken down and lost in the digestive process before being absorbed into the bloodstream. But this methyl group is what increases the potential for liver damage at high doses and gives "testosterone" a bad reputation. Methyl testosterone was used primarily for men until more effective forms became available. The commercial products for women—Estratest, Premarin-MT combination (now off the market)—have generally been higher doses of MT than most women can use on a daily basis without having negative effects.

Micronized natural testosterone. Micronized means that the hormone particles are small enough to survive digestion and be absorbed into the bloodstream. Micronized testosterone is made from building blocks in soybeans and wild yams, similar to the process used for estradiol and progesterone. The chemical precursors are extracted, purified, and synthesized into *testosterone USP,* which is *identical to the molecules made in the human body.* Compounding pharmacists can take testosterone (T) USP and make pills, creams, gels, injections, or implants in almost any dose that may be needed. Currently, in the United States, a micronized testosterone patch in a dose designed for women is in clinical trials for FDA approval. This patch is using the same technology that has made estradiol patches available, but it is not yet on the market. The testosterone patches (Androderm, Testoderm) and gel (AndroGel) are *far too high in their doses for women to use.* Do not try to use *men's* products for your own testosterone replacement.

Background on Important Pros and Cons with Estratest

Estratest has become much more popular in recent years with increased awareness of the importance of testosterone for women, but there are problems with this product, *particularly if you are struggling with weight gain.* Estratest contains esterified estrogens that are converted primarily to estrone and provide much less 17-beta estradiol, so it doesn't generally give you the best form of estrogen. Estratest contains the potent MT, in a dose that is usually more than most women need when taken every day. As a result, it often causes more negative side effects than micronized testosterone. (Concern about MT effects on the liver and potential to cause liver tumors has existed since the 1950s. The 1998 edition of the textbook *Testosterone: Action, Deficiency, Substitution,* published by Springer-Verlag, Berlin, has an important paragraph on page 299 that I think warrants mentioning here: *"Because of the side effects methyl testosterone should no longer be used therapeutically, in particular since effective alternatives are available. The German Endocrine Society declared methyltestosterone obsolete in 1981 and the German Federal Health Authority ruled that methyltestosterone should be withdrawn from the market. In other countries, however, methyltestosterone is still in use, a practice which should be terminated."*)

I find that women taking Estratest have more problems with increased appetite, sweet cravings, weight gain, facial hair, acne or oily skin, deeper voice, flare-ups of muscle pain, irritability, insomnia and feeling anxious or tense, loss of scalp hair (male pattern baldness), elevated total and LDL cholesterol, decreased HDL ("good") cholesterol, and elevated triglycerides and insulin (aggravating the body fat deposited around the waist).

Estratest illustrates a common problem with any fixed-dose combination medicine: there may not be enough of one and too much of the other for you to have exactly what you need of each one. In my opinion, these fixed-dose products do not allow for individualized adjustments of hormone therapies tailored to each woman. I prefer using each hormone separately to allow you to make changes in only one at a time, based on what you are experiencing, or taking into account interactions with other medications (such as antibiotics, asthma medications, etc.) and effects of situational stresses on your hormone metabolism.

Different Ways to Deliver Testosterone

Testosterone can be in pills, creams, gels, injections, or implants (pellets). Which way it is given will determine the amount absorbed; how fast the blood level rises and falls; how the hormone is metabolized to other forms such as dihydrotestosterone or others; whether you have a good, desirable response; what side effects you have; and whether there is a positive or negative effect on such things as liver enzymes, cholesterol, LDL, HDL, blood glucose, and so forth.

Here are some general pointers to consider:

◊ Rapidly absorbed forms of testosterone (gels, some types of cream, injections, sublingual troches) typically cause the fastest rise and fall in blood level. This means a greater chance of having headaches, irritability, edginess, muscle spasms, aggressive/angry feelings or anxious/restless feelings when the level is rising too quickly, and then losing the benefits when it falls too fast. The gels are the most rapidly absorbed, and many of my patients (even some men) have told me that they feel like they were hit by a Mack truck within five minutes of applying a testosterone gel. This is still true even if the dose is low, since the brain effects have to do with rate of absorption, not just the amount. As a result of these problems, I don't usually use these forms anymore.

◊ A slower-release form of testosterone, such as a sustained-release capsule or tablet, or a cream in a base that is more slowly absorbed, or a depot (slow release) injectable will all provide more gradual absorption and steadier levels over a longer period of time. These are the forms that I use more commonly, and I have these made up by compounding pharmacists in individualized doses.

◊ Injectable forms of several synthetic testosterone preparations are available, but these tend to give levels that are too high at the beginning and wear off unpredictably, so I don't use these for women.

◊ Implants (also called pellets) are not currently FDA-approved for women but are being used in some settings on an individual basis. We have seen a number of problems for women using these products, including erratic absorption and release, unpredictable "wearing-off" effects, and excessively high blood levels associated with masculinizing side effects (hair loss, acne, abdominal fat gain, negative lipid changes, increased insulin resistance). In addition, the implants have to be surgically inserted and removed, so you don't have the option of removing them on your own. For all these reasons, I don't recommend the implants.

⬦ My desire is for you to be in control of your hormone fine-tuning and have pills or a cream that you can choose to use or not use on any given day, based on how you are feeling.

⬦ Oral testosterone is changed by the liver in the first-pass effect before it is absorbed into the bloodstream. For some women, this causes no problems, and oral, sustained-release micronized testosterone works quite well to improve sexual interest, energy, bone density, and well-being. For other women, the oral form metabolized first in the liver may aggravate high blood pressure, fluid retention, and possibly lead to negative changes in the cholesterol profile, such as increased total cholesterol, lower HDL and higher LDL, and high triglycerides. If this happens, you can avoid these problems by changing from oral to transdermal (cream, or patch, when available), because this is absorbed directly into the bloodstream and bypasses the liver first-pass effect.

Find Your Optimal Dose: Comparisons by Type and Route

Each woman responds to testosterone differently, so the dose *has* to be carefully individualized. Most women need only very small amounts of testosterone to achieve its benefits. Especially if you have been gaining abdominal fat, serum levels should be checked to make sure that your estradiol is optimal and that you are not getting too much testosterone.

It is important to understand that which *way* you take testosterone will determine the dose range that is appropriate. Oral doses are typically higher than nonoral forms since some of the active hormone is lost in the process of absorption and liver metabolism. If you are using a cream or gel, a rule of thumb is a concentration about one quarter to one tenth of an oral dose to adjust for the greater absorption into the bloodstream with this route. This dose recommendation for testosterone is comparable to what the FDA approved for other ovarian hormones: estradiol 1.0 mg oral = 0.1 mg patch, or one tenth the oral dose; natural progesterone (Prometrium) oral = 200 mg/day; progesterone cream (Crinone 4 percent) delivers 40 mg every *other* day or 20 mg/day average, again one tenth the oral dose.

Recommendations of 1 percent and 2 percent testosterone creams or gels are much *too high* for most women, since this concentration means 10 mg/gram or 20 mg/gram of cream per day. A 1 percent cream concentration translates to an *oral* dose of somewhere between 25 to 100 mg a day (double that for a 2 percent cream). The actual conversion from gel/cream to oral is affected by type of testosterone being used and type of base. These are doses for *men;* you certainly wouldn't be taking this much oral testosterone! A more appropriate range of cream concentration for women would be 0.25 mg/gm (0.025 percent) to 1.0 mg/gm (0.1 percent, or one tenth of 1 percent) testosterone.

On average, I find that oral doses of 1 mg to 4 mg a day of natural micronized testosterone appear to work well for most women. These doses are lower than what has been used in the past for women, and are based on the physiologically natural range of testosterone production in women. When using a more appropriate *woman's* dose, we usually do not see the unwanted side effects associated with testosterone. I decide about dose increases based on how women tell me they feel, and what we are achieving in their serum levels. I generally do a serum testosterone level in the morning, twenty-four hours after the last dose, which shows whether the dose is giving levels that are too high for too long. If I want to know a peak level of testosterone, I check this about four to six hours after a dose to see if the dose is enough. In addition, I monitor fasting cholesterol and glucose to ensure that they remain in the desirable range after testosterone is added.

If you decide to take testosterone, remember that each woman's body is different. Trust *your* body wisdom, and what *you know* about how you feel. I prepared a table in chapter 7 that summarizes the benefits of adding testosterone, and I have also given you some pointers on what to look for to indicate too much or too little testosterone, or DHEA. Ask your doctor to take your blood level and work with you to adjust your dose to one that feels good for you. You and your physician need to be effective partners in the process of *maximizing* your benefits from hormone therapy and minimizing any undesirable side effects.

SUMMARY

We already have clear evidence of the important role that testosterone plays in boosting sexual vitality, improving muscle tone and strength, increasing bone density, and improving your overall well-being. Future research may lead to some interesting information about testosterone benefits for increasing metabolic rate and improving cognitive function, including memory. Now that we see all the roles testosterone plays in our health as both men and women get older, you can see why I have encouraged you to include it in your hormone-balancing program to restore your "hormone power."

TESTOSTERONE PRODUCTS

Micronized Testosterone ("Natural" or Bioidentical)
(Recommended)

No FDA-approved product for women yet; available from compounding pharmacies as USP testosterone, which can then be made into tablets, capsules, creams, gels, and injectables in whatever dose is needed.

Synthetic Testosterone-Estrogen Combined Products
(Not recommended for women with weight problems)

Estratest: regular strength oral tablet
    esterified estrogen   1.25 mg
    methyl testosterone   2.5 mg

Estratest HS: half-strength oral tablet
    esterified estrogens   0.625 mg
    methyl testosterone   1.25 mg

Depo-Testadiol:
    estradiol cypionate   2 mg (injectable)
    testosterone cypionate   50 mg

© 2001 by Elizabeth Lee Vliet, M.D.

BIRTH CONTROL PILLS: HORMONE OPTIONS TO EASE THE TURBULENCE OF PERIMENOPAUSE

Newer low-dose oral contraceptives (OCs), or birth control pills, are an excellent hormone-balancing option for premenopausal women who are still menstruating but beginning to have either health risks like bone loss or bothersome symptoms such as worsening PMS, hormonally triggered migraines, hot flashes, or fragmented sleep. "The pill" has been found to be not only *safe* for perimenopausal women, but to actually provide a number of important health benefits.

A June 1999 article in *OB Gyn News* had the following headline: "Prescribe OCs Until Age 52, Expert Advises." Dr. Patricia J. Sulak of the Scott and White Clinic in Temple, Texas, said, "OCs are one of the most important preventive health measures in all of medicine. There's no medicine that offers reproductive-age women more benefits; there's nothing out there that even touches OCs." Dr. Sulak went on to say that, "Women who don't stay on the pill have heavy periods and irregular periods, premenstrual syndrome, functional ovarian cysts, and they get endometriosis and fibroids. If they start the pill and stay on it except when they want to become pregnant and when breastfeeding, they don't have those problems. . . . The pill was really made for women over 35 . . . once you get over 35 your ovaries start acting up; 90 percent of women will develop irregular bleeding before they get to menopause."

Studies from several countries published in the mid-1990s showed a significant protective effect on bone density in women who used the OCs during perimenopause. Birth control pills help prevent osteoporosis in addition to providing a marked reduction in risk of both uterine and ovarian cancers. If you use an oral contraceptive in your premenopausal years, you typically do not experience the hot flashes and other symptoms that mark the endocrine transition to actual menopause. In addition, many women may not ovulate regularly in the decade before menopause, but the very erratic nature of ovulation means that you still need, and may want, contraception. I had one woman, age fifty-one, whose hormone profile confirmed that she had ovulated during her menstrual cycle, and she said (in a tone of shock and disbelief), "You mean I could still get *pregnant*? I thought I stopped ovulating a long time ago. The last thing I need in my life right now is a baby!"

Natural versus Synthetic

Because they are used to suppress the ovaries for contraception, all of the birth control pills in this country are made of synthetic estrogen (usually ethinyl estradiol) and one of several types of synthetic progestins. The natural progesterone and estradiol that we use for menopausal women to restore optimal hormone levels are not potent enough to reliably suppress ovulation and provide contraceptive effects. The synthetic hormones in birth control pills have gotten a bad reputation, but this is not always deserved. There are many medical situations, beyond need for contraception, in which these synthetic hormones can do a world of good, and prevent serious health problems from getting worse—such as endometriosis, fibroids, heavy bleeding, ovarian cysts, PCOS, severe PMS, menstrually triggered migraines, severe anemia, recurrent breast cysts—just to name some key ones.

So don't throw the baby out with the bathwater. Give some consideration to the possibility that birth control pills can help you at this time of life. The trick is to find one with the right balance of estrogen and progestin so it doesn't make headaches, low libido, depression, or weight gain worse.

Which Pills Should You Use to Avoid Making Weight Gain Worse?

BCP that are high in progestin (greater than 0.5 mg norethindrone or equivalent) and very low in estrogen (less than 30 mcg ethinyl estradiol) are more likely to cause increased appetite and weight gain. Pills with a better balance of ethinyl estradiol (30 to 35 mcg) to the progestin typically cause less appetite stimulation and weight gain. I have listed some of these above in the progestin discussion, but three good ones are Ovcon 35, Modicon, and Ortho-Cyclen.

Two other birth control pills, Yasmin and Diane 35, both contain the optimal amount of estrogen with a progestin that actually is an "antiandrogen." This means these two pills are especially good for women with acne and middle-body weight gain. Diane 35 is not available in the United States but has been a very successful birth control pill for about twenty years in Canada, Mexico, Europe, Australia, and New Zealand. It has been especially helpful for women with PCOS, many of whom have gone to overseas sources for this medication. Yasmin is similar to Diane 35 and is newly available in the United States, so this may be an effective option for women who have gained weight with the high progestin content of other birth control pills. Don't give up just because you had problems with one birth control pill—small changes in the chemical makeup can make huge differences in the types of side effects that occur.

CHANGING FROM BIRTH CONTROL PILLS TO MENOPAUSE HORMONE APPROACHES

How do you decide when to change over to the usual postmenopausal hormone options? Why is it even necessary to make a change to another hormone regimen if the oral contraceptives are working well? The second question is simpler to address: It is important to make the change because even the low-dose oral contraceptives contain more estrogen and progestin than is generally needed for postmenopausal use. Conversely, keep in mind that doses of hormones for menopause are not enough to provide contraception for the premenopausal women who still ovulate and could become pregnant. After menopause, since your follicles have been depleted and you no longer ovulate, contraception is no longer an issue; you can use the bioidentical human hormones that are more "natural" and have even fewer side effects than the low-dose birth control pills.

Your transition to a postmenopausal hormone plan is best done with the assistance of a knowledgeable health professional to help prevent any unwanted effects from stopping oral contraceptives abruptly or from differences in potency between birth control pills and the natural hormones.

Chapter 14

BALANCING YOUR
THYROID, ADRENAL, AND INSULIN HORMONES FOR WEIGHT LOSS

RESTORING OPTIMAL THYROID BALANCE: TREATMENT APPROACHES

Types of Medicines

Now you must be ready to ask, "What thyroid medication is best if I need to take it?" This is an important issue, particularly in women with weight problems. I hear from my patients that there is lots of debate on the Internet about this one! Is it better to take synthetic pure T4 (Synthroid, Levoxyl, and generics) or a mixed, animal-derived T4-T3 blend (such as Armour thyroid)?

"Natural" versus "synthetic." The "natural" buzzword has also hit the thyroid hormone therapy arena as well as the menopause field. Remember, *natural* can mean "bioidentical," or it can mean that the substance comes from a biological source and is chemically different from the molecule made by your body. *Synthetic* can simply mean "made in a laboratory" to be identical to what your body makes, or it can also mean "chemically new" and unlike that which your body makes. It is crucial for you to know the difference and not get caught up in the marketing ploys.

When scientists had identified the exact molecular makeup of T4, they were able to create, or "synthesize," the bioidentical molecule of T4 in the laboratory. This led to the ability to make standardized commercial preparations of the T4 thyroid hormone that gave reliable results from batch to batch. Our commercial, pharmaceutical-grade thyroid products today (the brands Unithroid, Synthroid, Levoxyl, along with generics made by different manufacturers) are these bioidentical compounds even though they are made in a laboratory. These are "natural" for your body because they are identical to the T4 thyroid hormone made by your own thyroid gland. For most people, the T4 in these products will be converted by the thyroid gland and body tissues to adequate amounts of T3. For those in whom this conversion may not be taking place, we can restore natural, bioidentical T3 several ways, as I describe shortly.

Some people refer to "natural" thyroid, however, as the brand Armour thyroid, a blend of T4 and T3. It is called "natural" because it is derived from dessicated (dried) animal thyroid tissue. But in truth, this animal-derived blend of T3 and T4 is not the natural ratio found in the human body, so this product often provides more T3 than you need and not enough T4. Since it is a fixed-dose combination per grain of Armour thyroid, it means that it cannot be individually fine-tuned for your body needs the way T4 and T3 can be if used separately. My approach is to get the best balance for your body of each one, not use a fixed ratio natural to a pig or cow that doesn't reflect what you need.

I have two additional concerns about Armour thyroid, since it is animal derived. One is the rising concern about prion contaminants (viral-type particles) in livestock that can lead to lethal brain diseases. While the meat supply in the United States is considered safe, we don't always know the true source of animal tissue used for some of these products. I think this is a risk that you simply don't need to take when we have bioidentical thyroid hormone products that are not derived from animal tissue.

In addition, animal-derived hormones have the potential to be antigenic in humans, whether we are talking about thyroid, insulin, or ovarian hormones, and whether they come from cows, pigs, or horses. Antigenic means they can cause our bodies to form antibodies to the hormones and to our own endocrine glands. This was one of the early problems recognized decades ago with the animal-derived insulin given to diabetics, and also with the allergies to horse-serum when this was used as a base for many medicines in the past. Most of these problems have been resolved with the development of synthetic human insulin and medicines not given in a horse serum base. Similar problems occurred with animal-derived thyroid products when they were all we had and therefore used more widely.

Synthroid, Levoxyl, Unithroid and the generic brands of levothyroxine (T4) do not have any animal residue and therefore do not cause the problems of stimulating antibody production. I have seen too many women develop high levels of both types of thyroid antibodies when they take animal-derived thyroid products long term, so I prefer not to use Armour thyroid for this reason. This is an especially significant problem for women with weight difficulties, in whom we need to have optimal thyroid effects on metabolic pathways and muscle tissue, as well as avoid triggering antibodies that "block" effective function of the thyroid gland and thyroid hormones.

One of the reasons some practitioners recommend Armour thyroid is that it contains T3 as well as T4. This is not really a valid reason to use the animal-derived product today, as I explained above. We have better options available to provide T3 if you need this hormone in addition to T4. For over fifteen years, I have used a pure, hypoallergenic, sustained-release form of T3 compounded by Belmar Pharmacy in Lakewood, Colorado, to help those people who don't appear to properly convert T4 to T3 and have low T3 levels even on the right amount of T4. Cytomel is a commercial T3 product that has been in use in the United States for several decades. It can be effective, but it has a very short duration of effect, which means some people experience too much T3 stimulation soon after taking it, and then feel a "crash" when it wears off. I used Cytomel in the past when I didn't have access to a longer-lasting preparation, but my patients often didn't like the "rise and fall" feeling they had with it.

I use the compounded sustained-release T3 from Belmar instead of the commercial ones primarily for the following reasons: it isn't animal derived and doesn't trigger antibody formation; I can get it made in a time-release preparation to give desired effects over the course of the day; I can get doses made up to be as low or as high as a particular woman needs, rather than being limited to the few commercial strengths available; and I can individualize the doses of both T4 and T3 to give the right balance, since they aren't "fixed" in one tablet.

Safe Ways to Start

Too much thyroid too fast will commonly cause rapid heartbeat, palpitations, headaches, anxiousness, irritability, or insomnia. These symptoms also are occurring in women whose estradiol is too low, so if thyroid is added too quickly before estradiol is optimal, it can feel a little like someone just poured gasoline on your fire! Heart-racing-mind-racing-not-sleeping-head-pounding is no fun way to feel. You can see that it is important to start with a low dose and gradually increase it to avoid these problems.

I typically start a woman on one of the T4 products, at half of the lowest commercial dose, for about two weeks. I encourage her to observe how she feels, and then we work together to increase gradually based on her brain-body responses, as well as how her TSH is responding. My goal is to have a TSH in the range of 0.5 to 2.0. Then, if she still is having symptoms of low thyroid function and the free T3 is still low, I may add T3 starting with a very low dose (5 mcg is a usual dose) and again, increasing very slowly. Sometimes, if it feels to her like 5 mcg is too much at once, we may decide to split the tablet in half, and have her take half in the morning and half at lunchtime. If you take T3 much later than lunchtime, it may cause restless sleep due to overstimulation of the brain pathways.

It becomes a little more complicated when working with the ovarian and thyroid hormones, since they affect each other in a variety of ways. I prefer to stabilize the ovarian hormones with whatever approach a woman prefers, and *then* work with the thyroid balancing—unless the TSH is so high that the hypothyroidism simply must be treated right away. It can be quite a juggling act, and I often find I have to combine our "science" (lab tests) along with a lot of "art" (clinical judgment and listening to the woman) in order to decide what to do.

Thyroid hormone replacement is clearly a complex topic and I can't give you all the "specifics" in this short space. These are the highlights of some crucial issues I think are important for you to address in talking with your physicians, particularly if you have been struggling with stubborn weight gain or problems losing excess weight in spite of exercise and healthy eating. There are a lot of ways to fine-tune and optimize thyroid replacement to help you feel better and be able to be successful with all your other weight-loss strategies.

RESTORING OPTIMAL CORTISOL BALANCE: TREATMENT APPROACHES

A lot of women come to our center for evaluation, and they often have been put on hormone medications to treat "low cortisol" and "low DHEA" without ever having appropriate tests of all their ovarian hormones, or the reliable tests for cortisol and DHEA, or even complete tests of thyroid function. There are serious consequences to taking cortisone (cortisol) or DHEA hormones if these are not really what you need. I described many of these complications in chapters 7 and 9 for you to review if these have slipped your mind (*a common experience for us at "mental pause," yes?*). Especially if you are overweight, make sure that you have *all* of the gold-standard tests done, as I outlined in chapter 11, before you let someone prescribe cortisone (Cortef, and others) or DHEA for you.

What to Do If Cortisol Is Really Low

Adrenal insufficiency (AI), or Addison's disease, is a serious metabolic illness that can cause death if not evaluated and treated properly. If you have a documented low serum cortisol along with electrolyte imbalances and other laboratory findings suggestive of Addison's, or AI, I urge you to see an endocrinologist who has experience with these disorders. You want to make certain that you don't have other hormone imbalances, and there are additional tests that normally should be done to confirm the diagnosis and identify any possible causes. You will want a physician who also has experience in the various medicines that are used to replace the inadequate adrenal production of cortisol, such as hydrocortisone or cortisone acetate, and who is knowledgeable about side effects and problems that can occur.

It can be dangerous to take over-the-counter "adrenal support" supplements, or "adrenal glandulars," if you have had only saliva tests or "kinesiology" testing to check for low cortisol and adrenal insufficiency. I have seen many women over the years who have been told that they have "adrenal exhaustion" based on these unreliable tests, but then when serum cortisol assays were done at the proper times of day, they actually had *high* cortisol reflecting the stress response from other hormone imbalances. High cortisol has many adverse effects on your body (see chapter 9), especially to cause more weight gain. So you certainly don't want to take it unless you really need it.

Furthermore, adrenal glandulars sold in health food stores are animal derived, with the same potential problems I described above. Taking "adrenal support" products may actually suppress your own adrenal hormones further, or could add to the problem of *high* cortisol, making you fatter.

What to Do If Cortisol Is High

Adrenal or pituitary *disease* causing high cortisol is actually less common than a number of more mundane causes that include everything from life stress to loss of optimal estradiol, other illnesses, infections, chronic pain, surgeries, loss of optimal thyroid function, biological depression, high-progestin birth control pills, medications such as decongestants and steroids used to treat asthma and arthritis, to name some of the most common ones.

These problems will be treated best by addressing the underlying cause, such as changing medications or improving your "stress relief" strategies. Cortisol will usually return to normal when these other problems have been corrected. We typically find that if the cortisol is elevated because of thyroid disorders or menopausal loss of estradiol, then the cortisol will come back to normal once we have restored estradiol and/or thyroid balance. But if it doesn't, then we explore further medical evaluation and treatment options.

If cortisol is high due to a suspected adrenal disease such as Cushing's syndrome, or to a pituitary disorder, your physician will likely suggest further testing such as a DST, described in chapter 9. If the DST shows morning or afternoon cortisol higher than 5 µg/dl the day after you take 1 mg of dexamethaone, then I recommend you have a thorough evaluation for Cushing's disease. This will involve further tests, such as serum ACTH, twenty-four-hour urine for urinary free cortisol, and a CRH test as well as possible MRI of the pituitary if indicated. Once a specific adrenal or pituitary cause is identified, treatment can then be individualized and directed to that cause.

RESTORING OPTIMAL INSULIN BALANCE: TREATMENT APPROACHES

Nutrition First: Your Hormone Power Plan MAP

There is no way around this point: Sound meal plan balance, as I describe in chapters 15 and 16, along with eating smaller meals throughout the day provide the *cornerstone* of your Meal Action Plan, or the "MAP" to your destination of lower insulin levels and improved insulin sensitivity. You simply can't get there without this step. I have described the MAP in detail in later chapters, so I won't say any more about it right now.

Second Step: Step Out and Exercise

Low-to-moderate-intensity exercise, such as walking, acts as an "invisible insulin" that serves to facilitate delivery of glucose to the muscles and lower the tendency to have *high* glucose levels in the bloodstream. This in turn decreases the insulin outpouring from your pancreas in response to all that glucose floating around. Simple brisk walking is one of the best things you can do for yourself on many mind-body levels, but it is an absolutely critical component to reduce the deadly consequences of insulin resistance. Even if you just walk for five to ten minutes a few times a day to start out, you will see some improvements in your glucose tolerance and your energy level. Once again, you can't get to your health destination without adding more physical activity—so stay tuned and I'll tell you in chapter 18 how to get started.

Optimizing Ovarian Hormones

Many doctors prefer to recommend insulin-sensitizing medications next, but I think this overlooks the key role of the ovarian hormones in improving your insulin response, as I have already described in earlier chapters. So, I really think the next important step to reducing insulin resistance is getting your estradiol, progesterone, testosterone, and DHEA back into a healthy, optimal balance as I have already described. If you are overweight, have glucose intolerance or insulin resistance, or have actual diabetes, then I recommend you focus on using the natural bioidentical hormone preparations I describe in chapter 13.

If you are dealing with insulin excess, here are a few key points to refresh your memory. The patch form of estradiol gives the best results to improve insulin sensitivity, based on many well-done international studies published in the last few years. If you have a uterus and need to prevent endometrial hyperplasia, a nonoral natural progesterone such as Crinone will cause fewer adverse effects on blood sugar swings and insulin production.

Try to avoid using hormone preparations that can make glucose intolerance and insulin resistance worse. This includes mixed estrogens (for example Premarin, Estratab/Estratest, Cenestin), synthetic progestins (Provera, MPA), and progestin-dominant combination products such as Prempro, Premphase, CombiPatch, Femhrt. Don't use over-the-counter progesterone ("wild yam") creams or high progestin birth control pills (for example, Loestrin, Alesse, Mircette) if you are overweight, insulin resistant, or diabetic. If you have further questions about these key points, review chapter 13.

Consider Insulin-Sensitizing Medicines

Glucophage (metformin), Avandia (rosiglitazone), Actos (pioglitazone), are several medicines available today that work to improve your insulin sensitivity and reduce the health risks that go with excess insulin. We have used these quite successfully at *HER Place* for many midlife women ("Syndrome Xers") and our younger PCOS patients who have the metabolic abnormalities I have been describing. While we emphasize the strategies I just listed above, there are many women who also need these medicines to get the insulin resistance under control and be successful with weight-loss efforts. In turn, being able to lose weight helps decrease many of the risk factors for both diabetes and heart disease.

Because the multiple health risks of PCOS and Syndrome X are so severe, I think there are clearly times when these medicines are necessary, even though we need to monitor their use carefully to avoid side effects. Our approach is to start with lower-than-usual doses, and increase very gradually. This way, bothersome side effects have been relatively uncommon. "Start low, and go slow" is our motto for just about all the medication approaches we are using.

SUMMARY

The good news is that there are a lot of very effective medication options today to help you reach your goal of improved thyroid, cortisol, and insulin balance. Another plus: The more you can achieve stable glucose, insulin, and cortisol levels with your meal plan, exercise, healthy hormonal balance, and when appropriate, other medication options such as metformin, the less you will need antidepressant or antianxiety medicines to improve mood, decrease anxiety, and improve your energy and sleep. This means you have fewer side effect risks and lower medication costs. So, take charge, use these suggestions, and get started on reclaiming your "hormone power" and your health!

Chapter 15

BALANCING
PROTEIN, FAT AND CARBS
TO REV UP YOUR ENGINES

I have been fit and I have been fat. I have tried almost every diet that came out. I know how hard it can be to overcome a weight problem. I struggle with it, just as you do.

The Meal Action Plan (MAP) I have created for this book and describe in chapter 16 draws from many experiences: my professional education and review of the current medical studies on obesity and metabolism, my study of the complex hormone interactions in a woman's body and how these affect weight gain, my study of nutrition since I was a teenager, and my life experience as a woman struggling with excess weight since childhood.

I can tell you with certainty that the balance in what you eat at each meal and snack makes a huge difference in such critical aspects as our daily energy level, memory, mood stability, concentration and ability to focus, how well we sleep . . . along with the obvious effects on body weight and body fat composition. My "hormone power" MAP is designed to provide a balance of protein, fat, and carbohydrates that will work *with* your midlife fat hormones, not against them, and make it easier to lose excess fat.

FOOD: YOUR "FUEL" FOR ENERGY, POWER, AND ZEST

Let's take a closer look at these food types and what they do. Proteins, fat, and carbohydrates are called our *macronutrients* because we need them in larger quantities for our bodies' daily energy, growth, and repair to take place. Vitamins and minerals, discussed in the next chapter, are called *micronutrients* because they are needed in such small quantities each day.

As you read about the macronutrients, keep in mind that glucose is the basic molecule that becomes the body's primary fuel. Glucose, which can be made from carbohydrates, protein, or fat, combines with oxygen in the cells and is "burned" to generate the energy to run the cells of our body. To the body, glucose is like gasoline for your car. Neither your car nor your body can run without adequate fuel to "burn" with oxygen to make energy.

MACRONUTRIENTS

Carbohydrates

Carbohydrates are the body's primary "quick-start" fuel and are quickly converted into glucose. In fact, when you eat a cracker, the starch is already being converted to sugar in your mouth while you chew it. Based on how quickly they are converted to glucose, carbohydrates are classified as *simple* (very rapid conversion to glucose, with a corresponding rapid rise in insulin production) or *complex* (slower rate of conversion to glucose, less stimulation of insulin release). Complex carbohydrates include *whole* grains, vegetables, and fruits; they are also a good source of dietary fiber: soluble fiber (such as pectin) and insoluble fiber (cellulose, like the "strings" in celery). Simple carbohydrates include "starches" like breads, potatoes, pasta, simple cereals; fruit juices, sweets, alcohol, soft drinks; and some high-sugar fruits like bananas.

In contrast, proteins and fats are more slowly metabolized to glucose and help to stabilize our energy needs over several hours after a meal. The brain needs steady glucose, so our food intake needs to be balanced and timed in such a way that the brain receives a steady supply of this important nutrient. Look at figure 15.2 to see how you can achieve this balance and timing for optimal results. If you are getting too little food, or go too long between meals, it leaves you feeling "foggy" because your brain isn't getting a steady supply of the most efficient fuel it needs to function optimally.

When I was in my twenties, women's magazines talked about cutting out the "fattening" carbohydrates. A decade or so later, we heard "carbs are good, it's the excess fat we put on them that is bad." This idea focused on the belief that excess fat on your body came from the excess fat on your plate: all the sour cream, butter, oils, and mayonnaise that were added to foods like baked potatoes or pasta or salads. While there was some truth to this, the excess weight gain has more to do with the higher calorie consumption (plain potato, 100 calories; potato with sour cream, bacon bits, and butter, 500 to 600 calories) than the type of food consumed.

Now we hear a lot about carbs being "bad." So what's the real scoop? Should you follow the low-to-no-carb school, or the high-carb/low-fat school? How do you know who or what to believe with all the conflicting claims? Part of the answer depends on your body size and build. If you are slender and already at your ideal body weight and composition, you probably don't really have to worry too much about which way you go—stay with what is working for you.

However, if you are one of the millions of women who find themselves losing their waist at midlife it becomes crucial for you to really concentrate on the right type and amount of carbohydrates in your overall meal plan. Continued high intake of carbs—especially the simple carbs such as breads, pastas, fruit juices, alcohol, and sweets—will overstimulate production of the fat-storing hormone, insulin, leading to increasing body fat.

If you have a thyroid disorder and you restrict your carbohydrates too much, you will end up sending "starvation" signals to the brain, which in turn sends signals to the thyroid gland to push more of your active thyroid hormone, T3, into the protein-bound form that makes it inactive. Less free T3 is a protective response to slow down your metabolism and preserve your body's fuel reserves (fat) if you were *really* starving. But if you are a midlife woman who is just trying to lose excess body fat, the *last* thing you want to do is slow down your metabolism!

I find that most diet books don't even mention this effect on the thyroid balance, and it is a critical point for women to understand since it is one reason that diets such as the Atkins Diet that overly restrict carbohydrates don't work as well long term for women, who have a much higher rate of subtle thyroid disorders. Having *some* carbohydrates in your overall diet is important, but notice I said the right *type* and right *amount.* Let's look at what that would be.

For most midlife women, *carbohydrates should make up only 35 to 40 percent* of your daily food intake. Carbohydrates provide four calories of energy per gram (half as calorie dense as fat), but they actually require the body to expend more energy to utilize them as a fuel source. The best source of carbohydrates at this stage of life are complex carbohydrates—whole grains, whole fruits, and whole vegetables. Choosing complex carbohydrates over simple carbs will provide slower rise in blood sugar, less of an "insulin surge," a lower peak blood sugar, a slower fall in your blood sugar, more gradual absorption of the other nutrients, more fiber, and a healthy feeling of fullness so you won't have the desire to overeat. Complex carbs don't tend to overstimulate insulin production, which is helpful because as we get older and fatter, our cells don't respond to insulin as well and more of our calories are turned into fat. It is essential to have a balance of proteins and fats at each meal to prevent the "blood sugar swings" from carbs alone, and to provide a feeling of fullness (satiety) over more hours, and sustain energy levels longer.

Proteins

Protein sources in the diet are broken down to provide the 28 amino acids that serve as the basic building blocks for the body to then make its own proteins for our growth, to repair body tissues, and to fight disease. Proteins are also metabolized to glucose to provide our daily fuel for energy, growth, and repair. Some amino acids also serve as building blocks for neurotransmitters and pain-relieving chemicals such as endorphins and enkephalins.

Proteins also provide 4 calories per gram as energy for the body. The conversion of proteins to glucose is slower than making glucose from carbohydrates, so proteins in our meals serve to keep blood sugar (glucose) levels steady over three to four hours, compared to the one to two hours from carbohydrates. This is why a healthy balance of protein—about 35 percent of your food intake—is important at every meal. Both protein and carbohydrates are crucial elements of your "eating well" plan to maintain energy, concentration, memory, stable mood, and a normal metabolic rate throughout the day.

Amino acids are classified into two categories: those the body can make and do not have to be included in the diet (about 80 percent), called *nonessential* amino acids, and those amino acids the body cannot make itself and must get in the diet (20 percent), called, *essential* amino acids. The nine essential amino acids are leucine, isoleucine, lysine, tryptophan, methionine, valine, histidine, threonine, and phenylalanine. These essential amino acids have specific jobs ranging from pain relief to helping the cells use oxygen more efficiently

Complete proteins are those foods from animal sources that contain all nine essential amino acids, such as meat, fish, chicken, eggs, and cheese. Since these protein foods also contain higher amounts of fat, select ones that are lower in fat: lean meats, low-fat cheeses, poultry without the skin, egg whites in place of a whole egg, etc. If you do not eat animal protein, you need to combine plant-derived proteins in such as way that you get complete proteins, since plant sources lack one or more of the nine essential amino acids. For example, beans combined with rice make a complete protein source, but keep in mind, this combination also provides a great deal of starch at one time, which tends to overstimulate insulin release.

Fats

Fats are made up of chains of many units of fatty acids hooked together. During digestion, these links are broken to release the separate fatty acids into the bloodstream. Fatty acids are ultimately digested to glucose, but it takes the body a long time to do this step. The complex digestion pathways for fats and fatty acids give a very slow rise in glucose levels following a meal, and a very slow fall in glucose an hour later. In this way, fats help provide satiety, or a sense of fullness, over several hours. We don't get hungry as quickly after eating a meal with the proper amount of fat to keep glucose levels steady longer.

Fats are further classified into saturated (animal fat), monounsaturated, and polyunsaturated (derived from vegetable sources). The right balance of fat is crucial to help absorb fat-soluble vitamins and to provide the essential fatty acids that are used to make a variety of hormones—including estrogen, progesterone, and testosterone produced by the ovaries. If you cut back on fat in your diet too much, it will cause a premature decrease in production of your ovarian hormones, leading to early menopausal-type symptoms. A new finding from the Nurses Health Study, published in *Circulation* in February 2001, showed that women with extremely low fat intake (less than 20 grams per day) were about *twice* as likely to have suffered a particular type of stroke called an *intraparenchymal hemorrhage*. This type of stroke is less common than those due to blockage of blood vessels—called ischemic stroke. The increased risk of intraparenchymal hemorrhagic stroke was seen primarily in women with high blood pressure, which is common in overweight women. It may be that extremely low fat diets plus high blood pressure leads to structural weaknesses of blood vessels in the brain, which causes them to rupture.

For these reasons, I don't think overly low fat diets are desirable for women, but neither am I giving you license here to throw away all concerns about eating fat, particularly the unhealthy ones. "Trans" fats, such as the partially hydrogenated margarines and spreads popular today, are especially unhealthy for women with our midlife hormone changes that add to our diabetes and heart disease risk.

Fats have nine calories per gram and are therefore the most concentrated energy source for our bodies, which means we need only small quantities each day. Most people don't realize that all fats (whether vegetable oils, olive oil, butter, margarine, or lard) have *twice* as many calories per gram as carbohydrates and protein (9 cal/gm versus 4 cal/gm for protein and carbs). While olive oil is a "better" fat than, say, butter, because it is unsaturated, both olive oil and butter have the identical number of calories per gram or per serving. So don't go dipping your bread into the olive oil dish!

Although fat is the most calorie-dense type of food we eat, foods that are high in fat don't take up space in the intestinal tract like high-fiber foods do, so we often don't realize how much fat (and calories) we have eaten. It is dramatic how much more dietary fat Americans eat now than was true at the turn of the century: 45 percent now versus 28 percent to 30 percent in 1900. Diets that are too high in fat and are not balanced with proper amounts of carbohydrates and proteins slow down the gastrointestinal tract motility, contributing to more constipation, distention of the tummy, and feeling generally fat and miserable, especially the second half of the menstrual cycle.

My MAP for midlife women recommends no more than 30 percent

dietary fat, a level consistent with the ADA and American Heart Association (AHA) diets. I encourage you to focus on the unsaturated, plant-derived oils and fats for your limited added fats, and the rest of your fat each day will be in the protein sources. This approach will keep you pretty well on target with the 25 to 30 percent percent fat goal. My sample meals plans in chapter 16 are designed to carry out this recommendation.

A primary source of unwanted dietary fat for most Americans is the hidden fats, especially the "trans" fats, such as partially hydrogenated fats in soft margarine and in processed foods. These hidden calories often sabotage our best weight-loss efforts. Watch the food labels to help you detect these hidden fats. They are everywhere: cereals, salad dressings, prepared soups, frozen meals, cream-based pasta sauces, donuts and cookies, non-dairy creamers for coffee, commercial pizzas dripping with cheese and pepperoni, French fries, and those big yummy-looking commercial "bran" muffins. There's probably a day's worth of sugar and fat in each one and certainly not much bran. It helps to learn where the fats are hidden in various foods and gradually cut back every day to reach the level I have recommended in this meal plan. There are now several good paperback guides to fat content available. Use these to identify items that contain more fat than is desirable, and then you can pick lower-fat choices

One gimmick to watch for is the *low-fat* and *fat-free* food items now filling the shelves. The fat has been removed but it has been replaced by simple sugars that give excess calories with little nutritional value. All this sugar plays havoc with blood sugar levels and insulin surges, which makes you store more fat and also causes fluctuations in your energy levels. Plus, when that box of cookies is labeled "fat free," we feel it is okay to eat more! Be honest—have you ever eaten the whole box in one sitting? While it may be fat free, it certainly isn't calorie free, and it is a sure way to increase insulin production and make more body fat.

Figure 15.1 shows how these groups of foods affect the rate of rise in your blood sugar, how high it goes, and how rapidly it falls. Then in Figure 15.2, I show you how to blend the three food groups of your MAP for better stability in your glucose and insulin over the day. Use this food MAP as you work with the meal plans in the next chapter, and you'll be on your way to reducing your "middle spread and mental pause." You will also feel more energetic!

Figure 15.1
BLOOD SUGAR (GLUCOSE) CHANGES WITH VARIOUS FOODS

FOOD TYPE	BLOOD SUGAR CHANGES: PEAKS/FALLS	COMMENTS
Simple Carbohydrates (sweets, alcohol, rice, potatoes, white flour pasta/bread and crackers, soft drinks, candy, desserts, fruit juices, and some high-sugar fruits such as bananas)	Peak (10–25 minutes) 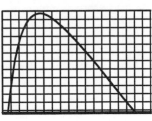 Baseline normal blood sugar level (70–100 mg/dl)	*Simple carbohydrates and sugars* cause a rapid rise, followed by a sharp fall in blood sugar (i.e., a blood sugar "swing"). This fast rise in glucose causes a rapid, high burst of insulin release from the pancreas to help the glucose move from the blood *into* cells to be used as fuel, or stored as fat.
Complex Carbohydrates (C) (whole fruit, vegetables, beans, starches, whole grains)	Peak (1½–2½ hours) 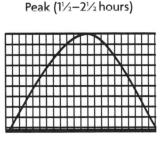 Baseline glucose	*Complex carbohydrates (C)* cause a slower rise and more gradual fall in blood sugar, and a slower release of insulin that means less will be stored as fat and more will be used as fuel. The insulin released is still higher than with proteins or fats.

© 1985, revised 1995–2001 by Elizabeth Lee Vliet, M.D.

Figure 15.1 (continued)
BLOOD SUGAR (GLUCOSE)
CHANGES WITH VARIOUS FOODS

FOOD TYPE	**BLOOD SUGAR CHANGES: PEAKS/FALLS**	**COMMENTS**
Proteins (P) (meat, cheese, fish, poultry, milk, eggs, tofu, tem- peh, etc.)	Peak (2–4 hours) 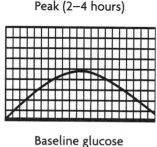 Baseline glucose	*Proteins (P)* are more complex to digest, result- ing in a much slower rise and fall in blood sugar. Total rise in glucose is not as high as with carbohy- drates. Protein foods keep glucose levels more even, and cause less rise in insulin.
Fats (F) (butter, mar- garine, lard, olive oil, mayonnaise, vegetable oils, salad dressings)	Peak (3–6 hours) 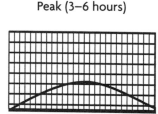 Baseline glucose	*Fats (F)* take much longer to digest (approximately 8 to 12 hours), and cause a lower, slower rise in glucose. Fats keep blood sugar steady longer and don't cause an insulin "surge."

Figure 15.2
BALANCING YOUR P-F-C FOOD MAP

Dr. Vliet's
Your Hormone
Power Meal Plan → Protein 35%
Fat 30%
Carbohydrate 35%

For effective fat loss, your
meal action plan for each
meal and snack should be:

P-F-C = 35%-30%-35%

Example:
turkey + mayo+whole
grain bread+lettuce+fruit

This combination of protein, fat, and complex carbohydrates (P-F-C) helps keep your blood sugar steady throughout the day. This balance also minimizes the *excess release* of insulin that makes it harder for you to lose excess body fat.

In the food MAP below, notice that snacks, with the same ratio of foods, are timed to cause a *beginning rise* in glucose again as the level is *falling* from the previous meal. This meal-snack spacing sustains your energy level more consistently over the day, improves your memory and concentration, improves stability in your mood, as well as revs up your *metabolic rate,* and leads to *more effective "burning" (loss) of body fat for fuel* rather than storing fat.

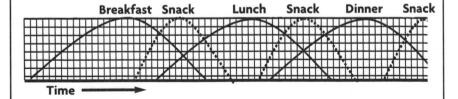

Breakfast Snack   Lunch   Snack   Dinner   Snack

Time ━━━━▶

© 1985, revised 1995–2001 by Elizabeth Lee Vliet, M.D.

BALANCING YOUR FOOD INTAKE

Remember, low-fat, high-carbohydrate diets make you fatter by causing more swings in blood glucose and stimulating more insulin production by the pancreas. More insulin production in turn tends to drop the blood glucose even lower, and faster, as well as push the body toward storing more fat. More body fat then makes more insulin resistance, so it is another of those terrible vicious cycles.

To *avoid overstimulating insulin production* and have optimal, steady glucose stability through the day, follow this P-F-C MAP. While the exact optimal balance may vary slightly from one woman to another, this range helps lower excess insulin levels, thereby preventing insulin-glucose imbalances that make you store more food as fat instead of being burned for energy.

YOUR P-F-C MAP

Protein	35%	(range 30 to 35 percent)
Fat	30%	(range 25 to 30 percent)
Carbohydrates	35%	(range 35 to 40 percent)

To further *decrease* overstimulation of insulin with meals, I also recommend that you focus more on foods that are not as quickly converted to glucose. These are called *low glycemic index* foods because they give a less rapid rise in blood glucose and more stable levels over time. *High glycemic index* foods are those that are quickly converted to glucose, causing a rapid rise in blood sugar and a surge of insulin release. Examples include bananas, fruit juices, alcohol, candy, cookies, crackers, white flour pasta and breads, and sweets, to name a few. There are helpful paperback pocket guides available that list many different foods by glycemic index.

WATER AND OXYGEN: THE OFTEN FORGOTTEN, ESSENTIAL ELEMENTS

Healthy water intake and oxygen delivery to your cells are two elements that are vital to good health and to effective weight loss. They are available and free, yet most people forget about them!

Water

Water provides the fluid that bathes the outside of our cells and maintains the environment inside the cells that allows everything to work properly to sustain life. One of the most common nutritional "deficiencies" is not getting enough water to drink each day. Chronic mild dehydration causes problems with all of the cellular machinery, including those pathways that help you lose weight as well as those involved in building healthy muscle and connective tissue. Diet-induced "brain fog" is made markedly worse if you are mildly dehydrated and the brain doesn't have the fluid it needs for optimal function. So drink eight to ten 8-ounce glasses a day!

Oxygen

We take breathing for granted, and don't realize that oxygen is one of the essential "nutrients" to sustain life. You can go without water and food for days. Without oxygen, brain death occurs in as little as four minutes! Oxygen is needed to carry out all of the chemical reactions in the body that keep us alive and make our metabolism work properly to burn fat.

Long, slow, deep breaths provide a fresh supply of oxygen and help clear out the excess carbon dioxide that is a byproduct of the body's cellular metabolism. Stress management techniques that utilize diaphramatic breathing and activities such as yoga teach our body how to breathe better for better oxygen exchange.

WHEN YOU EAT IS IMPORTANT, TOO

For women going through those maddening hormonal changes such as with PMS or PCOS or perimenopause, we need better balance in protein, fat, and carbohydrate to maintain steady energy levels and improved brain clarity over our busy days. So you need to pay attention to *when* you eat, as well as *what* you eat.

For example, your blood sugar normally hits the "afternoon slump" between 3:00 to 4:00 P.M., leading to more fuzzy thinking, low energy, and problems concentrating. Then you feel ravenous and tend to overeat to compensate. Planning a balanced P-F-C snack according to my MAP above will help you overcome the slump, maintain mental sharpness, and keep you from eating everything in sight.

You also need to have most of your food intake during the day when you are more active and your metabolic rate is higher. Eating less at night as your metabolism is slowing down to rest will help avoid excess body fat storage at night that sabotages your fat-loss efforts. Your goal should be to consume the majority of your calories, about 60 to 70 percent, before your evening meal at dinnertime.

And remember, plan your exercise one to two hours after eating, when your glucose levels are higher and will sustain your energy needs during exercise. Low-to-moderate-intensity exercise, such as walking, acts as your "invisible insulin" that serves to facilitate delivery of glucose to the muscles and lower the tendency to have *high* glucose levels in the bloodstream. It also decreases the problem of insulin resistance.

And most importantly, *don't skip meals, especially breakfast.* You need the metabolism-boosting effect of food in the morning to get your body engines going. If you skip meals, you typically will have more anxiety, mood, and cognitive changes that are characteristic of the brain effects of marked glucose fluctuations due to hyperinsulinemia, aggravated by falling estradiol and stress, whether you call them "fibro-fog" or the "fuzzies."

I know, you say you don't have time for breakfast. I struggle with eating right myself, and I am not perfect. Like most of you, I have too many things to do and too little time to do them. But, I will tell you this. I am very careful not to skip meals, especially during the workday when I need to be alert and able to function at my best. I make sure to have a good breakfast. If I don't, I really pay the price in terms of "mental pause," depleted energy, feeling irritable, and having more muscle pain. Even if it is something quick and simple, there are ways to get a healthy start to your day. In chapter 16, I have given you some quick solutions to "the breakfast problem." You simply must get in the habit of eating properly to start your day, or you will not be successful in losing excess fat.

HOW MUCH YOU EAT

"How is the way I eat really going to help me lose weight . . . I know all I have to do is cut down the calories, right?" That's not the full picture for women. In fact, if you cut the calories too low, you again give your body a signal that you're in "starvation mode" and your metabolism slows down. Sometimes, as strange as it sounds, you actually have to *increase* your calories to lose weight effectively.

I can hear you now: "No way, I know if I eat more than eight hundred calories a day, I will gain weight." It turns out that is not correct. You do need more calories so that your body will effectively burn fat for fuel. My meal plan in chapter 16 is designed to give you enough calories each day so that your body won't thwart you by holding onto its fat stores. If what you are doing now isn't working, I suggest you try what I recommend and see if it makes a difference. After all, you have to eat. You may as well try eating in a way that just might help you rev up your metabolic engines so you can lose weight more effectively.

Paying Attention to Portion Sizes

America has become the land of plenty: Plenty of overweight people (more than half our population), plenty of sugar (more than 150 pounds per person per year), plenty of fast food (growing at the rate of 7 percent per year in number of fast food restaurants), plenty of eating out (almost 40 percent of our total food dollars are spent now on eating out, double the amount in 1970), and plenty of super-sized portions (in some cases, portion sizes for restaurant meals, snacks, and convenience foods have increased over 100 percent). King-size, super-size, jumbo, super-jumbo portions abound everywhere, and all those extra calories go right to our middle-spread fat padding.

For example, a normal bagel size used to be two to three ounces, or about the size of a hockey puck. Specialty bagel shops today make bagels five to seven ounces, about the size of a softball, which is equivalent to about four slices of bread. Yet people have been sold the idea that because bagels are low fat you can eat as many as you want. The calories mount up and pack pounds onto your waist.

A normal, healthy serving of meat or fish is about three to five ounces (the size of the palm of your hand, not including your fingers), but most restaurants serve portions of twleve, sixteen, even twenty-two or thirty-six ounces for one meal! No wonder we are a nation of obese people. As you can see, even a twelve-ounce portion of meat or fish is too large, making enough for about three or four normal-sized servings. If you want to succeed in losing excess body fat, you really need to work on training your eye for proper portion sizes. The list below summarizes some helpful comparisons to help you get a mind's-eye picture of what size serving of food you should be choosing.

> Computer mouse = one medium baked potato
> One regular-size bar of soap = one 3 oz. serving of meat, chicken, or fish
> Hockey puck = one bagel or one serving of rice, pasta, or grains
> Four dice = 1 oz. serving of hard cheese (1 protein equivalent)
> Tennis ball = 1 serving of fruit
> Golf ball = 1 serving of peanut butter (2 tablespoons)
> Two cassette tapes = 2 servings of bread

ALCOHOL: YOUR WEIGHT LOSS SABOTEUR

Women who drink alcohol on a regular basis often don't realize how this can be a saboteur of your weight-loss efforts. First of all, alcohol provides loads of extra calories, particularly in rum punches and margaritas. These calories are "nutritionally empty." They simply make you fatter without any benefit. Alcohol is also metabolized quickly, causing a rapid rise in blood glucose that, in turn, stimulates more insulin release, adding to the problem of insulin resistance. In addition, regular alcohol intake leads to higher triglycerides, an independent risk factor for heart disease in women. This isn't a pretty picture, is it?

Alcohol is also an independent risk factor for breast cancer. In fact, it is a greater risk factor for breast cancer than anything that has been found with estrogen, yet you don't hear much about the alcohol connection in the popular media. In studies from Italy, researchers found that daily alcohol intake contributed to a twelvefold greater risk of breast cancer compared to the risk in women who did not drink alcohol. When we say an "independent" risk factor for breast cancer, we mean that the increased risk is not due to other confounding variables such as total calories, fat, fiber, and vitamins.

Age at which you begin drinking is an important component of this risk factor: Drinking alcohol before age thirty increases breast cancer risk, regardless of alcohol consumption patterns later in life. The main effect of alcohol on breast cancer risk seems to be in the vulnerable time of breast development during puberty, as we are finding with fat in the diet. Doesn't it just make sense to reduce or eliminate alcohol? It is one factor you can control.

THE PROBLEM WITH SOFT DRINKS

Women tell me that they are cutting out dairy products, especially milk, for fear of the fat. What do they replace milk with? Typically, it's soft drinks, whether regular or sugar- and caffeine-free. Bad choice. All soft drinks contain high levels of phosphates, which attach to the calcium and magnesium ions in the digestive tract and increase the loss of both minerals from the body. Calcium and magnesium then move from the bones to maintain adequate blood levels, which are needed for normal nerve and muscle function. So the more soft drinks you consume, the more calcium and magnesium you lose. Caffeine, as a diuretic, adds to this mineral loss.

Think about it. Low-fat milk has *fewer calories* than a regular soda, and rather than leaching calcium from your bones, skim milk provides both calcium and protein and gives you a healthy between-meal snack that has no fat. I have been drinking skim milk for so long that even 1% milk now tastes too rich.

Regular soft drinks not only leach these minerals from your bones, they are also loaded with sugar. A twelve-ounce non-diet soft drink contains about seven to eight teaspoons of sugar. This becomes a real problem when you drink five or six sugared sodas a day, because you end up with almost half your total daily calories coming from a source without any nutritional value. Plus, you overstimulate the insulin pathways. Even if you drink the sugar-free ones, you are still getting artificial sweeteners whose sweet taste contributes to excess stimulation of insulin that leads to more fat storage.

FOOD AS MEDICINE

Food really is one of our most fundamental medicines for healing. We can't make serotonin in the brain to help lift our moods if we don't take in adequate tryptophan, as one example. We can't make the hormones that run our bodies without fat. We can't make immunoglobulins without enough protein. In this chapter, I have focused on eating for "wellness of being" rather than a "diet." Diets don't work ... for weight loss or for much of anything else. What you really need is a "fat loss and wellness" eating plan to get healthy fuel to all of your body cells and tissues so that you may have better metabolism, balanced energy levels, better quality sleep, fewer mood swings, less pain, better muscle repair, and, ultimately, reduced risk of serious diseases like diabetes.

Gradual changes are key. I don't want you to do anything drastic, because that doesn't work for the long run. Some suggestions to get started are simple ones: If you are not eating enough, start increasing to healthier amounts. If you are overeating, start decreasing the portions gradually. If you are eating junk foods, start letting go of one unhealthy thing each week and replace it with something better for you. Spread your meals and snacks over the whole day to avoid low-energy periods and snack cravings. If you aren't feeling well now, just focus on these few steps. Then slowly incorporate more changes, as you feel ready. See . . . it doesn't have to be so bad.

KEEP A THREE-DAY FOOD DIARY

We have consistently found that when our patients are feeling better and their hormones are back in balance, they are then able and motivated to make additional changes in their eating patterns. You will get there, too. For now, evaluate your eating habits to see if there is room for improvement. Take an honest look at what you eat. Write down every single thing that you put in your mouth for three days. Then compare what you are eating with the meal plan recommendations that follow. Can you find some healthy changes you have already made? Good. Now add to your list three or four new ones, changes you are ready to make *now.*

STRATEGIES FOR FEELING BETTER

My goal is to help you find dietary approaches with meal plans that help you recapture your sense of well-being and "zest." I find that it is frequently difficult to get women to accept that something as "simple" as changing the way they eat can have a profound impact on the way they feel—their mood, energy level, clarity of thinking—*but it does!* Chapter 16 provides your MAP to effective meal balance, and the following suggestions are helpful beginning steps.

First, you have to decide that you really *want* to change. To paraphrase an old Hebrew proverb: Change is not difficult. It is the *resistance* to change that is hard. Commit now to really giving it your best effort for long enough to see a difference. Pay attention to these basics. These steps do make a big difference to help you improve energy and mind-body power. Before you ask your doctor for medication to lift your mood and energy, or rush out for an herbal "fix," make certain you try these basics first.

DR. VLIET'S STRATEGIES
FOR FEELING BETTER

◇ Avoid simple sugars. (You know what I am talking about: all those sweets that just seem to stick to your fingers!)

◇ Reduce "white stuff"—white flour pasta, breads, potatoes, white rice, etc. Focus on whole grain options for your carbohydrate selections.

◇ Reduce salt. It contributes to bloating, making you feel fatter, and also adds to irritability and fatigue from the fluid retention that affects the brain as well as the body.

◇ Make sure that each meal and snack contains a balance of protein, fat, and carbs as outlined in your MAP.

◇ Cut out alcohol . . . it sabotages your weight-loss efforts, makes you feel headachy and sluggish as it is wearing off, and . . . it stimulates insulin and your appetite, making you eat more; then it impairs your judgment so you don't care that you are overindulging.

◇ Cut out excess caffeine . . . it makes you irritable, and it interferes with optimal fat-burning pathways! Limit yourself to just one or two cups of coffee or tea a day.

◇ Eliminate nicotine . . . same reasons as caffeine.

◇ Divide your total food for the day into five or six smaller meals to keep glucose steady, rev up your fat-burning pathways, keep your energy up, and improve mood and mental clarity.

◇ Frequent small meals and elimination of simple sugars will reduce those ravenous "sweet cravings."

◇ Take healthy choices to work or with you when you travel.

◇ Cut out artificial sweeteners and diet drinks and drink water or plain sparkling water instead.

◇ Make sure you drink at least 64 ounces of water a day for adequate hydration.

© 2001 by Elizabeth Lee Vliet, M.D.

> **Chapter 16**

YOUR MEAL ACTION PLAN—

THE MAP FOR STARTING YOUR JOURNEY

If you started out to drive from New York to San Francisco, you would probably get a current map to show you the way. You would not likely want to rely on one from the 1970s, since there have been a lot of new roads constructed since then. Likewise, you need a food MAP for your weight-loss journey that has the latest updates relevant to women's bodies, not one based on men's needs. If you are going to be successful at losing excess body fat during the times of "hormonal challenges" that we women face, then you will need a *new* food MAP based on turning women's fat-storing hormones into fat-burning ones. That's what my Meal Action Plan, or MAP, is designed to do.

My MAP features a higher protein intake than some current programs, but it should not be considered a high-protein, high-fat diet similar to the popular ones currently in fashion, such as the Atkins Diet. The truly high protein diets restrict carbohydrates so much that the lower activity of T3 thyroid hormone makes your metabolism even more sluggish. The trick is to have enough carbohydrate intake that your thyroid works properly, and you avoid that "draggy" feeling that occurs with highly restricted carb intake, but without having so much carbohydrate that you overproduce insulin. It is a balance that is unique to women's needs—research done on men doesn't apply well here!

So that my MAP will fit with other programs you may be using, I have used the concept of building blocks or *exchanges* as used by the American Diabetes Association (ADA) and the American Heart Association (AHA). An *exchange* is simply a group of foods with similar nutritional value that you can swap, or exchange, for one another based on what you most like to eat or have available in your area. For example, if you don't like broccoli, this vegetable serving (exchange) may be swapped for a serving of another vegetable that you prefer. I have listed these food groups in the table that follows. You can find a more detailed exchange list in booklets from the ADA. Think of these building blocks, or exchanges, as ways you can customize the meal plan for your tastes, since you can exchange an apple for a pear or an apricot, and you can swap your servings of meat for a comparable protein equivalent in eggs or cheese.

The majority of the fat in my meal plan will come from your protein intake, and the total daily fat is comparable to that recommended in the ADA and AHA diets, about 27 to 30 percent a day. As a result, you will notice that I do not recommend adding many additional fat building blocks, or exchanges, beyond what is included in the protein group. In the sample meal plans, you will see that I have tended to use fruits that have a lower glycemic index to minimize insulin overshoot and offer you more quantity and fiber for each fruit exchange. Try to focus on eating whole fruits instead of fruit juice in order to avoid excess stimulation of insulin release.

If you summarize the daily intake in each food group, you will see that, although my meal plan is lower in carbs than the ADA suggests, I have still met the minimum recommendations of the American Cancer Society for five to six servings of fruits and vegetables a day to reach desirable levels of fiber, vitamins, and antioxidants.

Since many of you are working outside the home as well as the "home management jobs" you do each day, you may want to use shortcuts that help you incorporate this meal balance into your daily life. For example, you may take the basic meal ingredients and combine them into your favorite stew receipe that simmers in the Crock-Pot while you are at work. Or you may want to buy bags of salad greens already washed and cut into pieces. The trick is to make these meals work for you and your family.

YOUR HORMONE POWER PLAN: SAMPLE MEAL PLANS

	Percent	1600 calories/day		1800 calories/day	
		Calories	Grams	Calories	Grams
Protein	35%	577	131	630	157
Fat	30%	495	50	540	60
	25%	412	42	450	50
Carbs	35%	577	131	630	158
	40%	660	150	720	180

DR. VLIET'S DAILY RECOMMENDATIONS
35% protein = 144 grams
30% fat = 55 grams
35% carb = 144 grams

ADA plan (for comparison)
21% Protein = 80 grams
27% Fat = 45 grams
52% Carb = 195 grams

USING THE SAMPLE MEAL PLANS

The exchanges given on the leftmost column provide you with flexible meals you can plan yourself. You don't have to get stuck in a rut eating the same things day after day. Take breakfast, for example. Select skim milk or plain nonfat yogurt, one slice of whole grain bread or half a bagel, and for the proteins, choose one of these: ¾ cup cottage cheese, or 3 eggs, or 3 ounces of ricotta cheese, or 3 ounces of turkey/lean beef/fish (such as smoked salmon). Choose fruit such as 2 ounces of orange juice or 4 ounces of tomato juice. You may use 1 teaspoon of reduced-fat butter or ½ teaspoon regular butter on toast for the ½ fat exchange. Or a combination: 1 ounce nonfat cream cheese and 2 ounces smoked salmon (lox) on half a bagel. If you substitute one whole egg with two egg whites, you will reduce the protein-derived fat by 5 grams, which may be added back as one teaspoon of butter on toast.

© 2001 by Elizabeth Lee Vliet, M.D.

YOUR HORMONE POWER PLAN: SAMPLE MEAL PLANS

Breakfast

	Protein grams	Fat grams	Carb grams	Calories
3 protein (low fat)	21	9	0	165
½ fat exchange	0	2.5	0	22
1 bread	3	1	15	80
1 milk, skim	8	0	12	90
½ fruit	0	0	7.5	30
Totals	**34%**	**30%**	**36%**	**387**

Lunch

	Protein grams	Fat grams	Carb grams	Calories
5 protein (low fat)	35	15	0	275
½ fat	0	2.5	0	22
2 bread/starch	6	0	30	140
2 vegetable (nonstarchy)	4	0	10	50
½ fruit	0	0	7.5	30
Totals	**33%**	**32%**	**35%**	**537**

Afternoon Snack

	Protein grams	Fat grams	Carb grams	Calories
1½ protein (low fat)	10.5	4.5	0	82
1 fruit	0	0	15	60
Totals	**30%**	**28%**	**42%**	**142**

(continued on next page)

YOUR HORMONE POWER PLAN: SAMPLE MEAL PLANS

This plan means that over 60 percent of daily calories are consumed prior to dinner, which helps prevent more fat being stored at night.

Dinner

	Protein grams	Fat grams	Carb grams	Calories
4 protein (low fat)	28	12	0	220
½ fat	0	2.5	0	22
1 bread	3	1	15	80
2 vegetable (nonstarchy)	4	0	10	50
1 fruit	0	0	15	60
½ milk	4	0	6	45
Totals	**33%**	**29%**	**38%**	**477**

Bedtime Snack

	Protein grams	Fat grams	Carb grams	Calories
1½ protein (low fat)	10.5	4.5	0	82
½ milk	4	0	6	45
Totals	**46%**	**35%**	**19%**	**122**

YOUR HORMONE POWER PLAN: SAMPLE MEAL PLANS

YOUR HORMONE POWER PLAN DAILY SUMMARY

1600 Calorie Meal Plan*

	Protein grams	Fat grams	Carb grams	Calories
Daily Totals:	141	56	149	1645
Total Percents:	35%	30%	35%	100%

1800 Calorie Meal Plan†

	Protein grams	Fat grams	Carb grams	Calories
Daily Totals:	154	61	164	1800
Total Percents:	35%	30%	35%	100%

*I really do not recommend decreasing daily caloric intake below 1600 calories for most women. Cutting calories too low simply makes your metabolism slow down even more and makes it harder for you to lose excess fat. Your body will hang on to all it has, because it thinks you are in a famine! Keeping your daily calories *above* the level of your resting metabolic rate will help jumpstart your metabolism and rev up the metabolic rate if you are currently eating less than this amount.

†Women who weigh more than 190 to 200 pounds will need to eat more calories to provide adequate energy throughout the day and avoid making their metabolism slow down even more. To increase from 1600 to 1800 calories per day, I suggest adding 1.5 protein exchanges (lean or low-fat proteins) and 1 bread exchange during the day, such as for a midmorning snack. Or, you may add 1 bread/starch exchange to breakfast, and the 1½ meat exchanges to dinner.

© 2001 by Elizabeth Lee Vliet, M.D.

EXCHANGES, OR BUILDING BLOCKS FOR YOUR MEALS

PROTEINS

The proteins are meats and meat substitutes. This group is divided into groups, based on fat content, which in turn affects the calories and fat grams, as shown in the chart.

One building block, or *exchange*, provides:

	Protein grams	Fat grams	Carb grams	Calories
Very lean meat or meat substitutes	7	0–1	0	35
Lean meat or meat substitutes	7	3	0	55
Medium-fat meat or meat substitutes	7	5	0	75
High-fat meat or meat substitutes	7	8	0	100

The serving size for one building-block unit, or one exchange, is as follows:

Meat, chicken, fish:	1 ounce
Hard cheeses:	1 ounce
Soft cheeses (cottage, ricotta, farmers):	¼ cup
Egg:	1 whole egg or two egg whites (no yolk)
Egg substitutes:	¼ cup
Peanut butter:	2 tbsp (medium-fat meat group)
Soy milk:	1 cup
Tempeh:	¼ cup
Tofu:	4 ounces or ½ cup
Beans, peas, lentils:	½ cup cooked, counts as one very lean meat *and* one starch exchange

© 2001 by Elizabeth Lee Vliet, M.D.

EXCHANGES, OR BUILDING BLOCKS FOR YOUR MEALS

FATS

One building block, or *exchange*, provides:

> 5 grams of fat
> 0 grams of carbohydrate
> 0 grams of protein
> 45 calories

Sample foods: all oils, salad dressing, mayonnaise, butter, cream, margarine, sour cream, coconut, bacon, avocados, olives, nuts, seeds, tahini paste, shortening/lard/fatback/salt pork.

If you use a reduced fat version of butter, margarine, sour cream, mayonnaise, or salad dressing, this means you may increase the serving size as shown below to give the same total fat content.

The serving size for one building-block unit, or one exchange, is as follows:

Regular butter/margarine:	1 teaspoon
Whipped butter/margarine:	2 teaspoons
Reduced-fat butter/margarine:	3 teaspoons (1 tablespoon)
Regular sour cream:	2 tablespoons
Reduced-fat sour cream:	3 teaspoons (1 tablespoon)
Regular mayonnaise/salad dressing:	1 teaspoon
Reduced-fat mayo/salad dressing:	3 teaspoons (1 tablespoon)

EXCHANGES, OR BUILDING BLOCKS FOR YOUR MEALS

CARBOHYDRATES

Bread/Starch Group

One building block, or *exchange*, provides:

> 15 grams of carbohydrate
> 3 grams of protein
> 0 grams of fat*
> 80 calories

*Some starchy foods that are prepared with fat count as 1 starch exchange plus 1 fat exchange: e.g., biscuits, corn bread, crackers, croutons, granola, muffins, pancakes, bread stuffing, taco shells, and waffles.

Sample foods: breads, cereals, grains, starchy vegetables (potatoes, beans, corn, green peas, yams, winter squash), crackers/snacks, beans, lentils, black-eyed or split peas.

© 2001 by Elizabeth Lee Vliet, M.D.

EXCHANGES, OR BUILDING BLOCKS FOR YOUR MEALS

CARBOHYDRATES

Vegetable Group

One building block, or *exchange*, provides:

> 5 grams of carbohydrate
> 2 grams protein
> 0 grams fat
> 25 calories

Sample foods: artichokes, asparagus, green beans, beets, broccoli, brussels sprouts, cabbage, carrots, cauliflower, celery, cucumber, eggplant, green onions, dark greens (collard, kale, mustard, turnip, spinach), kohlrabi, mushrooms, okra, onions, pea pods, peppers, radishes, salad greens, sauerkraut, spinach, summer squash, tomatoes, turnips, water chestnuts, watercress, zucchini

Fruit Group

One building block, or *exchange*, provides:

> 15 grams of carbohydrate
> 0 grams of fat
> 0 grams of protein
> 60 calories

Sample foods: apples, apricots, bananas, blackberries, blueberries, cantalope, cherries, dates, figs, grapefruit, grapes, honeydew, kiwi, mandarin oranges, mango, nectarines, oranges, papaya, peaches, pears, pineapple, plums, prunes, raisins, raspberries, strawberries, tangerines, watermelon

EXCHANGES, OR BUILDING BLOCKS FOR YOUR MEALS

MILK

Milk and milk products contain protein, carbohydrate, and fat building blocks. The amount of fat a particular type of milk contains will determine both the fat grams and the total calories.

One building block, or *exchange*, provides:

	Protein grams	Fat grams	Carb grams	Calories
Fat free (skim milk, nonfat yogurt)	8	0	12	90
Low fat (1% milk, low-fat yogurt)	8	3	12	100
Reduced fat (2% milk)	8	5	12	120
Whole milk	8	8	12	150

The serving size for one building-block unit, or one exchange, is as follows:

Milk (cow, goat, or kefir)	1 cup
Buttermilk	1 cup
Evaporated milk	½ cup
Yogurt	¾ cup
Fat-free dry milk	⅓ cup powder

Rice milk is considered a starch exchange, and soy milk is considered a medium-fat meat (protein) exchange.

YOUR HORMONE POWER PLAN:

SAMPLE MEALS

DAY 1

Breakfast

1 egg
½ cup regular cottage cheese sprinkled with ½ cup bran cereal
8 oz skim milk
2 oz grapefruit or orange juice

Poach or hard boil egg, or prepare scrambled using nonfat cooking spray. Drink 8 oz of decaffeinated hot beverage or water with breakfast.

Lunch

5 oz cubed, cooked chicken
1 large whole wheat pita bread, cut in halves
Leaf lettuce, dark green
1 cup raw cauliflower
1 whole tangerine
1 Tbsp reduced-fat salad dressing
1 Tbsp nonfat yogurt

Mix chicken with nonfat yogurt, season to taste. Stuff chicken salad and lettuce into two pita bread halves. Use salad dressing as dip for raw cauliflower. Peel and eat tangerine on side or add to pita sandwich. Drink 8 oz of water with meal and additional 8 oz throughout early afternoon.

Midafternoon Snack

½ cup cottage or ricotta cheese
¾ cup fresh berries

Mix berries with cheese if desired. Drink 8 oz of water.

Dinner

4 oz prime rib
1 small potato, baked
1 cup sautéed onions, mushrooms, green peppers
1 fresh peach, sliced
1½ Tbsp reduced-fat sour cream
4 oz milk, skim or 1%

Grill or bake prime rib. Sauté vegetables in nonfat cooking spray. Spread sour cream on baked potato. Enjoy sliced peach on side or as dessert. Drink 8 to 16 oz of water with meal.

Bedtime Snack

4 oz milk, skim or 1%
1.5 oz sliced beef left over from dinner

Drink additional 8 oz of water and keep cup of water by bedside.

DAY 2

Breakfast

2 oz turkey, white meat, no skin
1 oz cheese
1 slice whole wheat toast
8 oz skim milk
½ orange, sliced

Melt cheese over turkey and toast. Drink 8 oz of decaffeinated hot beverage or water with breakfast.

Lunch

5 oz lean hamburger or turkey burger
1 whole wheat roll
Leaf lettuce, dark green
1–2 tomato slices
½ cup raw cucumber slices
½ cup raw carrots
2 dried apple rings
1 Tbsp reduced-fat mayonnaise

Drink 8 oz of water with meal and additional 8 oz throughout early afternoon.

Midafternoon Snack

2 Tbsp peanut butter
1 sliced Granny Smith apple

Drink 8 oz of water

Dinner

4 oz fish, baked or grilled cod, flounder, haddock, trout
½ cup brown rice
½ cup mixed vegetables
1 cup dinner salad
1 cup fresh raspberries
1 Tbsp reduced fat salad dressing
4 oz milk, skim or 1%

Drink 8 to 16 oz of water with meal.

Bedtime Snack

4 oz milk, skim or 1%
1.5 oz cheddar cheese, low fat
1 Tbsp salsa

Drink additional 8 oz of water and keep cup of water by bedside.

DAY 3

Breakfast

2 oz lox, smoked salmon
1 oz cream cheese, reduced fat
½ bagel, whole wheat
½ cup canned pineapple or ⅜ cup fresh
8 oz skim milk

Spread cream cheese on toasted bagel and top with smoked salmon. Serve with fresh fruit on the side. Drink 8 oz of decaffeinated hot beverage or water with breakfast.

Lunch

Chef Salad:
    2 oz turkey, chopped
    1 oz ham, chopped
    1 oz shredded cheese, low fat
    1 egg, hard boiled, sliced
    10 whole wheat crackers, no fat added, or two slices whole grain toast
    2 cups leafy greens and choice of vegetables
    1 tangerine—peeled
    1 Tbsp reduced-fat salad dressing

Mix the above ingredients in bowl, add salad dressing, enjoy fruit in salad or on the side. Drink 8 oz of water with meal and additional 8 oz throughout early afternoon.

Midafternoon Snack

15 peanuts
½ mango or papaya or 1 small whole apple

Drink 8 oz of water

Dinner

4 oz roast beef
½ cup peas, cooked
Dinner salad with 1 cup raw vegetables
1 Tbsp reduced-fat dressing
1 cup unsweetened berries of your choice
4 oz nonfat yogurt

Mix berries with yogurt for dessert. Drink 8 to 16 oz of water with meal.

Bedtime Snack

4 oz milk, skim or 1%
1 Tbsp sesame or sunflower seeds

Drink additional 8 oz of water and keep cup of water by bedside.

DAY 4

Breakfast

3 oz lean breakfast ham, or Canadian bacon or turkey sausage
3 Tbsp wheat germ
1 cup nonfat plain yogurt
½ cup fresh berries

Cook ham with nonfat cooking spray. Mix berries, wheat germ, and yogurt.
Drink 8 oz of decaffeinated hot beverage or water with breakfast.

Lunch

3 oz turkey, sliced, white meat, no skin
2 oz cheese, sliced, low fat
Salsa
2 flour tortillas
8 grapes or ½ apple

Layer turkey, cheese, and salsa on tortillas, heat in microwave to melt cheese
then roll and eat. Enjoy fruit on the side. Drink 8 oz of water with meal and
additional 8 oz throughout early afternoon.

Midafternoon Snack

9 almonds, raw
½ fresh pear

Drink 8 oz of water.

Dinner

2 eggs
1 oz cheese, shredded
1 oz lean ham, chopped
1 small potato, roasted, chopped
1 cup chopped mushrooms, green peppers, onions, tomatoes
½ fresh pear
½ tsp olive oil
4 oz milk, skim or 1%

Dinner omelet: Cook two beaten eggs in pan with oil, add cheese, ham, potato,
and vegetables, fold in half and serve. Enjoy second half of pear from afternoon
snack on side. Drink 8 to 16 oz of water with meal.

Bedtime Snack

4 oz milk, skim or 1%
1.5 oz cheese

Drink additional 8 oz of water and keep cup of water by bedside.

DAY 5

Breakfast

½ cup cooked oatmeal, add:
2 Tbsp (4 halves) chopped walnuts
½ small apple, chopped
8 oz skim milk or buttermilk

Drink 8 oz of decaffeinated hot beverage or water with breakfast.

Lunch

Make a lentil stew by cooking lentils with the following vegetables and seasonings in a Crock-Pot. Each serving should contain:

1 cup cooked green or red lentils
½ cup cooked carrots
½ cup cooked tomatoes
¼ cup chopped onions
bay leaves, chopped, salt and pepper to taste

3 oz cheddar cheese
1 kiwi, sliced or ½ orange

Melt cheese on top of stew. Enjoy fruit on the side. Drink 8 oz of water with meal and additional 8 oz throughout early afternoon.

Midafternoon Snack

1½ oz low-fat string cheese
1 small apple

Drink 8 oz of water

Dinner

4 oz broiled shrimp scampi with 1 tsp whipped butter
½ cup cooked brown rice
½ cup cooked spinach
½ cup cooked broccoli
4 oz nonfat yogurt over 1 cup fresh raspberries, for dessert

Drink 8 to 16 oz of water with meal.

Bedtime Snack

4 oz milk, skim or 1%
9 almonds, raw

Drink additional 8 oz of water and keep cup of water by bedside.

DAY 6

Breakfast

½ cup egg substitute
1 oz shredded cheese, low fat
1–2 Tbsp salsa or picante sauce
½ cup shredded wheat cereal or 1 slice whole wheat toast
4 oz tomato juice
8 oz skim milk

Pour egg substitute into pan with nonfat cooking spray. Add shredded cheese to cooked eggs and salsa as desired. Drink 8 oz of decaffeinated hot beverage or water with breakfast.

Lunch

3 oz boiled ham
2 oz sliced cheese, low fat
2 slices whole grain bread
1 tsp mustard
1 cup fresh broccoli flowerets
2 whole, fresh apricots
1 Tbsp reduced-fat salad dressing

Make sandwich with mustard, dip fresh broccoli in salad dressing, and enjoy fruit on the side. Drink 8 oz of water with meal and additional 8 oz throughout early afternoon.

Midafternoon Snack

½ cup cottage cheese, low fat
16 grapes, halved, or 1 small apple, chopped

Add grapes or chopped apple to cottage cheese. Drink 8 oz of water.

Dinner

4 oz salmon, grilled or baked
Dinner salad
½ cup mixed vegetables
½ cup unsweetened applesauce
1 Tbsp reduced-fat dressing
4 oz nonfat yogurt

Drink 8 to 16 oz of water with meal.

Bedtime Snack

4 oz skim milk
2 Tbsp peanut butter, natural style
1 slice toast or 4 whole grain crackers

Drink additional 8 oz of water and keep cup of water by bedside.

DAY 7

Breakfast

3 oz chipped beef
1 slice whole wheat toast
½ orange
1 tsp whipped butter
1 tsp flour
4 oz skim milk or ½ cup yogurt for chipped beef

Make cream sauce for chipped beef by melting 1 tsp whipped butter in sauté pan, stir in the flour and heat about 1 minute, then slowly add ¼ to ½ cup skim milk or yogurt and stir until smooth. Add in the chipped beef, heat, and spread over toast. Drink any remaining skim milk. Drink 8 oz of decaffeinated hot beverage or water with breakfast.

Lunch

5 oz canned salmon, drained
¼ cup celery, chopped
½ cup onion, chopped
¼ tsp dill, chopped
2 slices whole grain toast
1 cup cooked mixed vegetables
2 small apricots
1 Tbsp reduced-fat mayonnaise

Add dill, onions, and celery to salmon to taste, mix in mayonnaise and spread on toast. Enjoy vegetables and fruit on the side. Drink 8 oz of water with meal and additional 8 oz throughout early afternoon.

Midafternoon Snack

1½ oz hard cheese, reduced fat
1 small apple or pear

Drink 8 oz of water.

Dinner

4 oz grilled lamb loin with rosemary
½ cup cooked wild rice
½ cup cooked broccoli
½ cup cooked carrots
1 tsp whipped butter
2 small plums
1 tsp whipped butter for rice
4 oz skim milk

Drink 8 to 16 oz of water with meal.

Bedtime Snack

4 oz skim milk or yogurt
1½ oz sliced chicken left over from dinner or 1½ oz cheese

Drink additional 8 oz of water and keep cup of water by bedside.

DAY 8

Breakfast

3 egg omelet with chopped tomatoes and/or mushrooms and peppers
1 slice whole grain rye toast
½ orange, sliced
1 tsp whipped butter
8 oz skim milk or buttermilk

Spread low-fat butter on toast. Drink 8 oz of decaffeinated hot beverage or water with breakfast.

Lunch

5 oz canned tuna, drained
¼ cup celery, chopped
½ cup onion, chopped
½ cup plain nonfat yogurt
½ cup bean sprouts
2 slices whole wheat bread, toasted
2 dried peach halves

Tuna salad: Add yogurt to tuna, mix in vegetables and spread on toast. Layer with bean sprouts. Drink 8 oz of water with meal and additional 8 oz throughout early afternoon.

Midafternoon Snack

1½ oz low-fat string cheese
1 small apple

Drink 8 oz of water

Dinner

4 oz chicken breast, chopped
½ cup each chopped celery, onions, carrots
½ cup pineapple chunks, in unsweetened juice, drained
10 almonds, chopped
½ cup plain nonfat yogurt
½ cup cooked brown rice or couscous
1 tsp curry powder, or more to taste

Mix chicken, vegetables, pineapple, almonds, yogurt, and curry to taste. Serve couscous on side. Drink 8 to 16 oz of water with meal.

Bedtime Snack

4 oz milk, skim or 1%
1½ oz curry chicken left over from dinner

Drink additional 8 oz of water and keep cup of water by bedside.

DAY 9

Breakfast

3 oz skim mozzarella cheese
1 slice whole grain toast
4 oz tomato juice
4 oz skim milk

Melt mozzarella over toast. Drink 8 oz of decaffeinated hot beverage or water with breakfast.

Midmorning Snack

½ cup plain yogurt, low-fat or nonfat

You may add 1 Tbsp fruit spread (no sugar added), or ¼ cup chopped fresh fruit.

Lunch

3 oz canned tuna, drained, mixed into 2 oz melted cheese
1 cup whole grain pasta
½ cup chopped broccoli, season to taste
1 small kiwi or fig for dessert

Drink 8 oz of water with meal and additional 8 oz throughout early afternoon.

Midafternoon Snack

2 Tbsp peanut butter (natural)
1 small apple, sliced

Drink 8 oz of water

Dinner

4 oz roast lamb
½ cup cooked pumpkin or winter squash
1 cup cooked snow peas
½ tsp butter for vegetables
½ cup vanilla yogurt served over ¾ cup canned mandarin oranges (water pack)

Drink 8 to 16 oz of water with meal.

Bedtime Snack

4 oz skim milk
1½ oz low-fat cheese

Drink additional 8 oz of water and keep cup of water by bedside.

DAY 10

Breakfast

3 oz herring, uncreamed or smoked
1 slice whole wheat toast
1 tsp reduced-fat butter
1 cup plain nonfat yogurt
½ cup fresh berries

Chop and mix berries with yogurt, spread low-fat butter on toast. Drink 8 oz of decaffeinated hot beverage or water with breakfast.

Lunch

3 oz turkey, sliced, white meat, no skin
2 oz cheese, sliced, low fat
1 whole wheat bagel (small)
1½ tsp reduced-fat mayonnaise
Leaf lettuce, dark green
1–2 tomato slices
6 fresh cherries

Assemble bagel sandwich with the above ingredients, enjoy fruit on the side. Drink 8 oz of water with meal and additional 8 oz throughout early afternoon.

Midafternoon Snack

1½ oz string cheese, low fat
1 kiwi

Drink 8 oz of water

Dinner

4 oz chicken, baked or grilled, white meat, no skin
⅓ cup baked beans or beans of your choice
1 corn on the cob, steamed
1½ tsp reduced-fat butter
4 oz milk, skim or 1%

Cook chicken with nonfat cooking spray or basted with water/fruit juice mixture. Drink 8 to 16 oz of water with meal.

Bedtime Snack

4 oz milk, skim or 1%
9 almonds, raw

Drink additional 8 oz of water and keep cup of water by bedside.

DAY 11

Breakfast

1 egg or 2 egg whites, scrambled
1 oz lean Canadian bacon
1 slice whole wheat toast
1 Tbsp 100% fruit spread
½ tsp butter or 1 tsp whipped butter
8 oz skim milk or ¾ cup yogurt

Spread fruit spread and butter on toast. Drink 8 oz of decaffeinated hot beverage or water with breakfast.

Lunch

Tuna salad:
 5 oz water pack tuna, drained
 ½ cup celery, chopped
 ¼ cup onion, chopped
 ¼ cup green or red pepper, chopped
 ½ tsp cilantro, chopped
 ½ tsp dill
 ½ tsp celery seed
 1½ tsp reduced fat mayonnaise
 1 Tbsp nonfat yogurt
2 slices whole wheat bread
½ cup each raw carrots, broccoli
1 small plum or ½ small apple
1½ tsp reduced fat mayonnaise

Mix mayonnaise and yogurt, add to tuna, vegetables, and spices. Drink 8 oz of water with meal and additional 8 oz throughout early afternoon.

Midafternoon Snack

1½ oz low-fat string cheese
1 small apple

Drink 8 oz of water

Dinner

4 oz grilled chicken with rosemary
½ cup cooked brown rice
½ cup cooked yellow squash
½ cup cooked Brussels sprouts
1 tsp whipped butter
4 oz nonfat yogurt
1 cup fresh raspberries

Serve yogurt over berries for dessert. Drink 8 to 16 oz of water with meal.

Bedtime Snack

4 oz milk, skim or 1%
1½ oz low-fat string cheese **or**
1½ oz sliced chicken left over from dinner

DAY 12

Breakfast

3 scrambled eggs
1 slice whole wheat toast
1 Tbsp 100% fruit spread
1 tsp reduced-fat butter
8 oz skim milk

Spread fruit spread and low-fat butter on toast. Drink 8 oz of decaffeinated
hot beverage or water with breakfast.

Lunch

4 oz roast beef, sliced
1 oz provolone cheese
2 slices whole grain bread
½ cup bean sprouts
1 Tbsp low-fat mayonnaise
½ cup carrots sticks
1 small peach

Roast beef sandwich with bean sprouts and cheese. Enjoy carrot sticks and
peach on the side. Drink 8 oz of water with meal and additional 8 oz throughout early afternoon.

Midafternoon Snack

⅜ cup cottage cheese
1 small apple or 12 grapes

Drink 8 oz of water.

Dinner

4 oz broiled lobster
½ cup cooked wild or brown rice
½ cup cooked spinach
½ cup cooked asparagus
1 tsp whipped butter (for lobster); add lemon if desired
1 small pear, steamed
4 oz nonfat yogurt with dash of cinnamon and nutmeg

Drink 8 to 16 oz of water with meal.

Bedtime Snack

4 oz yogurt or skim milk
1½ oz left over beef (from lunch) or lobster (from dinner)

Drink additional 8 oz of water and keep cup of water by bedside.

DAY 13

Breakfast

¾ cup ricotta cheese, with maple flavor added
1 slice whole grain toast
½ small banana, sliced into ricotta cheese
8 oz skim milk

Spread cheese and banana on toast. Drink 8 oz of decaffeinated hot beverage or water with breakfast.

Lunch

5 oz swordfish, broiled, with lemon, capers, and ½ tsp whipped butter
1 dinner roll
½ cup cooked rice with ½ tsp whipped butter
½ cup carrots
½ cup spinach
1 small peach or nectarine

Drink 8 oz of water with meal and additional 8 oz throughout early afternoon.

Midafternoon Snack

1½ oz low-fat cheese
1 small apple

Drink 8 oz of water.

Dinner

Clams Marinara:
　　　4 oz canned fresh clams
　　　½ cup tomatoes
　　　¼ cup onions
　　　¼ cup celery
　　　¼ cup mushrooms
　　　½ tsp olive oil for sauce
　　　½ cup cooked whole grain pasta
　　　Italian seasoning to taste
1 sliced kiwi

Simmer clams, vegetables, and oil for sauce; pour over pasta. Drink 8 to 16 oz of water with meal.

Bedtime Snack

8 oz skim milk, or yogurt
1½ oz sliced chicken or turkey

Drink additional 8 oz of water and keep cup of water by bedside.

DAY 14

Breakfast

½ cup cooked oatmeal, add:
1 Tbsp raisins
6 almonds, chopped
½ cup cottage cheese
8 oz skim milk or nonfat buttermilk

Mix raisins, almonds, and cottage cheese with oatmeal for a hearty breakfast cereal. Drink 8 oz of decaffeinated hot beverage or water with breakfast.

Lunch

4 oz lean ground beef
½ tsp olive oil to brown meat
1 cup cooked spaghetti with marinara sauce
1 oz Parmesan cheese, grated
1 small apricot

Add browned meat to marinara sauce and serve over spaghetti. Sprinkle with Parmesan cheese. Drink 8 oz of water with meal and additional 8 oz throughout early afternoon.

Midafternoon Snack

1½ oz low-fat cheese
1 small apple

Drink 8 oz of water.

Dinner

4 oz roast pork loin (spread with Dijon mustard if desired)
½ cup cooked, mashed sweet potatoes
½ cup cooked Brussels sprouts
½ cup cooked asparagus
½ tsp butter
1 small pear
4 oz skim milk

Drink 8 to 16 oz of water with meal.

Bedtime Snack

4 oz milk, skim or 1%
9 almonds

Drink additional 8 oz of water and keep cup of water by bed.

Chapter 17

BALANCING
VITAMINS, MINERALS, AND SUPPLEMENTS FOR WEIGHT LOSS

Vitamins and minerals are called *micronutrients,* because we need very small amounts each day, not because they are "micro" in importance. They are essential to our survival because they are vital catalysts for all the chemical pathways our body uses to convert food into energy. Most of us don't really eat a "balanced diet" these days, and even if we did, we still wouldn't get all the vitamins and minerals we need just from our food. Soils in which foods are grown are often depleted of needed minerals, and vitamins are frequently processed out of foods or lost in cooking. You can be overweight and actually malnourished.

Stress also increases the body's demands for the vital "micro" nutrients and antioxidants. Without them, stress causes chemical changes that lead to cellular damage throughout the body. And what woman in the United States today doesn't live a high-stress life? If you want your "fat-burning" plan to work, you must take the right amount of vitamins and minerals each day. As you read further, keep in mind that taking supplements means learning the proper balance to make them work—too much of one vitamin may reduce the absorption and effectiveness of another.

TYPES OF SUPPLEMENTS OR "MICRONUTRIENTS"

CATEGORY	WHAT THEY DO
Vitamins	Serve as coenzymes or catalysts for most crucial chemical reactions in the body. Essential to life.
Minerals	Needed for balance of body fluids, serve as cofactors and catalysts in chemical pathways involved in most body functions such as the formation of bone and muscle, proper nerve conduction, making the enzymes that catalyze reactions to make everything from immune cells to hormones.
Antioxidants	Compounds (some are vitamins, some are minerals) that combine with the free radicals (oxyradicals), destructive "scavenger" molecules that cause cell damage and death if they build up in excess amounts. Accumulation of free radicals as we age is what is thought to be a major factor in the development of degenerative diseases such as atherosclerosis, arthritis, cancers, and heart disease.
Phytochemicals	Biologically active substances found in many plants that help protect against abnormal cell growth (such as cancers), improve disease resistance, and help decrease free radical damage. Examples are flavinoids (citrus fruits), indoles (cruciferous vegetables), saponins (many beans), p-coumaric acid and lycopenes (tomatoes), sulforaphane (broccoli), and PEITC or phenethyl isothiocyanate (turnips).

PRACTICING SAFE SUPPLEMENT USE

First, an important warning: As a result of the Dietary Supplements Health and Education Act of 1994, the FDA is no longer allowed to oversee the supplement industry the way it watches over quality, safety, and effectiveness of prescription and over-the-counter medications. This means that consumers in this country have no agency to provide regulatory oversight to ensure the quality and safety of what you are getting when you take herbs and supplements. Recent reports on herbal products in the United States found contamination of lead, arsenic, pesticides, and other adulterants, and that many products don't even contain what the label says. This is in contrast to Germany, where herbs and other types of supplements have been used as medicinal agents for years, and are overseen by the German Commission E. This is a government agency that checks the safety, purity, and effectiveness of herbs and other supplements that are marketed as having therapeutic benefits. Products have to meet the standards set by Commission E before they can be sold as medicinals in Germany.

How can you determine a product's safety and that it contains what it is supposed to? One resource that is now available is *ConsumerLab,* an organization that conducts detailed analyses of supplement products to help consumers know which brands actually provide what the label says they do, and are free of known contaminants. Check out their Web site, *www. consumerlab.com,* for the current list of products being tested, as well as those that have successfully passed the detailed laboratory analysis. This at least gives you more confidence in the purity of brands you decide to use.

There are now thousands of vitamin and supplement products on the market, which can vary enormously in quality and reliability as well as price. The most expensive is not necessarily the best, so shop carefully.

WHAT HELPS WITH WEIGHT LOSS?

A variety of vitamin combinations have been reported to help improve the success of weight-loss programs, but there are few controlled studies showing clear-cut benefits. In addition to the essential vitamins and minerals, various diets claim that certain supplements will help with weight loss.

What's hype and what's helpful? I'll try to give you a balanced perspective on this subject. My goal is to give you a list of vitamins and minerals that are known to be involved as cofactors in the chemical reactions that have to take place for healthy metabolism. Then you can be sure you are getting these essential ones in the right amounts for optimal effects. Further in this chapter, I will address popular weight-loss supplements, particularly ones to avoid. I will also give you a list of prescription medicines that are likely to increase appetite and make you gain weight.

B Vitamins

Most of the B vitamins are involved as cofactors for the energy-generating, fat-burning metabolic pathways in our bodies, and they are crucial for carbohydrate metabolism. They also critical cofactors in the brain pathways to make serotonin and other mood and metabolism-regulating neurotransmitters.

B vitamins are quickly depleted when you are under stress, including the stress of dieting, so a B complex vitamin supplement is important when you start your weight loss program. The B vitamins include thiamine (B_1), riboflavin (B_2), niacinamide (B_3), pantothenate (B_5), pyridoxine (B_6), cyancobalamin (B_{12}), and folic acid, and they have similar deficiency symptoms such as low energy, muscle fatigue, depression, insomnia, headaches, and anorexia. I have described more specifics in the chart on the following pages.

I have found it is better to supplement the *B complex vitamins as a group* in a balanced supplement rather than taking just vitamin B_6, because the B complex needs to be present in the proper balance and ratio in order to work optimally. There are now a number of very good commercial vitamin formulas that have been designed to provide the B vitamins with folic acid. I suggest you avoid products derived from brewer's yeast, since many women are already having "yeast" problems, especially if they are insulin resistant and glucose intolerant.

YOUR B VITAMINS

B Vitamin	Function
Thiamine (B$_1$)	Required for carbohydrate metabolism.
Riboflavin (B$_2$)	Involved in metabolism of carbohydrates, fats, and proteins. Aids in utilization of oxygen by cells.
Niacinamide (B$_3$)	Needed to metabolize food into energy, essential for release of energy from fats, carbohydrates, and proteins
Pantothenate (B$_5$)	Involved in release of energy from fats, carbohydrates, proteins, and synthesis of fats, cholesterol, steroid hormones, and phospholipids.
Pyridoxine (B$_6$)	Required for amino-acid metabolism as well as lipid and carbohydrate metabolism. Involved in making dopamine and serotonin, inhibits prolactin metabolism, involved in metabolism of estrogen by the liver and may help relieve PMS symptoms.
Cyanocobalamin (B$_{12}$)	Important in red blood cell production, DNA synthesis, and maintenance and growth of nerve fibers.
Folic acid	Plays major role in intracellular metabolism and DNA synthesis

© 2001 by Elizabeth Lee Vliet, M.D.

YOUR B VITAMINS

Dietary Sources	Suggested Daily Dose
Enriched grain and grain products such as cereals, brewer's yeast, rice bran, wheat germ, legumes, nuts, meat, pork	1.0–2.0 mg
Milk, meat, eggs, nuts, enriched flour, and green vegetables	1.0–4.0 mg
Nutritional yeasts, meats, fish, eggs, green vegetables, legumes (including peanuts), enriched cereals, potatoes	13–20 mg
Meats, legumes, whole grain products, wheat germ, nuts, vegetables, seeds, brewer's yeast, eggs, milk	5–10 mg
Cereal grains, legumes, vegetables, liver, meat, and eggs	25–30 mg if taking BCP 50–100 mg for PMS
Found only in animal foods, meat, poultry, eggs, fish, milk	50–100 mcg
Spinach, okra, asparagus, legumes, beef liver, orange and tomato juice, fortified cereals and breads	400 mcg

© 2001 by Elizabeth Lee Vliet, M.D.

MINERALS THAT MANAGE
THE METABOLIC PATHWAYS

Magnesium

Magnesium is a critical mineral for metabolic pathways, nerve cell conduction, muscle contraction, and bone growth/formation, and it has an independent role in regulating blood pressure. It appears to be an important factor in reducing migraine headaches and heart attacks because it helps prevent spasms of the blood vessels throughout the body, especially in the coronary (heart) arteries. In the brain, magnesium is a cofactor in the production of mood-regulating chemical messengers such as dopamine, which regulates appetite. Magnesium helps prevent, and possibly relieve, irritable, depressed moods that occur commonly with PMS and perimenopause and may also be associated with weight gain. Several B vitamins require magnesium as a catalyst to make these vitamins biologically active in the body. Magnesium also is a cofactor for the chemical reactions to build protein for growth and repair of muscles and tissues. The pathways for the body to make its energy compounds are also dependent upon magnesium.

Optimal intake of magnesium and zinc (which I will discuss next), as well as regular deep breathing, improves oxygen flow to the tissues, which helps your fat-burning pathways work more efficiently. Magnesium is also important in preventing free radical damage to cells. When magnesium is low, we lose this protective effect. Low magnesium is also a trigger that generates more free radicals leading to cell damage and aging effects. Getting an optimal amount of magnesium also decreases your risk of diabetes. Overall, this mineral is crucial if you are trying to lose excess body fat.

Magnesium and Estrogen. Estrogen enhances magnesium uptake and utilization by the body's soft tissues and by bone, which is another factor helping women have lower rates of heart disease and bone loss when both estradiol and magnesium are in balance. With decline in estrogen, we also lose our ability to absorb and use magnesium optimally, which aggravates the problems that come with loss of estrogen: high blood pressure, weight gain, greater bone loss, more migraines, insulin resistance, and increased risk of heart disease.

There is a flip side of this coin that you need to keep in mind: If you are on supplemental estrogen and your magnesium intake is too low, the estrogen shifts more of the magnesium into the soft tissues and bone, with a resulting decrease in serum magnesium. This imbalance not only causes more muscle spasms and cramps, but it also means you may be at higher risk to develop a blood clot because a shift in the calcium-to-magnesium ratio favors coagulation. If you are taking calcium and are on estrogen, it is critical that you also get enough magnesium each day.

Magnesium Robbers. Women have low magnesium intake for several reasons. Drinking soft drinks daily—diet or regular—prevents absorption of magnesium and calcium since the phosphates (and phosphoric acid) in these beverages bind up magnesium and calcium and make them insoluble. The glutamate (MSG) and aspartate (Nutrasweet) added to soft drinks increase the body's need for magnesium as well.

Other factors that deplete our magnesium are high coffee consumption, excess catecholamine effects (e.g., from stimulant medications), and excess glucocorticoid effects (cortisone medications, and stress). People with Type A personality have also been found to deplete magnesium stores more rapidly.

Getting Adequate Magnesium. The average American woman gets only about 100 to 200 mg a day of magnesium from her diet, and the RDA for magnesium is 400 to 600 mg daily. I urge my patients (and I do it myself) to take 200 to 300 mg of magnesium supplement every morning and 200 to 300 mg every evening. A side benefit of optimal estradiol and optimal magnesium is that I no longer have those awful chocolate cravings that used to drive me crazy.

Taking magnesium and calcium at least two times a day provides better absorption and more even levels throughout the twenty-four hours. The calcium amount should be about twice the amount of magnesium in the morning and evening, with your remaining calcium taken in the middle of the day at lunchtime. The 2:1 ratio of calcium intake to magnesium intake is important for proper balance.

I recommend magnesium capsules with easily absorbed magnesium powder, such as the Twin Lab brand. I've found absorption is poor with hard tablets and caplet forms. There are many good brands, and it is important that you choose one that works for you and use it daily. You may also find a liquid form is well absorbed and less irritating to the GI tract.

Magnesium's importance is often overlooked, and physicians often haven't paid enough attention to the importance of optimal magnesium intake to help treat weight problems, as well as other problems like muscle pain/spasms, fibromyalgia, PMS, headaches, high blood pressure, depressed mood, anxiety, and a host of other woes that plagues us at midlife.

Zinc

Zinc is as important as protein in the normal processes of growth and maintenance of body tissue, particularly the brain and nervous system. It plays an important role in DNA and protein synthesis, helps to regulate your blood sugar, aids in formation of healthy collagen (in skin and connective tissue), and plays a role in normal immune function. Zinc is also needed for optimal ovarian function, is a helper for some twenty enzymes, and is involved in the action of insulin, the utilization of vitamin A, and the healing of wounds. In addition, it helps decrease the spread of pain sensations.

One reason that many Americans, especially women, don't get enough zinc is that we have cut down on animal foods that are rich sources. Many plant sources, such as whole grains, now have reduced zinc content due to soil depletion from modern farming methods or from the refining and processing of foods. In addition, plant sources of zinc are affected by how high the *phytate* (phytic acid) content of the plant is, since this compound interferes with the absorption of several critical minerals (calcium, magnesium, iron), particularly zinc.

Animal foods and seafood are good sources of zinc. Plant sources include whole grains, with pumpkin seeds being a particularly rich source. The recommended intake is 15 mg per day for the average adult. Generally, two servings of lean animal protein per day are sufficient. Vegetarians are more likely to have inadequate zinc intake, particularly if they eat a diet high in soy products as a main source of protein, because soybeans have the highest *phytate* content of any grain or legume. Soybeans are more resistant than other beans and grains to the beneficial effects of long, slow cooking as the usual approach to reducing phytates, which allows better absorption of important minerals. Only a long process of fermentation, such as involved in making miso and tempeh, will significantly decrease the amount of phytates present in soybeans. So if you are a vegetarian relying on soy foods as your primary source of protein, you risk having significant deficiencies of several important minerals unless you take appropriate supplements.

If you feel you may not be getting enough zinc, a safe dose range for zinc is 10 to 25 mcg daily. Zinc supplements come in several forms: arginate, picolinate, or citrate. If you add zinc supplements, be careful not to take too much, since excess doses cause other problems. Large doses of zinc may interfere with copper absorption across the intestinal wall, so check your multivitamin to see that it contains 1.5 to 3 mg of copper, and take it at a different time of day relative to when you take the zinc. I suggest taking your multivitamin (with its copper) in the morning and zinc at night.

Absorption of zinc depends on adequate dietary intake of tryptophan and B_6. A deficiency of either will impair zinc absorption. Supplementing with chromium can be useful to aid in zinc absorption and help keep blood glucose more stable throughout the day. Current studies have shown that 200 mcg of chromium once or twice a day is reasonable and has not shown any adverse effects. Higher doses can be toxic, so don't overdo it. If you are overweight and have shown clinical symptoms of glucose intolerance, adding chromium supplementation with zinc may be helpful as an addition to optimal hormone balance and a properly balanced diet.

Manganese

Manganese is another often overlooked mineral. Manganese deficiencies are associated with osteoporosis, chronic depression, chronic pain, blood sugar problems, and allergies. Manganese is involved in a number of enzyme pathways needed for the utilization of the B vitamins, vitamin E, and vitamin C, as well as the pathways of energy metabolism, glucose regulation, and immune function. Manganese is also is essential to the process of forming T4 (thyroxine) by the thyroid gland, and helps regulate pituitary function, pain, and mood. In addition, manganese is a component of the antioxidant enzyme superoxide dismutase (SOD), which controls superoxide free radicals formed in the body during cellular metabolism. SOD helps prevent the buildup of excess superoxide radicals that causes cell damage.

Dietary deficiencies of this mineral are more common today due to several factors: soils depleted of manganese, diets high in simple sugars, high-fiber and high-soy diets containing *phytates* that bind up the manganese and prevent its absorption, and soda beverages that contain phosphorus, which impairs manganese absorption. An excess of calcium and iron supplements will also impair manganese absorption.

Manganese is widely available in many plant foods. Examples include nuts, whole grains, raisins, spinach, carrots, broccoli, green peas, oranges, apples, tea leaves, and wheat bran. When wheat is milled to make white flour, most of the mineral is lost and is not added back even in the white flours marked "enriched." The body loses about 4 mg of manganese a day, so it must be replaced daily by diet or with supplements. You will get most of the manganese you need in a good multivitamin and a diet rich in the above foods. I don't think it is necessary to take additional manganese supplements if your multivitamin includes manganese.

MAINTAINING STRONG BONES WHILE LOSING WEIGHT

We've just read about the importance of magnesium and manganese in your overall health, but there are some other vitamins and minerals important for bone health while you are losing weight.

Calcium

Calcium is something we hear a lot about in maintaining bone, but it is also critical in metabolism-, mood-, and sleep-regulating pathways, and for normal muscle function. The sad part is that even with so much emphasis on calcium, the average calcium intake for American women is still too low at only 450 milligrams a day. Low calcium also makes weight loss more difficult. The recommended amount for premenopausal women is 1,000 to 1,200 mg daily, and for postmenopausal women not taking estrogen, 1,500 mg daily.

Cutting back dairy products to lose weight is one reason for low calcium intake. We are drinking more diet beverages instead of milk. So, not only are we replacing an important source of calcium, the phosphates in sodas prevent proper absorption of the calcium we are getting. Dairy products are still the richest dietary calcium sources, but there are other sources as well. Vegetables contain much less calcium per serving, and the fiber in vegetables serves to decrease the amount of calcium absorption. If you don't eat dairy products, it really is important to supplement calcium every day.

I caution you to *avoid* calcium products made from *oyster shell or dolomite.* These have been found to be contaminated with toxic heavy metals, such as lead, mercury, and arsenic. Calcium citrate is promoted as being better absorbed, but studies have not consistently confirmed this. Since calcium citrate has less elemental calcium per tablet, you have to remember to *take more tablets* daily. Another option is Tums (a pure calcium carbonate antacid). You may laugh at this, but bioavailability studies of Tums have shown it is readily absorbed and well tolerated. Tums contains no aluminum, so it is safe to take daily. It's inexpensive and easy to carry in your handbag, so there's no excuse for not taking your calcium.

Calcium absorption can be checked by a twenty-four-hour urine test of calcium excretion. This may be appropriate if you are not responding to bone-rebuilding therapies (medication, exercise, hormones, and supplements) or if there is greater bone loss than expected based on the other lab tests. I look at two things with this test. First, very low urinary calcium tells me you're not absorbing calcium very well and may need additional calcium in the diet, or a better estradiol level to help absorb calcium, or additional tests to find out why. Second, very high urinary calcium tells me you are excreting more than you are absorbing, which typically occurs in women when estradiol levels are low.

One question my patients often ask me is, "How do we get enough calcium without getting constipated?" I'll almost guarantee you that if you are getting enough magnesium, which is a very effective natural laxative, you won't have to worry about constipation from your calcium! Remember, the time-tested constipation remedy, Milk of Magnesia, is based on magnesium's ability to stimulate the intestines. Too much magnesium quickly causes diarrhea, so you have a clear indication of getting too much, and when to cut back.

Vitamin D

Vitamin D deficiency may be more common than previously thought. A 1999 study found that about half of the women hospitalized for hip fracture at Brigham and Women's Hospital in Boston between 1995 and 1998 had laboratory evidence of vitamin D deficiency with levels below 30 nmol/L. The authors suggested that restoring vitamin D to optimal levels may reduce the risk of future fractures and may also help the healing of current hip fractures.

VITAMIN AND MINERALS "BONE BUILDERS"

Mineral	Function
Magnesium	Critical for metabolic pathways, muscle contraction, bone growth/formation, and blood pressure regulation
Zinc	DNA and protein synthesis, growth and maintenance of body tissue, blood sugar regulation, and collagen formation
Manganese	Needed for vitamin B, E, and C utilization, energy metabolism, glucose regulation, forming T4, and immune function
Calcium	Maintaining bone-, metabolism-, and sleep-regulating pathways, and normal muscle function
Vitamin D	Aids absorption of calcium from intestinal tract, regulates calcium excretion from kidneys, helps prevent osteoporosis and fractures
Boron	Important in bone metabolism and reduces calcium and magnesium excretion

© 2001 by Elizabeth Lee Vliet, M.D.

VITAMIN AND MINERALS
"BONE BUILDERS"

Dietary Sources	Suggested Daily Dose
Bran cereal, beans, brown rice, nuts, spinach, seafood, whole wheat breads	400–600 mg
Animal foods and seafoods, whole grains	10–25 mg
Nuts, whole grains, raisins, spinach, carrots, broccoli, green peas, oranges, apples, tea leaves, and wheat bran	RDA in multivitamin should be sufficient
Dairy products, leafy greens, broccoli, calcium-fortified fruit juices	1,000–1,200 mg premenopausal 1,500 mg postmenopausal not on estrogen
Milk, eggs, fish, fortified breakfast cereals	400 IU
Vegetables such as green peppers and tomatoes	RDA in multivitamin should be sufficient

Make sure you are getting at least 400 IU of vitamin D daily, and if you already have significant bone loss, ask your doctor to check your blood level of Vitamin D to ensure proper absorption. Vitamin D deficiency is clearly a *preventable* cause of osteoporosis and fractures.

Boron

Boron is a trace mineral that is important in bone metabolism and helps reduce excretion of calcium and magnesium. It is found in a variety of vegetables such as green peppers and tomatoes. Just to be sure, make certain that your multiple vitamin also contains boron. Too much boron is not good either, so make certain you are not taking multiple supplements that give you an excess cumulative amount.

◇ ◇ ◇

So, don't forget your minerals. Just to review, the most important minerals for women experiencing hormonal problems and at risk for bone loss are magnesium, zinc, calcium, vitamin D, manganese, and boron. These minerals play crucial roles as cofactors and catalysts in building bone; in regulating sleep, pain, and mood; and in muscle health and repair. These minerals are absolutely important to us, but you don't have to take the more expensive *colloidal* (fine particles suspended in a uniform medium) versions . . . regular capsules or tablets are readily absorbed by most people unless there is an underlying disease affecting the gastrointestinal tract. In that case, you may want to consider a liquid form.

ANTIOXIDANTS:
WHAT THEY DO, WHERE THEY ARE

All of the cells and tissues of your body are constantly subjected to highly reactive and unstable molecules termed *free radicals* that cause cell damage as they build up. These hostile free radical molecules are a normal byproduct of life, and chemical changes in the body, as well as environmental sources (smoke, ionizing radiation, air pollution, chemicals, toxic heavy metals, and oxidized [rancid] fats). Free radicals by their very chemical nature promote a chain reaction of cell damage by forming more free radicals that, in turn, chemically alter important biological molecules your body needs to function. The function of antioxidants is to protect biomolecules from oxidative damage. Eating food with plenty of natural antioxidants, and taking appropriate antioxidant supplements, helps prevent this type of cell damage.

Research is continuing to find that much biological damage and diseases are induced and/or mediated by injury from free radicals. Inadequate intake of antioxidants is associated with higher risks of cancer, cardiovascular disease, arthritis, cataracts, and many other degenerative diseases. Many good studies confirm that antioxidants help to prevent these and restore health. In addition, antioxidants play a key role in the metabolic pathways that are involved in weight regulation. So make sure you get plenty of the following in your diet!

Beta-carotene

This antioxidant is found in dark yellow vegetables such as carrots, pumpkin, winter squash, sweet potatoes; dark green vegetables such as collard greens, kale, spinach, Swiss chard, broccoli; fruits such as cantaloupe, mango, papaya, and apricots.

Vitamin C

This vitamin is found in fruits such as oranges, grapefruit, cantaloupe, mango, kiwi, papaya, guava, strawberries; vegetables such as broccoli, bell peppers, Brussels sprouts, cabbage, tomatoes, spinach, kale, and potatoes. Higher intake also decreases risk of gallstones in women.

Vitamin E

Vitamin E is found in nuts such as walnuts, almonds, hazelnuts, peanuts, sunflower seeds; oils such as wheat germ oil, vegetable oils; vegetables such as asparagus, broccoli, Brussel sprouts, corn, sweet potato, peas and beans (legumes); grains such as whole wheat, oats, whole grain cereals.

Vitamin E plays a significant antioxidant role counteracting damaging free radical effects, including ones generated from excess glucose. Vitamin E reduces glucose levels and improves insulin sensitivity, amoung other functions. I recommend supplementing with *natural vitamin E,* a superior alternative to the synthetic version. Although more expensive than the synthetic, it is worth spending the extra money in this case. Look for "d" in the name to identify natural vitamin E. For example, d-alpha-tocopherol. Synthetic vitamin E is identified with a "dl."

Selenium

The selenium content of foods grown in soil varies a great deal due to the variability of the mineral in soil in different regions. It is found in vegetables such as broccoli, tomatoes, onions; in grains such as bran, wheat germ, whole grain products;and in fish and poultry

RECOMMENDED DAILY INTAKE OF ANTIOXIDANTS

Beta carotene:	10,000–25,000 IU
Vitamin C:	1,000–2,000 mg
Vitamin E:	400–800 IU (natural form, d-alpha tocopherol)
Selenium:	100–200 mcg

SUPPLEMENTS CRITICAL TO A SUCCESSFUL WEIGHT-LOSS PROGRAM

Coenzyme Q 10

This is an antioxidant, vitaminlike compound that plays a critical role in the energy and oxygenation pathways throughout the body, and it declines as we get older. It has effects similar to vitamin E but is thought to be an even more powerful antioxidant. There is evidence that it helps to improve overall immune function, helps with chronic persistent pain, and helps lower blood pressure and improve cardiovascular response in people with congestive heart failure (CHF).

CoQ10 is found in oily, deep-water fish such as salmon, sardines, and mackerel, but also in spinach and peanuts. There are many "CoQ10" products available now, but quality varies enormously and oral absorption is not always reliable. Since it is an oil-soluble compound, oral forms are better absorbed if taken with a meal containing oily or fatty foods, such as salmon or other cold-water fish. Daryl Spence, R.Ph., (Spence Pharmacy, Ft. Worth, Texas) indicates that oral CoQ10 is poorly absorbed and recommends a sublingual form that can easily be compounded in higher doses with a physician's prescription, or you may want to consider a 50 mg sublingual product from Food Science Laboratories, or VitaLife.

Essential Fatty Acids

Although these are technically considered macronutrients, I am going to discuss them briefly here since so many women now take these as supplements. The body needs a certain amount of the right kind of fat for critical life functions, such as to make hormonelike messengers called prostaglandins, to provide cholesterol as a building block for the steroid hormones (your three estrogens, testosterone, progesterone, and adrenal steroids such as cortisol), to maintain normal nerve conduction and brain function, and for the essential processes of building new cells and repairing cellular damage. Fatty acids are the building blocks the body uses to make necessary fats. The essential fatty acids (EFAs) are ones the body cannot make and must be supplied by foods and/or supplements. There are two categories of EFAs.

Omega-6 Fatty Acids. These include linoleic acid (LA) and gamma linolenic acid (GLA). GLA serves as a precursor for the body to form unsaturated fatty acids, which are important in making cell membrane structures, serving as cellular energy messengers, and to make eicosanoids, another group of important chemical messengers involved in pain, inflammation, immune control, and other functions. Omega-6 fatty acids can be found in raw nuts, seeds, legumes, and unsaturated vegetable oils (borage oil has the highest content). GLA is also found in evening primrose, grapeseed, and sesame oils.

Omega-3 Fatty Acids. These are alpha linolenic acid (ALA) and eicosapentaenoic acid (EPA). Good sources include fish oils—salmon, mackerel, and sardines contain the highest amounts per ounce; vegetable oils such as canola, flaxseeds and flaxseed oil, walnuts and walnut oil. Avoid taking a very large amount of these supplements, which can lead to excess production of "bad" eicosanoids that can increase joint and muscle pain. If you take fish oil supplements, avoid ones that have been heat processed (destroys the EFAs), but do look for ones that have been distilled in a special process to remove contaminates.

I recommend you try to get your EFAs from the food you eat and the rich sources I have identified. However, if you are taking these supplements, balance is crucial. If you take GLA supplements, it is important that you also take EPA as well. The ratio of these two EFAs is important in determining the balance of production of "good" versus "bad" eicosanoids—a balance that is especially important for those trying to lose weight. To improve balance of the "good" eicosanoids, you should need doses of GLA (omega-6 EFA) only in the range of 1 to 10 mg accompanied by 50 to 500 mg of EPA (omega-3 EFA). Figure that the amount of EPA should be about fifty to a hundred times the amount of GLA used.

SUPPLEMENTS AND WEIGHT-LOSS PRODUCTS TO AVOID

The plethora of weight-loss products all with miraculous claims is mind-boggling—and scary. Many of these are dangerous and may complicate underlying medical problems. Don't be misled by the word *natural* when looking for remedies for weight loss. Herbs may be "natural" plants, but many have toxic effects on the heart and liver as well as other side effects, just as some medications may have. Just because compounds are *natural* to plants does not necessarily they are *natural* for humans. This is the same reasoning I used in talking about the horse-derived estrogens, remember? The ones of most concern to me are: ephedra (ma huang), over-the-counter stimulants (phenylephrine, phenylpropasolamine), adrenal glandulars, thyroid glandulars, and ginseng.

Many of the following herbs are used in weight-loss supplements or herbal remedies. I strongly urge you to read the labels before taking any of these products, and do not use any products containing the following herbs.

Herbs

Known to cause acute liver injury, chronic hepatitis, cirrhosis, and/or liver failure: chaparral, comfrey, coltsfoot, germander, margosa oil, mate tea, mistletoe and skullcap, Gordolobo yerba tea, pennyroyal (squawmint) oil, pyrrolizidine alkaloids, aflatoxins, *Amanita phalloides,* Jin Bu Huan (a Chinese herbal product), and others.

Known to increase heart rate, blood pressure (dangerous in people with cardiovascular disease): ephedra (Chinese name: ma huang), excessive amounts of caffeine (not generally shown on labels, but a common adulterant in "tonics"), and others.

Known to cause kidney damage (acute interstitial nephritis and/or renal failure): *Tung Shueh* pills found to be adulterated with an anti-inflammatory agent, *mefanamic acid,* not shown on the label; aristolochic acid; products adulterated with phenylbutazone.

Additional Cautions

St. John's Wort should not be taken with prescription antidepressants (may lead to serotonin excess syndrome), with birth control pills (leads to loss of contraceptive effectiveness), or prescription hormones (decreases effectiveness by 50 percent or more).

Do not take *melatonin* on a nightly basis, as it may cause clinical depression, weight gain, headaches, and elevated cortisol levels in women.

I do not recommend over-the-counter *DHEA*. Most doses are more than women need and can cause weight gain, acne, facial hair, loss of scalp hair, irritability, restless sleep, and sweet cravings.

Soy has antithyroid effects, and may suppress ovarian hormone production in premenopausal women. If you already have thyroid disorders or ovarian imbalances, go easy on soy and other forms of isoflavones such as red clover.

Hormone Glandulars

I don't recommend the use of over-the-counter animal-derived "glandulars" (thyroid or adrenal) for weight loss. In fact, with current concerns about prions causing Mad Cow disease, I don't recommend using ground animal glands at all since we don't know the source of these products.

Whether you use over-the-counter glandulars or prescription thyroid medication, excess thyroid pushes your TSH too low, creating a *hyper*thyroid state. This causes heart arrhythmias and more rapid breakdown of bone and also causes the remaining bone to be more brittle.

Why would you take over-the-counter glandulars or excess thyoid medications? Some health practitioners, newsletters, and Internet sites promote use of thyroid hormones for weight loss based on symptoms of low basal body temperature. This is dangerous for midlife and menopausal woman who are also experiencing loss of estradiol and testosterone that regulate bone metabolism and cardiovascular health. There are now very effective and sensitive blood tests for measuring TSH and thyroid hormones, as well as tests for antibodies to the thyroid gland tissue and to your thyroid hormones. I urge you to work with your physician and follow the guidelines I have outlined in chapter 8 for appropriate thyroid dose adjustments.

Ginseng

Ginseng is often recommended as a "tonic" or energy booster in addition to its supposed effects on helping improve immune function to fight colds and flus. It is often used by women trying to lose weight in the belief that it will boost energy. But recent studies have found that it is no better than placebo and may actually merit some serious concerns. Ginseng can cause high blood pressure and should be avoided if you are already overweight.

WEIGHT-LOSS SABOTEURS

Here is a list of prescription medicines that can sabotage your weight-loss efforts. If you are taking any of these, I encourage you to discuss this with you doctor to explore more appropriate options. Keep in mind, one benefit of attaining a proper hormone balance, as we have discussed throughout this book, is that you may find you don't need some of these medications anymore.

PRESCRIPTION MEDICATIONS
THAT MAY CAUSE WEIGHT GAIN

⋄ **Beta blockers**—block conversion of T4 to T3; aggravate glucose intolerance and insulin resistance; increase risk of developing diabetes; and may cause depression, fatigue, and loss of sexual drive and ability to have orgasm.

⋄ **Tricyclic antidepressants**—these are older medications that all stimulate your appetite and impair insulin-glucose regulation. Serotonin reuptake inhibitors (SSRIs) are a better choice in the short run. Long term, SSRIs can also increase carbohydrate cravings and prolactin levels and cause weight gain. If this happens on SSRIs, ask your doctor to try a different antidepressant such as Wellbutrin.

◇ **Mixed antidepressants**—Serzone has adverse drug interactions with prescription hormones (lowers estradiol levels), and Remeron can make you sleepy and tends to cause
marked weight gain except at very high doses.

◇ **Mood stabilizers**—Depakote (valproate), Tegretol (carba-
mazepine), and Topamax (topiramate) can cause weight
gain and daytime drowsiness.

◇ **Diuretics**—avoid thiazide diuretics (HCTZ or hydrochloro-
thiazide, Dyazide, Maxide, and others) to alleviate the
fluid retention in the premenstrual week. These further
increase potassium loss, which may actually aggravate
PMS symptoms and impair metabolism. They also interfere with normal glucose balance and may increase cholesterol. Try spironolactone (Aldactone) instead if you
actually need a diuretic.

◇ **Lithium**—increases appetite and can cause hypothyroidism, leading to weight gain. It is appropriate for
true manic-depressive illnesses, but try to use the lowest
possible dose and monitor thyroid function carefully.

◇ **Antihistamines**—stimulate appetite, so if taken on a daily
basis for allergies, they may lead to weight gain. Try to just
take them when you have an allergy outbreak rather than
every day.

SUMMARY

Women who are trying to lose excess body fat need and deserve an integrated approach to their health care. Hopefully this chapter will help you
find the best combination of approaches for *you* and alert you to the ones
to avoid. As you begin, remember there are weight-loss saboteurs, both
with prescription medicines that may increase your appetite and add to
your weight gain, as well as herbal and other popular over-the-counter

supplements. You can become toxic on too many vitamin supplements, as well as by taking too much of a particular prescription medicine.

Women often tell me that herbal medicine is "more natural" and *therefore safer*. Herbs aren't *necessarily* "gentler" or "safer" than pharmaceutical products. For example, I have seen quite a number of patients, as well as myself, who have had allergic reactions or toxicity symptoms to herbal products, contrary to the reassurances of herbalists who have said herbs are "balanced" and don't cause allergic reactions. I also have patients who have had adverse reactions to prescription pharmaceuticals. The street runs both ways. If you are taking herbs to have a therapeutic effect, isn't it just possible that they can also have *side* effects? Whenever you are taking "medicinals," *no matter what the source,* there is the potential for benefit as well as the possibility of an undesirable reaction.

Remember, you may not need as much of such medicinals if you focus on all the components of *Your Hormone Power Life Plan* as I have outlined. There is no better medicine to add to good hormone balance than a healthy meal plan, proper vitamin-mineral intake, lots of water, plenty of oxygen, and *moving* the body.

Chapter 18

INTEGRATING
MIND, BODY, AND SPIRIT
FOR LIFELONG SUCCESS

In the previous chapters, I have talked about the importance of caring for the physical aspects of your health—knowing your height, blood pressure, body measurements, body composition, hormone levels, bone density, cholesterol profile and other metabolic tests; working with your physician to achieve your optimal hormone balance; and taking the time to provide your body with the right balance of healthy foods.

Your physical health is not the only dimension, however, that must be addressed to help you be successful for the long run. After all, life is rather like a marathon—you hope to have a long "run," pace yourself so you don't prematurely burn out, and finish strong. So as you look at what you need for lifelong success, your hormonal well-being and an effective meal plan are only the first two legs of the journey. Tapping into the "hormone power" that comes with physical activity and psychological hardiness will be crucial for you to achieve your goals. Putting all these pieces together will give you the best opportunity to fulfill this statement by Ashley Montague:

"The idea is to die young . . . as late as possible."

YOUR HORMONE POWER LIFE PLAN: TAPPING YOUR EXERCISE POWER

If you are struggling with a weight problem, I am sure the last thing you want to be told by another doctor is, "Just get out and exercise." Well, I am not saying *just* exercise. I *am* saying that physical activity is an *essential component* of an integrated weight-loss program for midlife women. Period. You cannot lose excess body fat without being more physically active, along with the right food balance and optimal hormone balance. I know. I have been there. There are hundreds of studies to show that regular exercise improves energy, muscle mass, metabolic rate, and the production of fat-burning, mood-lifting, fatigue-fighting, pain-relieving brain chemical messengers. Physical activity improves the function of every single part of your mind and body.

To lose fat you have two options: reduce your caloric intake or increase your caloric expenditure. You cannot decrease your caloric intake much lower than 1,400 to 1,500 calories daily without slowing your metabolism and getting fatter. So . . . you need to increase caloric expenditure . . . through more physical activity.

From the time I took up serious jogging/running in my first year of medical school in 1975, until 1989 with the last round of surgeries on my neck, I had been diligent about keeping up with exercise and maintaining a healthy body composition. Then I got off track, didn't exercise regularly for several years, and guess what? Those nasty pounds jumped out of hiding and right back onto my body. Darn. I thought I had them licked forever. There was *no* way around it. I had to get active again. I now spend about thirty to forty minutes, four to six days a week, either walking on the treadmill or swimming or doing my pool aerobics against resistance. I make an effort to walk up stairs instead of taking elevators. I look for ways to walk more during daily activities. Every little bit helps.

You can't do it all at once. You need guidance to begin at a level appropriate for you. You must start off slowly and increase your tolerance gradually as you build up stamina. This is crucial to prevent injuries and maintain your motivation. Consult your physician before beginning any type of exercise activities, and ask for a referral to a physical therapist or exercise physiologist to help you get started on an appropriate program.

I find that many overweight women have joint and body pain and are reluctant to exercise, afraid it will cause more pain. After four spine surgeries over the years, I have found just the opposite: If I pace myself and gear my workout to what my body can do safely, then I actually have less pain than I have if I don't exercise at all. As I shared with you in *Screaming to Be Heard,* the physical therapist found ways for me to exercise even though I was in a neck brace and couldn't lift a water pitcher. Many hospitals now have fitness programs and are a good place to start. This is especially important if you are significantly overweight and haven't been exercising, or if you have any type of pain syndrome. Be sure they have experience helping, and are willing to work with, people who have weight problems and other physical limitations.

Tips for Getting Started: Does It Have to Be "All or Nothing"?

Generally, *anything* is better than nothing. This is especially true with physical activity.

Some people resist exercising because there is also a perception that they must run X number of miles for X amount of time or there will be no benefits. This isn't true. You simply need to become more active in your usual daily life. This is more realistic, more likely to be implemented, and, therefore, more effective. Will that be enough? To begin with, yes. Over time, the amount of physical activity you need depends on your metabolism and how much excess fat you have to lose. Gradual increases in activity are very doable, so let's look at some tips to get started.

Tip #1: Walk more. No matter where, or how fast, just do it more. Walking helps stimulate your metabolism and helps your fat-burning pathways work more efficiently. You do not have to work up a sweat to benefit. Even if you walk for only five to ten minutes at a time, it helps. If you walk for ten minutes three times a day, that adds up to several hours a week and puts a meaningful dent in your couch-potato time. Walk *to* lunch. Pack a lunch and spend the rest of your lunch hour *walking, not sitting* in the office break room or a restaurant.

Tip #2: Don't fall into the food reward trap. Just because you have been "good" and increased your activity doesn't mean you can now eat anything you want. If you add activity and do not increase your food intake, you will see a steady loss of fat because you shifted to more calories *out* than calories *in.*

Tip #3: Boost metabolic rate with more muscle. Increased activity levels help jumpstart a sluggish metabolism. This occurs because more activity builds more muscles, which revs up your metabolism because muscles burn a lot more calories than fat. Having more muscle means a higher metabolic rate over the whole day, every day. You burn more calories not only when exercising, but also when you are watching TV, driving a car, and even when you are sleeping.

Tip # 4: Incorporate more activity into each day.
- ◇ Avoid elevators or escalators.
- ◇ Substitute manual devices for mechanical devices whenever possible.
- ◇ Walk to do your errands whenever possible.
- ◇ Avoid remote controls.
- ◇ Park further away from entrances and walk more.
- ◇ Stand more than you are sitting (if you can do a task at a counter, you will burn more calories standing than sitting).
- ◇ Walk for fitness at least a total of thirty minutes per day or one mile cumulatively (remember you can break this into segments).

Tip #5: Incorporate more strengthening activities into each day. The idea here is to look for the hard way to do things instead of the easiest.
- ◇ Rise from a chair without using your arms to assist.
- ◇ Lift heavier objects with one arm instead of two.
- ◇ Stand on one leg while waiting in line; alternate and use the other leg.
- ◇ Climb stairs using hand rails only lightly for balance, make your legs work harder.
- ◇ Sit down slowly using your muscles for control, rather than falling into the chair letting gravity do the work.
- ◇ Walk up and down stairs with exaggerated slow movements.

◇ Lift and lower objects slowly rather than swinging them using momentum to help.

◇ Don't rock your body to rise from a sitting position; use your abdominal muscles instead.

◇ Push down on floor with your toes while sitting. Release and repeat twenty times.

◇ Press your spine into the back of a chair while sitting. Release and repeat twenty times.

◇ Press legs together when sitting or lying. Release and repeat twenty times.

◇ Do abdominal tightening while riding in a car.

◇ Place hands, palms up, under your desk while you are sitting, and pull up against the desk several times a day.

◇ Push head back against high-backed seat, hold ten seconds, release, and repeat twenty times.

◇ Perform Kegel (pelvic floor) exercises any time, anywhere. No one will know why you are really smiling!

The "Lifestyle Approach" Grows Up and Becomes an Exercise Program

The "Lifestyle Approach" I outlined above is a good first step toward a more active life. An exercise program offers a more robust alternative. Once you've changed your habits, see progress, and feel better, you are ready for a more detailed plan designed to give greater results. Don't be intimidated. For the majority of the population, regardless of your current health, the benefits of exercise outweigh any potential negatives, if done correctly and at the proper level. Let me set the record straight, however, on some common exercise misconceptions.

Misconception: "Exercise increases your appetite. I'll eat too much if I work out."

Fact: Exercise actually decreases your appetite if you are working out within your aerobic heart rate range.

If your intensity is too high and you overshoot your aerobic range, you deplete muscle and liver glycogen stores, which makes you hungrier after a workout. If you stray, a slight increase in food intake is usually more than offset by two factors: calories expended by the exercise itself, and your increased metabolic rate for several hours after your workout is over.

Misconception: "The more you sweat, the faster you lose weight."

Fact: There is no benefit to excessive sweating, and it may be dangerous, particularly if you are on blood pressure medications or diuretics or are out of shape.

Don't wear "sauna suits" or excess clothes to increase sweating. You'll just get dizzy, faint, and light-headed and be losing only water weight, not fat.

Misconception: "Women shouldn't exercise during their periods. Now that I hit perimenopause, I have a period every two weeks, and I don't feel like exercising, so I get out of the habit."

Fact: There is no medical reason for not exercising during your period.

Physical activity actually helps the bloating and crampy feelings and lifts low moods that hit at this time. If your energy is lower, or the bleeding heavy, just take it a little slower than usual, or maybe do a little shorter workout. If you are bleeding more often, it's time to talk with a physician about options to smooth out the hormonal turbulence, control the bleeding, and better regulate your cycles.

Misconception: "In order for exercise to be effective, you have to work out every day, and I don't have time, so it won't do me any good."

Fact: You don't have to work out every day to see some positive changes.

Simply increasing your physical movement throughout the day, every day, will help your body burn more calories. Exercising at your aerobic heart rate range just three times a week for around twenty minutes each time will burn calories, stimulate your metabolism, and lead to more fat loss. Can't you make twenty minutes, just three days a week, an important time commitment for *you* in the midst of all you do for others?

Misconception: "Exercise has to be strenuous to lose weight and I hurt too much to do anything strenuous enough to do me any good."

Fact: Exercise does not have to be strenuous to be effective.

If you are overweight and out of shape, "really strenuous" exercise would probably put you above your aerobic range and would not be helping as much for losing fat. You will be surprised how quickly just simple walking will get your heart rate into the target range. This is all you need to do. Brisk walking for thirty minutes a day can burn up to fifteen pounds a year. Not bad.

Misconception: "Aerobic exercise is no better than any other form of exercise for weight loss."

Fact: Getting your heart rate to the aerobic range will speed up your metabolism better.

Increased metabolism from aerobic exercise also lasts four to eight hours after you stop exercising, so additional calories will be burned off long after you finish working out. Nonaerobic exercise, like housework or gardening or weight lifting, doesn't boost your metabolism to the same degree, but it will improve muscle mass and strength, which has the benefits I listed above.

WHAT ARE THE "AEROBIC HEART RATE" AND "TARGET HEART RATE RANGE"?

Aerobic heart rate is the number of heartbeats per minute that will increase the energy demands but still maintain enough oxygen delivery to combine with glucose and "burn" to provide fuel. If you work too hard and increase your heart rate above this level, you force the body to use "anaerobic" (i.e., without oxygen) pathways. Your *target heart rate range* (THR) is a heart rate between 60 to 85 percent of the heart's maximum capacity of beats per minute that will still allow it to pump blood to the body.

Your maxium heart rate is based on age: the older you are, the lower the number of maximum beats per minute. To calculate your target heart rate range, you can use this general formula to help you determine what your heart rate should be during exercise or physical activity. It's always best, however, to have your doctor give you a specific OK on these ranges since medications like beta blockers and some antidepressants may affect your heart rate.

CALCULATION OF
TARGET HEART RATE RANGE (THR)

$220 -$ age $=$ PMHR $\times$ 0.6 $=$ beats per minute for minimum THR

$220 -$ age $=$ PMHR $\times$ 0.85 $=$ beats per minute for maximum THR

Divide the number of beats per minute by 6 to get beats per 10 seconds.

Then take your pulse for 10 seconds while you are exercising to see if you have reached the target range between 60 and 85 percent of predicted maximum heart rate (PMHR).

© 2001 by Elizabeth Lee Vliet, M.D.

To make checking your THR easier, I suggest purchasing a heart rate monitor to wear during exercise. You can buy one locally at a sporting goods store or on the Web. These can be set to alert you when you drop below or go above your THR. One I recommend is the Polar Heart Rate Monitor. They have many models, from basic ones to those that allow you to download exercise information into your computer or even wear while swimming.

If you exercise *above* your THR (anaerobic exercise), you will be burning muscle glycogen instead of fat, which accumulates more lactic acid in the muscles, leading to stiff, sore muscles the next day. You will run out of "fuel" in the muscles, so you can't continue exercising very long. If you exercise *below* the lower limit of your THR, you are not stimulating the heart enough to improve cardiovascular fitness or to promote significant fat burning. Either way, if you are not exercising in your proper target range, you won't see the benefits you want and are less likely to keep up your program.

YOUR HORMONE POWER LIFE PLAN: **TAPPING YOUR EXERCISE POWER**

Aerobic Activities

When developing an exercise program, you need to ask yourself, "what activities do I *like* to do?" If you don't like it, you won't keep it up. Then think about *where* you are going to exercise. If it isn't convenient, you won't keep it up. If you like to walk, is there a nearby walking path, school track, or shopping mall? If you hate walking and love the music and "energy" of aerobics classes, you may want to consider joining a fitness center. This may also give you access to an exercise physiologist or certified personal trainer who can set up a program for you and show you how to monitor your progress.

Then think about with whom, and when, works better for your exercise needs. Do you like having the quiet time of exercising by yourself, or will you be more motivated to work out with a friend? Can you take your kids and the dog with you and make it a family outing? Are you a morning person, or do you feel better if you exercise at the end of the day? Regardless of *when* you exercise, remember to do a five to ten minute warm-up at the beginning of each session to gradually bring your heart rate up. Also remember to do five to ten minutes of cool-down at the end, to gradually slow your heart back to normal.

I recommend aerobic activities that are low impact to avoid injury to your joints. These include brisk walking (outside or on a treadmill indoors), swimming, water-walking, aqua-aerobics, bike riding, or stationary cycling. If you are overweight, it is especially helpful to do pool exercises because water helps support you and reduces strain on muscles and joints. Once you have increased your activity level, are comfortable with a general exercise routine, and reach a better level of fitness, you may be ready to adjust your workout routine to a higher intensity that will increase fat burning and maximize weight loss. You can do that very simply in several ways:

- ◇ Gradually increase your *frequency* of exercise.
- ◇ Gradually increase your *duration* of exercise.
- ◇ Increase the *intensity* of your exercise; for example, go from 60 percent to 75 percent of your PMHR. To continue effective fat burning with exercise, it helps to keep the intensity about in the middle of your predicted range.

Strengthening Activities

Aerobic activity improves cardiovascular fitness and increases the use of fat stores for fuel. Strengthening activities help to build more muscle mass and overall stronger bones and muscles. Strength, or weight, training, uses progressive resistance with machines or free weights. You can do these at home, in the simple ways I described earlier in this chapter; you can also purchase one of the excellent videotapes available for more intensive work-outs, or you can work with a trainer at a health club. Both aerobic and strength-training components work together to help you lose excess body fat and feel better about yourself.

Flexibility Activities

Flexibility, or the ease and degree to which a joint can move through a complete range of motion, helps prevent and reduce injury. Notice your cat or dog. They often stretch before they start moving. Stretching makes you more limber and helps improve circulation. Examples of activities that improve flexibility, balance, and strength are Tai Chi, Qi Gong, yoga, Callenetics, and Pilates. There are excellent videotapes available to help you start any one of these programs. I also highly recommend a book called *Stretching* by Bob Anderson. It describes ways to stretch all the muscle groups at many levels of difficulty and is well illustrated.

MEASURING IMPROVEMENTS

You will feel, and then see, progress after a few weeks. Remember that I said earlier you may not see loss of a lot of pounds on the scale, because you are replacing lightweight fat with heavier, denser muscle mass. What you will see, though, is that your clothes fit better. You will notice that you are sleeping better and awakening refreshed. Your resting pulse will start to decrease, another good sign of an improving fitness level.

Objective measures of your progress should be tracked in a chart that you keep in your health notebook. These include body measurements, BMI, body composition, WHR, resting pulse, and (if you insist) your weight. But you need to check these only once a month. Don't obsess over the numbers . . . just focus on feeling better.

As your fitness improves, you may need to increase the intensity of your aerobic training to stay in your THR range because you can do more work with less effort. For example, if you are walking, now start swinging your arms more, or add some small hand weights, or try race walking, or find a hillier course. If you are doing your walking on a treadmill, you can start gradually increasing the incline or the speed. Continue to monitor your heart rate and stay in your THR range.

MAINTENANCE

Remember, exercise is not a quick fix. You don't stop once you lose weight. Think of it like eating, breathing, sleeping, and drinking water. You need to do it on a regular basis. The good news is that once exercise becomes a habit, it will be easier to maintain your fitness than it was to start your new program. When you start to get discouraged or bored or tired of exercising, just remind yourself of how sluggish and lethargic you felt before you started your program. I know that if I do not do my pool exercises every day, I will pay for it in more neck and back pain, and more stiffness. Since I don't like being in pain, I get in the pool every day and do my workout. I *choose* to exercise so I can continue feeling good and have the energy I want to do my work and enjoy activities I love! And, if you have to miss a day or so, don't take too long a break or you may not *get back* to it! *Go for it!* You deserve to feel better and have a more fit body!

YOUR HORMONE POWER LIFE PLAN:
TAPPING YOUR MIND POWER

I have profound belief in, and respect for, the power of the mind and spirit in all aspects of health, disease, and the healing process. Indeed, these dimensions may be the most critical of all as we seek the "wellness of being" that is at the core of our human quest, instead of our cultural emphasis on doing and achieving. I know from a deep personal level and from my professional experience that healing in its fullest sense must include attention to our distressed spirits, not only our damaged bodies.

The body feels the pain of our soul and spirit, which your mind may block out of consciousness. Your mind and your thoughts affect your body in many ways, both chemically in the physical sense, and psychologically in how you see yourself. Our cells know and communicate things about us that are invisible to our eyes and ears. If our mind is permeated with negative thoughts, it is like sludge blocking the free flow of water in a creek.

Tapping into your mind power means getting in there and "mucking out the stables" of all the negative thoughts that sabotage your efforts to reach your goals. For women, one of the biggest saboteurs is a negative self-image. Feeling dissatisfied with, and even angry at, your body because you don't like how you look tends to rob you of the energy you need to move forward. Instead of struggling with the burden of your perceived inadequacies, use these thoughts as a foundation for change. Experience these feelings as a way out of the depths of pain from being overweight and unhappy with your body.

Think of this process of regaining your healthy body as one of moving from creating beauty in the cosmetic sense to creating the beautiful person of *you*. One who has known struggle and come out of the darkness into the light. One who has faced uncertainty and found her strength. One who accepts that none of us has a "perfect" body, and yet we are all beautiful in some way to those who care about us. Celebrate what is right, good, and wonderful about you as a person, and the wonderment of your body, no matter its current form.

YOUR HORMONE POWER LIFE PLAN:
COPING WITH CHANGE AT
"THE CHANGE OF LIFE"

For many women, midlife is a time of uncertainty as our roles and needs change. We are no longer who we were; yet we may not yet know who we want to become. As women, we face many changes throughout our lives: physical changes, role changes, emotional changes, spiritual changes. How you view change is a significant part of the challenge. Do you feel overwhelmed by changes in your life, or are changes exciting to you? Do you see them as challenges or threats, crises or opportunities?

One woman, moving from Norfolk, Virginia, to New York City on her own, described her feelings about this major change: "I feel a sense of petrified excitement!" Her words really hit me. In those two words—petrified excitement—she captured the essence of the mixture of emotions that often hits us when we have significant changes in our lives. Even positive changes create a stress response in our bodies as we adapt. The degree of impact on our health is dramatically intensified when we perceive changes as negative.

Having a sense of control over, and acceptance of, changes that come in our lives will enhance our inner strength and also facilitate a healthier view of self. Remember that if you focus on daydreaming about the person you would like to be, you end up wasting the time to enjoy being the person you are now. This can be a time to choose from many possibilities of actions, feelings, and thoughts. As a woman at midlife and beyond, you are moving from creating an "other" new life to creating *your* own new life, new goals, new priorities, new interests, new outlooks. But how do you choose? How do you focus? How do you get away from the "busyness" of daily life to really look at and reflect on all these questions?

FINDING YOU

"Knowing yourself takes time being with yourself."

This statement seems so obvious, and yet how often do we as women take the time to do it? In addition to the demanding careers each of us may have, we are giving to others day in and day out—as the twenty-four-hour-a-day mother, the attentive wife, the dutiful daughter, the dedicated community volunteer, the caretaker of the ill, the teacher of children, the social-political activist, the keeper of the calendar. Women are constantly "switching hats," as our multiple roles require that we dip into diverse areas of skills-insights-wisdom when new demands emerge. A man may have one primary career focus for his entire life. Women have many.

Do you really know who *you* are and what you want out of life? Do you really know *why* weight loss is important to you? Have you looked within to find out? Are you trying to meet someone else's ideal for what your body should look like, or are you doing it for you?

Your sense of self-worth and feeling of direction in your life is enhanced greatly by setting aside time to explore what is meaningful for you. Instead of investing everything in *doing* for others, this is a time to invest in *being* with yourself, getting to know the inner you, and what is important for your sense of soul purpose. This investment in you will nourish you for the years ahead.

Why not take time right now to write down the first six things that come immediately to mind as you read these statements:

1. I want to lose excess fat/weight because:
2. If I knew I only had six months to live, I would want to accomplish/finish:

Now, meld these two sets of answers in a way that fits for you. Use your imagination. Look at your lists. Are you trying to lose weight because of external forces? Or, do you see losing weight as a way to help you accomplish the items on your second list? I encourage you to take some time to answer these questions and start planning the second half of your life. Take a step outside any self-imposed limits. Take your own personal "sabbatical" to look a little deeper into your life and the aspects that you might want to change, improve, expand. Embrace solitude, take "me" time, meet a physical or intellectual challenge that is meaningful to you, go out and be in nature, whatever works for you.

> "You have to leave the city of your comfort, and go into the wilderness of your intuition. . . . What you'll discover will be wonderful. What you'll discover will be yourself!"
> —Alan Alda

YOUR HORMONE POWER LIFE PLAN: TAPPING YOUR STRESS MANAGEMENT STRATEGIES

Take a look at the ways that stress in your life aggravates your weight problems and makes it harder for you to lose excess fat. Stress plays a direct role in negatively influencing the chemical messengers that are out of balance and contributes to toxic weight gain as I described in chapter 9. In addition, stress saps our mental ability to focus on constructive solutions and explore new strategies for success. Stress keeps us stuck in our comfortable, and often unhealthy, patterns.

What are some simple, effective ways to break out of the vicious cycle of stress sabotaging your weight loss?

Strategy #1: Look for ways of reducing avoidable negative stresses, and look for ways of minimizing the adverse effects of unavoidable stresses.

Strategy #2: If stresses in your life can't be changed or eliminated, try working them out: Use deep breathing, walking, hitting tennis balls against a backboard, taking a plastic bat and beating up on a bed, or some other physical release form you like (that is still socially acceptable!).

Strategy #3: Learn the "relaxation response," popularized by Dr. Herbert Benson, but used for hundreds of years in many cultures. You can elicit the relaxation response using a variety of techniques: visualization, progressive muscle relaxation, self-hypnosis, autogenic conditioning, meditation and others. There are many good books and tapes available to guide you in using these approaches.

Strategy #4: Get a massage. This is an incredibly effective stress-management technique, especially during the premenstrual week. It improves relaxation; boosts endorphins; improves circulation; and decreases muscle tension, headaches, and back pain. Look for a registered American Association of Massage Therapy certified therapeutic massage therapist in your phone book. If you feel guilty about doing this for yourself, get your doctor to write a prescription for massage therapy for pain management.

Strategy #5: Try a personal coach or counseler to help you find more effective ways to deal with stress. It is amazing how much those outside, objective eyes can see things we miss when we are "up to our ass in alligators," as the saying goes. There are often a variety of counseling options through your health plan or through your workplace's employee assistance program. Getting an outside perspective on what you can do helps you feel more in control, which then decreases the body's "fight or flight" cortisol outpouring in response to stress. Too much cortisol adds fat to your middle, so you need to get the stress under control.

Strategy #6: Don't overlook major depression that saps your mental and physical energy and robs your spirit. Nearly everyone has occasional down, moody times or bouts of sadness and discouragement that may last for a short time. When do the "blues and blahs" become a major depressive disorder, requiring professional intervention and possibly medication treatment? When a black mood settles in and remains for several weeks, sapping your energy, appetite, interest in life and activities you usually enjoy, and altering your sleep, you may be clinically depressed and need to see a professional for evaluation and consideration of antidepressant medication. This is especially true if you feel so overwhelmed or sad that you are thinking about taking your life.

Clinical, or biological, depression is a medical illness that is caused by chemical imbalances in the neurotransmitter or "messenger" molecules in the brain. It is two to three times more common in women, with the gender differences beginning in puberty and ending after menopause. These rates are even higher in women who are obese, likely due to the many metabolic and hormonal factors I have been describing throughout this book. Lack of proper treatment not only causes untold suffering, lost productivity, and diminished quality of life, but is also a major risk factor in suicide. The lifetime risk of death from suicide in major depressive illness is greater than the lifetime risk of death from breast cancer. This is a tragic loss when we consider that treatment of depression is successful for 80 to 90 percent of sufferers, with proper diagnosis and careful use of medication.

Don't let yourself go without professional help if you have any of the symptoms I have described. This physical, or biological, form of depression is not likely to be cured by "talk" therapies alone. Proper medical diagnosis can identify this form of depression, rule out other medical causes for the symptoms, and prescribe medication to reestablish the normal chemical balance.

YOUR HORMONE POWER LIFE PLAN: FOOD FOR THE SOUL— TOUCHING YOUR SPIRITUAL SELF

In the sixth century B.C.E., Pythagorous wrote: "The physician's task is to teach men and women the physical and spiritual laws of life, and to live in accordance with God's purpose for them."

In the ancient arts of all cultures, and in the tradition of the physician as "healer," the emphasis had traditionally been on the whole person. This included addressing spiritual needs as well as physical and emotional needs. As the "science" of medicine evolved, in the last hundred years or so, the care of patients has become very compartmentalized. A variety of medical and surgical specialists attend to the physical body. Psychiatrists or psychologists attend to the needs of the mind. Our soul-spirit pain is turned over to ministers, rabbis, or priests for "treatment." Most commonly, none of these groups talk to each other for an integrated approach to the whole person. Ultimately, such partition of the mind, body, and spirit leads to artificial divisions that cannot lead to true healing and wellness.

Just as our bodies and minds change, our spirit grows in new directions as we move onward in our life journey. As we get older and wiser, we learn to cherish the considerable skills, insights, and wisdom we've accumulated, adapting to all of the changes that have occurred throughout our lives, weaving these experiences into our own unique tapestry. Sharing this with those around us gives our life meaning and purpose, a transcendence. Make time for this dimension of your life. Your survival, spiritually and physically, may well depend on your listening to your spirit calling to you to heed its needs.

Even with my emphasis on the importance of hormone connections in this book, I believe that we need a strong sense of faith and purpose in life as our foundation. On this base we can build a wellness lifestyle, and add medical approaches (hormones, medications, surgery) when needed. I know firsthand how important all of these are in achieving optimal health. I have sunk to the depths of despair during my own health crises, and have been forced to heed the call of my spirit to attend to that dimension in my healing journey. Be still . . . and listen to the unspoken messages of your body, as it calls you to pay attention to its needs and those of your battered spirit . . . you'll be guided on the steps to take toward healing and wholeness.

GO FORWARD NOW, FOR YOU

As you weave together the threads of *Your Hormone Power Life Plan* for you, remember balance can be achieved in different ways, with different techniques, for different individuals. The key is to weave and blend my suggestions of therapeutic approaches into your own tapestry. It is possible to find a way out of the hormonal haze and middle spread. Women like you have done it. Now it is your turn. Pay careful attention to healthy food, optimal hormonal balance, exercise, optimal vitamin and mineral supplements, and moving the body. Pump up your positive attitude. Find pleasure in your life. Use meditation and prayer. Make your choices from knowledge, not fear. In this book, I have provided you the information you need to be successful. Now it is up to you. Start with the options that feel right for you, trust your intuition, and begin. It's not too late to regain your health, zest, and vitality.

This time of life is not about losing weight just to be thin; it is about creating a healthy body and mind to carry you with strength into the years ahead. This book is not just about weight loss, it is about *health.* Your health. Your zest. Your energy. This book is about reclaiming your power over your life. Your life. Your power. Your power that comes when your body, mind, and spirit are whole and balanced again. Claim it.

> "You gain strength, courage and confidence by every experience in which you really stop to look fear in the face. . . . You must *do* the thing you think you cannot do."
> —Eleanor Roosevelt

> **"Don't compromise yourself. You are all you've got."**
> —Janis Joplin

GLOSSARY OF TERMS AND LIST OF MEDICAL ACRONYMS

LIST OF MEDICAL ACRONYMS

Hormones

E1–estrone
E2–estradiol
E3–estriol
T4–thyroxine (thyroid)
T3–triiodothyronine (thyroid)
FSH–follicle stimulating hormone
LH–luteinizing hormone
SHBG–sex hormone binding globulin
TSH–thyroid stimulating hormone
GH–growth hormone

Measurements

dl–deciliter
cc–cubic centimeter (1 cc = 1 ml)
mcg–microgram
mg–milligram
ml–milliliter (1 ml = 1 cc)
ng–nanogram
pg–picogram

Other Terms

BCP–birth control pill
BMI–body mass index
BMR–basal metabolic rate
BTL–bilateral tubal ligation
CHOL–cholesterol
CVD–cardiovascular disease
DEXA–dual energy X-ray absorptiometry
DA–dopamine
EPI–epinephrine
EFA–essential fatty acids
ERT–estrogen replacement therapy
FFA–free fatty acids
GABA–gamma aminobutyric acid

GLA–gamma linolenic acid
HDL–high density lipoprotein ("good" cholesterol)
HRT–hormone replacement therapy
IUD–intra-uterine device
LDL–low density lipoprotein ("bad" cholesterol)
NE–norepinephrine
NTx–N-telopeptide (bone breakdown product)
OC or **OCP**–oral contraceptive pill
PCOS–polycystic ovary syndrome (also abbreviated **PCO**)
PMS–premenstrual syndrome, more severe form called **PMDD**–premenstrual dysphoric disorder
SERMS–selective estrogen receptor modulators
ST–serotonin, also called **5-HT** (5-hydroxytryptophan)
TG–triglycerides

GLOSSARY OF TERMS

This is a glossary of medical terms I have used in my book. If you are going to take charge of your health, it will help for you to become informed about what these terms mean, so that you will understand terms used by your physician.

ABLATION: to remove, as in *endometrial* ablation–a surgical technique to remove as much as possible of the uterine lining (endometrium) to prevent heavy bleeding and reduce the risk of endometrial cancer.

ADRENAL GLANDS: Two small glands situated on top of the kidneys, which secrete steroid hormones (cortisol, aldosterone, DHEA) and the stress hormones epinephrine and norepinephrine (sometimes grouped together in common usage and called *adrenaline*).

AFFECT (AFFECTIVE): A term used to mean "mood" or range of emotional expression. "Affective" refers to emotional content or to disorders of mood.

ALOPECIA: Loss of hair that is excessive and abnormal. There are many medical, dietary, and lifestyle causes. Anorexia, bulimia and decline in ovarian and thyroid hormones are common causes in women.

AMENORRHEA: The absence of menstrual bleeding in a woman who has not gone through menopause; may be due to prolonged stress, thyroid disorders, excessive exercise, eating disorders, premature ovarian failure, and others.

AMINE(S): Compound(s) that contain a nitrogen atom, found in foods.

AMINO ACIDS: Chemical molecules found in foods that serve as the "building blocks" for the body to make its proteins. *Essential amino acids* are those that the body cannot synthesize and that must be included in the food we eat. Dietary protein containing all of the essential amino acids is "complete protein" and can be obtained from animal/dairy products and also by combining any three of the following: nuts, grains, seeds, or legumes at one meal.

ANABOLIC: A term meaning "to build up," as in the *anabolic* phase of metabolism, a process of using nutrients to build larger molecules that are used by the body for growth, repair and healing. See also *catabolic* and *metabolism.*

ANABOLIC STEROIDS: Hormones that stimulate the growth of bone and muscle (lean body mass) and have male ("virilizing") effects on body chemistry and shape.

ANDROGENS: A group of hormones that produces masculine effects on the body. This group of hormones is produced by both the adrenal glands and the gonads (testes in males and ovaries in females). Androgens are produced in much smaller amounts in women compared to men. Androgens decrease with aging in both men and women, but after menopause the levels of androgens in women are higher relative to the amount of estrogen that remains. This change in balance of androgens to estrogen produces the characteristic body changes (waist area fat, hair growth on face and chin, etc.) seen in older women.

ANDROGENIC: An adjective used to describe substances (natural or synthetic) that produce masculine changes in the body: stimulating male pattern hair growth (or loss), oily skin, acne, deepening of the voice, increased appetite, increased muscle mass, increased bone mass, and increased total cholesterol with lower HDL.

ANDROSTENEDIONE: An androgenic hormone produced by the ovaries, testes, and adrenal glands; excess levels in women (such as in PCOS) lead to unwanted facial hair, acne, infertility, body fat gain around the middle of the body, oily skin, and other masculinizing effects.

ANGINA: Pain in the arm, neck, or chest caused by lack of blood supply (ischemia) to the heart.

ANTIBODIES: Protein substances produced by the body (or transferred from a mother to infant during pregnancy) that react with foreign substances called antigens as part of our immune process. Antibodies are made to foreign tissue such as grafts, bacteria and viruses; antibodies may also be produced against our own body organs (thyroid, ovary, etc.) in the autoimmune disorders.

ANTIGEN: A substance that triggers the formation of antibodies to stimulate an immune reaction; may be introduced from external sources (bacteria, viruses, etc.) or formed within the body.

ANTIOXIDANT: Substances such as vitamins A, C, and E, beta-carotene, and selenium, which protect the cellular structures from oxidative damage caused by free radicals.

ATHEROSCLEROSIS: Artery-clogging deposits formed by cholesterol, fibrin and "sticky" platelets; a major cause of heart attacks, strokes, angina, and other cardiovascular disease.

ATROPHY: Wasting or thinning of tissues or organs.

BENIGN: Non-cancerous or nonmalignant.

BIOAVAILABLE: A substance, often carried in the bloodstream, that is unattached to carrier proteins and therefore able to bind to special receptor sites on cells throughout the body. The amount of a compound or hormone that is "bioavailable" is also called "active" or "free fraction."

BIOFLAVINOIDS: Substances found in plants along with vitamin C that exert a beneficial effect upon the walls of the blood and lymphatic vessels.

BIOIDENTICAL: A molecule that is exactly the same makeup and configuration as those made by the body. Hormones that are "bioidentical" may be made in the laboratory from building blocks found in plants, but end up with the same chemical structure as the hormones made by body organs such as the thyroid and ovary. Bioidentical hormones are often called "natural" hormones, but "natural" may also refer to a biological source (such as the horse) that produces molecules different from those made by the human body. Bioidentical is a more correct term than "natural" when referring to the types made by the human body and pharmaceuticals that are designed to duplicate ones made by the body.

BISPHOSPHONATES: A group of medications that prevent excess bone break-down, and stimulate the formation of healthy new bone. Examples are Fosamax, Actonel.

BODY MASS INDEX (BMI): A scientific way of determining body composition. It is calculated according to the formula BMI = weight (kilogram)/height squared (meters). The normal BMI for women ranges from 20 to 25 kg/m^2 and many hormonal and menstrual problems can be overcome by keeping weight in the normal range.

BONE RESORPTION: The normal process of bone break-down or "remodeling" that occurs throughout our lives to allow healthy strong bone to replace older, brittle bone. Resorption can lead to osteoporosis if the bone building process slows down too much, and breakdown (or "withdrawal") of bone exceeds bone formation.

BOUND HORMONE: Hormone that is circulating in the bloodstream connected to a carrier protein (such as sex-hormone binding globulin, SHBG or corticosteroid binding globulin, CBG), and therefore is not "free" to be biologically active at cell receptor sites. See also *free hormone*.

BREAKTHROUGH BLEEDING (BTB): Irregular vaginal bleeding or spotting occurring in women when they are taking oral contraceptives or postmenopausal hormone therapy.

CALCIUM: A crucial mineral involved in maintaining normal bone strength/density, and normal nerve and muscle function.

CALCITONIN (Thyrocalcitonin): A hormone produced in the thyroid gland that regulates calcium balance in the body.

CANCER: A malignant growth/tumor with rapid multiplication of abnormal cells which may spread to and invade distant body parts.

CARDIOVASCULAR DISEASE (CVD): Disease of the heart, arteries, veins, and capillaries that make up the circulatory system.

CATABOLIC: A term meaning "to break down," as in the *catabolic* phase of metabolism, a process of breaking nutrients into smaller molecules that are either utilized by the body for growth and repair, or excreted through the skin, lungs, kidneys and bowels. See also *anabolic* and *metabolism.*

CAT SCAN: A computerized X ray of consecutive sections of the body, which is used to look for tumors, masses, and other abnormal structural changes inside the body.

CELL: The basic unit of structure of all animals and plants that carries out the physical functions of life processes, either by itself or working together with other cells making up organs.

CELLULITE: Fatty deposits resulting in a dimply or lumpy appearance of the skin. It is gradually lost with proper fluid intake, exercise, and overall weight loss.

CERVIX: The opening of the uterus that projects into the vagina. It is also called the mouth of the womb. Some women report that the penis thrusting against the cervix during intercourse leads to greater sexual stimulation and more intense orgasm, which may be a reason to leave the cervix if a woman needs to have the uterus removed.

CHOLESTEROL: An important body molecule that is the precursor for the body to make sex hormones, adrenal hormones, and other molecules. It is found in the blood in three forms: high density lipoprotein (HDL), which *protects* against plaque formation in the arteries (atherosclerosis); low density lipoprotein (LDL), which *promotes* plaque formation (atherosclerosis); and very low density lipoprotein (VLDL), also a plaque promoter. Cholesterol is produced in the liver even when dietary intake is lowered, and it is found in all animal fats and oils (butter, milk, meat, cheese, etc.).

CIRCADIAN RHYTHM: The regular, rhythmic pattern of changes in biological activity and function that occurs over the course of a day. Examples of circadian rhythms are our sleep–wake cycle, the daily cyclic variation in cortisol and melatonin secretion, among many others.

CLIMACTERIC: The span of years in a woman's life when hormone levels are gradually decreasing, leading to changes in body shape and function ultimately ending in the last menstrual period.

CLOTTING FACTORS: Substances carried in the bloodstream that promote coagulation (the process of clotting), such as prothrombin; thrombin; thromboplastin; calcium in ionic form; and fibrinogen. Clotting can be retarded by cold, smooth surfaces, and other substances. Clotting is hastened by warming or by providing a rough surface (such as plaque inside arteries). Medications may be given to promote or decrease clotting.

CLITORIS: The female equivalent (embryologically) of the penis. It is a small bulb found at the top of the vulva, just below the pubic bone, and is covered by a hood of tissue. It contains erectile tissue and nerve endings that are very sensitive to stimulation and enhance a woman's sexual arousal and orgasm. Clitoral nerve endings become less sensitive at menopause with declining hormone levels.

CLUSTER HEADACHE: A severe and intense headache, more common in males, which lasts several hours and may recur frequently over a six- to eight-week period.

COMBINED ORAL CONTRACEPTIVE PILL (OC): A contraceptive pill containing both female sex hormones, estrogen and a synthetic progestin. (To contrast the *combined* OC, there are also progestin-only contraceptives (Micronor is an oral tablet; Norplant and Depo-Provera are long-acting implants/injectables).

COMPLEX CARBOHYDRATES: Carbohydrates are macronutrients that provide a quick energy source. Complex carbohydrates refers to those found occurring naturally "complexed" with fiber, minerals, and other nutrients (such as grains, whole fruits, vegetables). They are more slowly absorbed and utilized than processed or refined carbohydrates (sweets, pasta, white bread).

CONJUGATED ESTROGENS: A mixture of estrogens, chemically different from those made in the human female ovary, that may come from animals (Premarin, horse), or plants (Cenestin).

CORPUS LUTEUM: The yellow-colored, progesterone-producing sac that is formed within the ovary from the remains of the follicle after it has released its egg at ovulation.

CORTICOSTEROID: A number of steroid hormones produced by the cortex of the adrenal gland. Cortisol is an example. Also known as "glucocorticoid," "steroid."

CORTISOL: An adrenal cortical hormone (glucocorticoid), usually referred to as our body's "stress" hormone because it prepares the body to respond to emergencies or stresses. It is closely related to cortisone in physiological effects.

CORTISONE: A steroid compound made naturally by the adrenal glands and also produced synthetically in laboratories for use as a drug. It has a powerful antiinflammatory effect, but may produce many adverse side effects with high levels over long periods of time.

CREATININE: The end product of creatine metabolism; found in muscle tissue, blood and urine. High levels may indicate excess muscle breakdown, for example, or advanced stages of kidney disease.

CUSHING'S SYNDROME (DISEASE): A group of symptoms and signs such as moon-shaped face, buffalo hump, and high blood pressure caused by excessive amounts of cortisone either produced by the adrenal gland or taken as medication.

CYSTIC ACNE: A skin disorder manifesting as blocked pores and pimples, many of which are blind cysts containing pus. It is a severe form of acne.

DAIDZEIN: Isoflavone compound (also called phytoestrogen) found in soy and other plants that has weak estrogenic effects.

DEXA (Dual Energy X-ray Absorptiometry): A highly reliable means of measuring bone mineral density using very small amounts of radiation. Recommended for women with multiple risk factors for osteopenia/osteoporosis, or women who want a baseline measure before beginning menopause.

DHEA: Dehydroepiandrosterone. One of the androgens ("male" hormones) produced in the adrenal glands and ovary in women. Excess levels cause facial hair, scalp hair loss, oily skin, acne among other changes.

DISOGENIN: A steroid compound found in wild yam and other plants that is used by pharmaceutical companies as a "building block" or precursor molecule to make bioidentical forms of human hormones such as progesterone and 17-beta estradiol. Disogenin in extracts of wild yam (found in skin creams) cannot be converted by the human body to progesterone or estradiol because we lack the necessary enzymes to do this.

DIURETIC: A substance, whether synthetic or natural, that stimulates the kidneys to excrete salt (sodium chloride) and water, thereby relieving fluid retention.

DIURNAL: Variation by time of day. For example, hormones in the body often are higher at one time of day and lower at another in a predictable pattern. Diseases may alter the normal diurnal pattern. An example: melatonin is normally highest at night (promotes sleep) and lowest in the bright sunlight of daytime. Melatonin that doesn't shut off properly in the daytime is considered a cause of seasonal affective disorder syndrome ("winter depression" or SAD).

DOPAMINE: A mood-elevating chemical messenger produced in the brain and body; it is also important in preventing Parkinson's disease, and as an inhibitory neurotransmitter preventing inappropriate milk secretion by the breast.

DOWN-REGULATION: A process in the brain and body in which the number (or function) of cell receptors are decreased. May occur as a natural process or due to medication effects.

DYSTHYMIA: A negative or unpleasant mood state or syndrome, less severe than major biological depression; often treated with psychotherapy rather than medication unless it persists.

ENDOCRINE GLANDS: Glands that manufacture and secrete hormones.

ENDOCRINOLOGIST: A medical specialist in diseases of the endocrine glands and their hormones; Endocrinology is the study and treatment of disorders of the glands and the hormones they secrete.

ENDOMETRIAL HYPERPLASIA: Abnormal degree of thickening of the lining of the uterus, usually due to excess estrogen effect with insufficient progesterone or progestin effect. If left uncontrolled, may lead over time to the development of endometrial cancer.

ENDOMETRIAL LINING: (also called ENDOMETRIUM): The lining of the uterus. This tissue grows under the influence of estrogen (*proliferative* endometrium), and thickens under the influence of progesterone each month (*secretory* endometrium) in the menstrual cycle. The fall in progesterone (or a progestin, such as Provera, Aygestin and others), triggers the secretory endometrium to "slough" and then be shed from the uterus in the monthly bleeding.

ENDOMETRIOSIS: The presence of small islands (implants) of endometrium lying outside of the uterus, scattered about the abdomen and pelvic cavities and many times stuck on the outside of the intestine and bladder. Endometrium tissue is normally found only *inside* the uterus, and menstrual blood is released to the *outside* of the body via the vagina. When these implants bleed at the time of menses, they cause severe pain because the blood is *released into* the abdomen and pelvis and acts as a significant irritant to other organs.

ENTEROHEPATIC CIRCULATION: Blood flow from the gastrointestinal tract to the liver and that prolongs the action of compounds such as estrogen and other hormones by allowing them to "recirculate" rather than being excreted in the stool.

ENDORPHINS (ALSO ENKEPHALINS): natural pain-relieving and mood-elevating compounds (peptides) produced in the brain, spinal cord and body to produce a morphinelike analgesia.

ENZYMES: Proteins produced by living cells that assist body functions by acting as catalysts in specific biochemical reactions. Enzyme catalysts are not themselves consumed in the reactions.

EPINEPHRINE (ADRENALINE): A chemical messenger made by the adrenal gland that prepares the body to handle emergencies called the "fight-or-flight" response. Epinephrine is also made in the laboratory to be used as a drug to treat severe allergic reactions, asthma, severe bleeding, and certain types of heart rhythm problems.

EQUINE ESTROGENS, EQUILIN: Estrogens derived from the pregnant mares' urine and used to make the animal-derived estrogen, Premarin. These estrogens are chemically different from the ones made by the human ovary. They have some effects that are similar to human estrogens, and some effects that are quite different from human estrogens. See chapter 5, 13, 15 for detailed explanations.

ESSENTIAL FATTY ACIDS: Fatty acids necessary for cellular metabolism, which cannot be made by the body, but must be supplied in the diet. Good sources are fish oil, oils from nuts and seeds, and evening primrose oil.

ESTROGEN: The group of three sex hormones produced by the gonads (ovary in women, testes in men), and by the adrenal gland. In women, the higher amounts of these sex hormones are responsible for the female characteristics of breasts, feminine curves, menstruation, pregnancy.

ESTRONE (E1): One of the human estrogens made by the ovary, adrenal gland, and body fat before menopause. It is the one found in higher amounts after menopause because it is still made by body fat and to a lesser extent, the adrenal glands. Estrone serves as a "storage" form of estrogen for the ovary to make the more active estradiol before menopause. High estrone levels are more associated with breast and uterine cancers, a good reason to maintain a healthy percent body fat and weight.

ESTRADIOL (E2, 17 beta estradiol): The primary estrogen produced by the ovary before menopause. It is the biologically active estrogen at the estrogen receptors and the most potent of all the natural human estrogens. Estradiol is involved in over 400 functions in a woman's body, and is the form of estrogen that is lost at menopause when the ovary follicles are depleted.

ESTRIOL (E3): The weakest of the primary human estrogens, it is produced in large amounts during pregnancy. It is barely detectable in the *nonpregnant* female body, so women do not normally have estriol present to a measurable degree on a continuous basis and it has not been shown to have bone, heart or brain preserving effects.

ESTRADIOL VALERATE: A more potent, synthetic estrogen, chemically different from the 17-beta estradiol produced by the ovary; used for menopausal hormone therapy in Europe for many years, but not used very often in the United States.

ETHINYL ESTRADIOL: A more potent synthetic estrogen used in birth control pills where the higher potency is needed (with the synthetic progestins) to adequately suppress the ovaries and provide reliable contraception. Not generally used in the United States for menopausal hormone therapy.

EVENING PRIMROSE OIL: The oil extracted from the evening primrose plant. It is a good source of the omega 6 fatty acids, in particular the essential fatty acid known as gamma linolenic acid (GLA).

FALLOPIAN TUBES: The tubes that carry the egg (ovum) from the ovary to the uterus. Fertilization of the egg occurs in the outer part of the fallopian tube.

FEEDBACK: The process by which products made in a series of reactions provide messages back to the beginning of the process to control further reactions. Feedback may be electrical, chemical or mechanical, or thermal. Example of a thermal "feedback" is the thermostat that controls your furnace. Chemical feedback occurs when hormone levels reach a critical level and feed back to the brain that no more is needed for awhile.

FEMALE SEX HORMONES: The two sex hormones produced by the female ovary and placenta during pregnancy, estrogen (see above for types) and progesterone.

FERTILIZATION: The union of the female egg (ovum) with the male sperm (spermatozoa), which occurs in the fallopian tube.

FETUS: A developing human from the end of the eighth week of pregnancy until birth.

FIBROCYSTIC: Development of dense, lumpy, ropy (fibrous) changes in tissue. About 60 to 70 percent of healthy women will have "fibrocystic" changes in their breasts, and this does not indicate a disease process. Similar changes may occur in muscle tissue in chronic pain syndromes.

FIBROIDS (FIBROMAS): Noncancerous growths of the uterus consisting of muscle and fibrous tissue. The medical term is leiomyoma, or sometimes just "myomas." The presence of fibroids tends to cause heavy, painful bleeding and cramps. At times they cause back pain, referred pain to the hip, or bladder pain and pressure with incontinence, depending on where the fibroids are found in the uterus.

FIRST-PASS METABOLISM: Breakdown of chemicals, medications, hormones, etc. by the liver as a first-step after being absorbed into the bloodstream from the gastrointestinal tract. First-pass metabolism can eliminate as much as 70 percent or more of an oral dose of a medication or hormone. This step is omitted when medications and hormones are absorbed directly into the bloodstream from the skin (patch or cream) or muscle (injection).

FOLLICLE STIMULATING HORMONE (FSH): A hormone secreted by the pituitary gland that reaches the ovaries via the blood circulation and stimulates the growth of ovarian follicles to form the egg that is released at ovulation. FSH above 10 to 15 occurs when the brain senses a decline in ovarian hormones, and levels of FSH greater than 20 are defined as menopausal. FSH also functions in men to stimulate the sperm-producing cells in the testes; high FSH levels in men indicate low levels of testosterone, sometimes called "andropause".

FOLLICULAR (PHASE): The first half of the ovarian hormone cycle leading up to the release of the egg at ovulation. Estrogen (estradiol) is the dominant hormone for this part of the cycle, and there is very little progesterone present.

FREE HORMONE: Hormone that is circulating in the bloodstream not connected to a carrier protein, and therefore "free" to be biologically active at cell receptor sites. See also *bound hormone.*

FREE RADICAL: "Scavenger" molecules that attack and damage body cells and tissues because they are so highly reactive. Antioxidant compounds in the body, such as vitamin E and C, bind up these free radicals and help prevent damage to cells.

GALACTORRHEA: The presence of milk or milky fluid in the breasts when not breast-feeding. It is usually a symptom of elevated prolactin, which may be caused by some medications (such as antidepressants) or by benign hormone-producing tumors (adenomas) of the pituitary gland.

GAMMA AMINOBUTYRIC ACID (GABA): An inhibitory neurotransmitter in the brain and nerves throughout the body; activation of this neurotransmitter produces a calming or anti-anxiety effect.

GAMMA LINOLENIC ACID (GLA): An omega-6 essential fatty acid that is used to synthesize prostaglandins. It has an anti-inflammatory effect in the body. Good sources: breast milk, evening primrose oil, borage plant oil, and black currant seed oil.

GENISTEIN: Isoflavone compound (also called phytoestrogen) found in soy and other plants that has weak estrogenlike effects. In some concentrations it acts to block estrogen receptors, while in other concentrations it may stimulate the estrogen receptors in certain tissues.

GLANDS: Body organs or tissues, generally soft and fleshy in consistency, that manufacture and secrete or excrete hormones, chemicals that exert their effects on target organs elsewhere in the body.

GLUCAGON: A hormone that rapidly breaks down glycogen stores in the liver and releases glucose into the bloodstream to raise blood glucose ("blood sugar"); serves as a counter-balancing hormone to the effects of insulin.

GLUCOCORTICOID: A group of hormones produced in the adrenal cortex that are primarily active in protecting against stress and in regulating protein and carbohydrate metabolism. These compounds (such as cortisone) tend to increase blood glucose, liver glycogen, and suppress the immune response and inflammatory response. Levels that are too high over time cause bone loss. See also *corticosteroid*.

GLUCOSE INTOLERANCE: Inability to properly regulate simple sugars (glucose), leading to glucose "swings" from high to low following ingestion of simple carbohydrates (such as sweets, fruit juices, soft drinks or alcohol) that are eaten alone, without adequate protein or fat to slow the absorption of glucose.

GYNECOLOGY: Surgical specialty of medicine that provides surgical and medicinal treatments for problems related to women's reproductive organs.

HALF-LIFE: A measurement of how long it takes for half of a substance to be lost or removed; for example, drug half-life refers to how long it takes for the concentration of a drug or hormone to be decreased by one-half due to metabolic breakdown or excretion. It is usually estimated that it takes five half-lives for a substance to be completely gone from the body.

HDL: See *cholesterol*.

HIRSUTISM: A condition of excessive facial and body hair (excluding hair on the scalp) and often in women is due to excess of androgens.

HOMEOSTASIS: A state of balance in the body; refers to the physiological processes that maintain body balance.

HORMONES: Chemicals produced by various glands that are then transported around the body to exert their multiple metabolic effects.

HORMONE RECEPTOR SITE: A "binding" or "docking" site in or on cells for hormones to connect in order to exert their actions. The hormone and its receptor create what is called a "receptor complex" that sends signals to the cell to carry out various functions.

HORMONE REPLACEMENT THERAPY (HRT): Technically, the administration of any hormonal preparations (natural or synthetic) to replace the loss of natural hormones produced by various glands (thyroid, ovary, testes, pancreas, adrenal, pituitary, etc.). HRT in *common* usage now refers to administration of female hormones (estrogen and progestin) after menopause.

HOT FLASH (FLUSH): Episode of vasodilation in skin of head, neck, and chest, accompanied by sensation of suffocation, sweating, feeling suddenly hot or cold. Occurs commonly during menopause due to falling hormone levels that trigger changes in the brain heat regulatory center.

HYPERTHYROIDISM: A condition caused by excessive hormone secretion of the thyroid glands that will increase the basal metabolic rate, increase heart rate and blood pressure, disrupt sleep, and may cause marked weight loss.

HYPOTHALAMUS: The "master conductor" or "control center" situated at the base of the brain regulates body temperature, thirst, appetite, sex drive, and all other hormonal glands. It releases hormones that travel directly to the pituitary gland and stimulate the release of pituitary hormones, which govern the other endocrine glands.

HYPOTHYROIDISM: A slowing of overall body metabolism due to deficiency of the thyroid hormone production or function. There are many diverse symptoms, but common ones include obesity, dry skin and hair, low blood pressure, slow pulse, sluggishness of all functions, constipation, depressed mood, muscle aches/weakness, hair loss, low energy, goiter.

HYSTERECTOMY: Surgical removal (abdominal or vaginal) of the uterus only. In common usage, women may say "hysterectomy" when both the uterus and ovaries have been removed or when just the uterus has been removed. The medical term for removal of the uterus and ovaries together is "hysterectomy with bilateral salpingo-oophorectomy (BSO)."

IMMUNE SYSTEM: The defense and surveillance system of the body that protects against infection by microorganisms and invasion by foreign tissues and substances. The immune system is made up of specialized blood cells (lymphocytes, B-cells, T-cells, etc.), blood proteins (antibodies), the spleen, thymus gland, lymph nodes, and bone marrow. Immune function is impaired with a variety of endocrine imbalances, such as menopause and thyroid disorders.

IMPLANT: A device that is surgically implanted into a part of the body for cosmetic or therapeutic purposes. Hormone-containing implants are sometimes used for contraception or for menopausal hormone replacement therapy, although I don't generally recommend them.

INFLAMMATION: A condition characterized by swelling, redness, heat, and pain in any tissue as a result of trauma, irritation, infection, or imbalances in immune function.

INSULIN: A hormone secreted by beta cells of the pancreas that regulates the level of glucose in the bloodstream, and moves glucose into cells where it can be used for energy (e.g. muscles) or stored as fat. Excess insulin production, and/or insulin insensitivity, is called "insulin resistance" and is associated with increased middle-body (male pattern) fat storage. Insulin medication is used to control high blood sugar in diabetes.

ISOFLAVONE: Chemical compounds found in a variety of plants (soy, red clover, etc.) that are weakly estrogenic in their effects and are often called phytoestrogens ("phyto-" meaning derived from plants). Common isoflavones that are being studied for their health effects are genistein, daidzein, biochanin, and formononetin.

IUD: Intrauterine device, an object inserted into the uterus, typically used for contraception, but may also be a means of delivering hormones (example: Progestasert progestin delivery system).

LDL: The "bad" artery-damaging form of cholesterol. See also *cholesterol.*

LIBIDO: Level of sexual desire, sexual energy, or drive.

LUTEAL (PHASE): The progesterone-dominant second half of the menstrual cycle, from ovulation until menses begin. The primary hormone of this phase is progesterone. It is also the time of the cycle when "PMS," food cravings, bloating, breast tenderness, constipation, depressed/irritable moods, fatigue and other "premenstrual" symptoms typically occur.

LUTEINIZING HORMONE (LH): A hormone produced by the pituitary gland that triggers ovulation and the egg release to become the corpus luteum. In men, LH stimulates production of testosterone by the testes and LH levels will rise in men with low testosterone.

MALE HORMONE: A hormone that promotes masculine characteristics in the body such as facial and body hair, acne, deepening of the voice, increased muscle mass, and increased libido.

MALIGNANT: Cancer, cancerous.

MELATONIN: A hormone produced by the pineal gland in the brain and is involved in regulating the sleep-wake cycle; levels rise during darkness and fall at daylight. Excess melatonin levels that fail to shut off during the day have been thought to cause seasonal affective disorder (SAD).

MENOPAUSE: The cessation of menstruation. The last period. May be natural (due to depletion of the ovarian follicles) or surgical removal of the uterus (without or with removal of ovaries). When the ovaries are gone or have lost their follicles, the body loses the hormones estradiol, progesterone, testosterone and much of the DHEA. The period of time leading up the menopause, when hormone production by the ovaries is decreasing, is called the *climacteric.*

MENSTRUATION: Monthly bleeding from the vagina in women from puberty until menopause, caused by shedding of the lining of the womb (uterus) if there is no fertilization of an egg.

METABOLIC HORMONES: Hormones that are involved in regulating cellular energy processes, synthesis of body proteins, and other functions involved in tissue growth and repair.

METABOLIC RATE: The rate at which the body converts chemical energy in foods into heat (thermal) and movement (kinetic) energy. Metabolic rate is governed by hormones from the thyroid, ovary, testes, adrenal, and pancreas.

METABOLISM: Chemical processes, regulated by hormones, utilizing the raw materials of food nutrients, oxygen, minerals, vitamins along with enzymes to produce energy for body functions such as growth, repair, healing. See also *anabolic, catabolic.*

METABOLITE: Any product of metabolism. Some metabolites are active and needed for other functions, and some metabolites may be toxic and need to be excreted. An example of a toxic metabolite is ammonia from the breakdown of protein; an active metabolite of progesterone has anxiety-relieving properties when it binds to the brain's GABA receptor.

MICROGRAM: One-millionth part of a gram. One thousandth of a milligram. The abbreviation on prescriptions is mcg.

MILLIGRAM: One-thousandth of a gram. The abbreviation on prescriptions is mg. See also *picogram, nanogram.*

MILLILITER: One-thousandth of a liter, or about 1 cc. The abbreviation on prescriptions is ml.

MINERALOCORTICOID: Hormones produced by the adrenal gland that primarily function to regulate electrolytes (sodium, potassium, chloride) and water balance in the body. An example is aldosterone.

MOLECULE: A chemical compound made up of different arrangements and types of atoms; a molecule is the smallest unit into which a substance may be divided without loss of its unique characteristics.

NANOGRAM: One billionth of a gram, abbreviated as ng.

"NATURAL" HORMONE: Bioidentical hormones are often called "natural" hormones, but "natural" may also refer to a biological source (such as the horse) that produces molecules different from those made by the human body. See *bioidentical.*

NEURON: A nerve cell, the structure and functional unit of the nervous system. Neurons function in initiation and conduction of electrical and chemical "nerve" impulses.

NEUROTRANSMITTERS: Chemicals that transmit messages from nerve cell to nerve cell in the brain, and between the brain and the tissues and organs of the body. Common ones referred to throughout this book are serotonin, dopamine, acetylcholine, GABA, norepinephrine.

NON-ANDROGENIC: Not causing masculine hormone effects in the body.

NOREPINEPHRINE (NORADRENALINE): A hormone produced by the adrenal gland, and certain areas of the brain that helps the body prepare for and cope with stress. It also has a mood-elevating effect, but levels that are too high may cause feelings of anxiety, raise blood pressure and cause insomnia. Epinephrine (adrenaline) is another "stress-hormone" produced by the adrenal gland with similar effects in some tissues and opposite effects in yet others.

NUCLEUS: The vital body inside cells that contains the genetic material (DNA) and is responsible for regulation of essential functions for cell growth, protein synthesis, metabolism, reproduction, and transmission of characteristics of a cell.

OOPHORECTOMY (OVARIECTOMY): Surgical removal of the ovaries.

ORAL: Indicating something is to be taken by mouth.

ORGASM: The physical and emotional release of sexual arousal tension; also called *climax.*

OSTEOBLAST: Cells that function to build new bone. These cells are stimulated by estradiol, testosterone and to a lesser extent, progesterone.

OSTEOCLAST: Cells that are responsible for resorption (breaking down) old brittle bone. Their action is regulated primarily by estradiol and teststerone to a lesser extent.

OSTEOPENIA: Loss of bone density that is not yet severe enough to be considered osteoporosis. Osteopenia will progress to osteoporosis if active measures are not taken to maintain bone (such as calcium, magnesium, exercise, and hormone therapy).

OSTEOPOROSIS: Loss of bone density (mass) due to loss of bone minerals and reduction of the normal bony architecture that provides strength to the skeleton. Causes bones to become porous, brittle and more easily broken.

OVA (OVUM): An ovarian follicle that has released to become the egg (ova) at ovulation. A ova that is fertilized with sperm becomes an embryo that develops into a fetus.

OVARIAN BLOOD SUPPLY: The blood carried to the ovaries via the ovarian arteries, which branch off from the uterine blood vessels. The ovarian arteries run alongside the fallopian tubes and may be injured or damaged with surgical procedures on the tubes (such as tubal ligation or hysterectomy even if the ovaries are not removed).

OVARIES: The female sex glands (gonads) located on each side of the uterus, which produce eggs and the female sex hormones (estrogen and progesterone), along with small amounts of testosterone.

OVULATION: The release of the egg from the ovary occurring around mid-cycle.

OVULATION PAIN: "Mittelschmerz" pain occurring at ovulation, which may be sharp and severe and last from a few minutes up to twelve hours.

PANCREAS: A gland situated behind the stomach that produces pancreatic juice (contains digestive enzymes such as lipase and amylase) and also the hormones insulin and glucagon, which function to regulate blood sugar and carbohydrate metabolism.

PARASYMPATHETIC NERVOUS SYSTEM: The part of the autonomic nervous system that regulates body relaxation and functions of growth and repair such as digestion. Its primary chemical messenger or neurotransmitter is acetylcholine.

PARATHYROID GLANDS: Located close to the thyroid gland, one of several small endocrine glands that secrete a hormone, parathormone, which regulates calcium-phosphorus metabolism.

PARENTERAL: A method of delivering substances (such as medications) directly to the bloodstream bypassing the digestive system and liver metabolism. Parenteral routes include: vaginal and rectal suppositories/tablets, sublingual tablets/capsules, transdermal (skin patch), subcutaneous (implant), intramuscular (IM) and intravenous (IV) injections.

PEAK LEVEL: The highest level of a hormone or medication that is reached after taking a dose or being produced by the body. ("Trough" level is the lowest point reached after a medication or hormone is taken or produced by the body).

PERIMENOPAUSAL: Time frame of several years prior to menopause when menstrual periods start to be skipped and continuing through menopause to the first few years just after periods stop. It has a variable age of onset and symptoms commonly include insomnia, mood changes, bone loss, cholesterol changes, disrupted sleep, hot flashes, and other phenomena. See also *premenopausal*.

PHARMACOKINETICS/ DYNAMICS: Study of drug absorption, delivery to tissues of the body, metabolism and excretion.

PHYSIOLOGICAL: Normal body processes and functions.

PHYTOESTROGENS: Plant(phyto) derived chemical molecules that may attach to the body's estrogen receptors and trigger certain estrogenlike actions; some of these compounds have estrogen-blocking actions (antagonists) that may or may not be desirable. Occur naturally in several hundred different types of plants, including soy, clover and a variety of grains.

PICOGRAM: One trillionth of a gram, abbreviated pg.

PITUITARY GLAND: A mushroom-shaped gland connected by a vascular stalk to the base of the brain. The pituitary gland manufactures hormones (FSH, LH, TSH, ACTH, prolactin, and others) that in turn control other hormonal glands, such as the thyroid, adrenals, and ovaries.

PLACENTA: The hormonal organ designed to provide for the nourishment of the fetus and the elimination of its waste products. It produces a number of hormones, such as progesterone and estriol, that have roles in sustaining pregnancy and adapting the mother's body to adjust to the increased physiological demands of pregnancy. It is formed in the uterus by the union of uterine mucous membrane with membranes of the fetus.

PLAQUE: A deposit of platelets, fibrin, calcium, cholesterol and other fatty substances that build up in arteries and cause clogging that leads to reduced blood flow and may cause angina, heart attacks, or strokes. The whole process of plaque buildup and artery damage is referred to as atherosclerosis.

PLASMA: The liquid part of blood and the lymph (minus the red and white blood cells) that contains proteins, clotting factors, and other chemicals such as glucose, hormones, etc.

PMS: see Premenstrual Syndrome.

POLYCYSTIC OVARY SYNDROME (PCO or PCOS): A disorder of the ovaries in which the usual female hormonal balance is altered, and there are excessive levels of insulin and male hormones accompanied by changes in body shape, hirsuitism, and irregular menstruation. It may also be triggered by stress, exposure to endocrine-disrupting chemicals, autoimmune illnesses, or weight gain. In PCO Syndrome, the ovaries have multiple small follicles or "cysts," which can be seen on an ultrasound scan of the pelvis. Other common features: truncal obesity, acne, glucose intolerance and insulin resistance, hypertension, infertility and changes in mood related to the hormonal imbalances.

POST-MENOPAUSE: The years following the end of menstruation and decline in production of ovarian female hormones (menopause).

POSTNATAL, POST-PARTUM: The time period after childbirth.

PRECURSOR: A substance ("building block") that is used to make another compound, hormone or medication. For example, cholesterol molecules are used as the building blocks for the body to make other steroid hormones, such as progesterone.

PREMATURE MENOPAUSE: Cessation of menses and decline of ovarian hormone production occurring before the age of forty-two.

PREMENOPAUSAL: The time leading up to menopause characterized by hormonal changes and irregular menstrual flow. It may begin as much as ten years before actual menopause, but more commonly occurs about four to five years before menopause. See also *perimenopause.*

PREMENSTRUAL SYNDROME (PMS): A collection of variable symptoms such as mood disturbance, headaches, abdominal bloating, etc. recurring on a cyclical basis in the week or two before menstrual bleeding. See also *perimenopause.*

PROGESTERONE: A steroid hormone produced by the corpus luteum (formed from the egg released at ovulation in the ovary) or placenta during pregnancy. Small amounts are also made by the adrenal glands. Responsible for secretory changes in uterine endometrium in second half of menstrual cycle to prepare the uterus to receive and nourish a fertilized egg. Progesterone also has many metabolic functions (e.g., increased appetite, promoting fat storage, etc.) designed help a mother's body change in ways that will support a pregnancy (*pro-gest*ation hormone = *progest*erone).

PROGESTIN: A group of hormones that have progesteronelike effects on the uterus and body; progesterone is correctly included in this larger class of hormones, but common useage usually means that "progestin" refers to synthetic compounds that are made in the laboratory and are chemically different from the natural ovary compound progesterone.

PROGESTIN-ONLY PILL ("mini-pill"): A contraceptive pill containing only a progestin such as norethindrone (Brand: Micronor and others). Unless it is given with estrogen to balance the unwanted side effects, the progestin-only pills are not recommended for midlife women due to the potential for adverse effects on cholesterol, glucose control and body weight. Progestin-only pills, implants or injections are not recommended for women with a history of depression, diabetes, headaches, hypertension or weight gain as progestins aggravate all of these problems unless estrogen is also given.

PROGESTOGENS: Natural or synthetic substances that have effects similar to the natural female hormone progesterone. Synthetic progestogens (called *progestins*) are commonly used in birth control pills and HRT to regulate menstrual bleeding. Examples are medroxyprogesterone acetate (Provera, Cycrin), norethindrone (Aygestin, Micronor), norethisterone, norgestrel, etc.

PROLACTIN: A hormone secreted by the pituitary gland that stimulates milk production in the breasts. At times other than nursing, high levels of prolactin may cause headaches, weight gain, depression and breast discharge (galactorrhea).

PROSTAGLANDINS: Chemicals manufactured throughout the body that exert a hormonelike effect and influence muscular (including the uterus) contraction, circulation, and inflammation. Release of prostaglandins in the uterus at the time of menstruation is a cause of menstrual cramps.

PSYCHOSOMATIC: Physical symptoms that are triggered by psychological and emotional causes and not due primarily to physical disease. This term is often misused when applied to women, as in "the cause isn't known so it must be psychosomatic, or stress-related."

PSYCHOTROPIC DRUGS: Drugs that act primarily on the brain to produce effects on mood, thinking, sleep, and other functions. Examples are sedatives, tranquilizers (antianxiety agents), antidepressants, antipsychotics, and analgesic and anesthetic agents.

PUERPERIUM: The period of time after childbirth required to return the reproductive organs to their pre-pregnant size and condition. This takes six to eight weeks.

RECEPTOR: See *hormone receptor*.

RECEPTOR ANTAGONIST (BLOCKER): A compound, hormone or medication that binds at a cell's receptor site but blocks the normal action of that receptor system. Examples are "beta-blockers" that block the normal action of the beta adrenergic receptors; tamoxifen that blocks the estrogen receptor of the breast and brain even though it will activate the estrogen receptors in the uterine lining (endometrium).

RECTAL: Pertaining to the rectum.

SEBACEOUS GLANDS: The tiny oil-producing glands in the skin. If they overproduce oil and/or become obstructed, pimples or acne will result.

SERMS: An abbreviation for a class of medications called selective estrogen receptor modulators. These drugs have both agonist (activating) and antagonist (blocking) actions at the body's estrogen receptors, depending on the particular organ. Examples are tamoxifen and raloxifen; both drugs *block* breast estrogen receptors, and *stimulate* estrogen receptors elsewhere (such as bone). Because they block important actions of estrogen, they are not a pure replacement for all of estrogen's actions in the body. Side effects of both medicines include hot flashes, formation of blood clots, pulmonary emboli, cataracts, and increased risk of uterine cancer (tamoxifen).

SEROTONIN (5-HT): A potent brain chemical that regulates sleep, mood, libido, appetite, pain, and repetitive thoughts and actions. Serotonin's chemical name is 5-hydroxytryptophan and it is made by the brain and body from dietary sources of the amino acid tryptophan (milk, turkey, whole grains, etc.).

SERUM: The fluid portion of the blood after coagulation has removed the cells, fibrin and fibrinogen.

SEX HORMONES: The male and female hormones produced from cholesterol by the testicles, ovaries, adrenal glands, and body fat: testosterone, estrogens, progesterone, androgens.

SEX HORMONE BINDING GLOBULIN (SHBG): A carrier protein in the bloodstream (made in the liver) that binds or carries estrogen, testosterone, progesterone to provide a reservoir of hormones ready for release into the free fraction to become the active form.

SLEEP APNEA: A serious sleep disorder characterized by multiple episodes of breathing stopping during sleep, and often accompanied by loud snoring. It increases in obesity, and in women as they lose their ovarian estradiol that helps regulate sleep. If undetected, leads to increased risk of further weight gain, depression, daytime fatigue, high blood pressure, heart disease, diabetes, stroke and premature heart attack. In men, it can cause impotence (difficulty with having an erection).

STEROID DRUGS AND HORMONES: The group of chemical substances that has a chemical structure consisting of multiple rings of carbon atoms. Cortisone (the drug), estrogen, progesterone, and testosterone (sex hormones).

STRESS (URINARY) INCONTINENCE: Loss of urine due to pressure on weakened bladder structures and supporting ligaments; this weakness occurs as a result of estrogen loss and damage during childbirth. Increased pressure on the bladder may come from coughing, sneezing, laughing, straining to lift objects, or prolonged standing.

STROKE: Brain damage resulting from diminished blood supply and oxygen (ischemia) to the brain; usually occurs as a result of a clot blocking the arteries.

SUBLINGUAL: Something (medication, hormones, allergy drops, etc.) given underneath the tongue to be absorbed into the bloodstream.

SUSTAINED (TIMED) RELEASE: A process in which a medication is prepared or formulated in such a way as to deliver small amounts over a longer period of time.

SYMPATHETIC NERVOUS SYSTEM: The part of the autonomic nervous system that prepares the body for stress through effects of the stress hormones it releases (e.g., by increasing oxygen to the tissues, increasing heart rate, blood pressure and glucose release, etc.). Its primary chemical messengers (neurotransmitters) are norepinephrine and epinephrine.

SYMPTOMS: Any physical or emotional change in the body that is perceived as distressing or painful. "Symptom" usually means a change that makes a person feel unwell. "Phenomena" is a word used to describe changes that don't necessarily cause distress.

SYNDROME: A group of symptoms and objective signs that typically occur together and serve to characterize a disease or disorder.

SYNERGISTIC: Substances interacting in ways that produce an effect *greater than* just adding the effects of the combined substances.

SYNTHETIC: Made by synthesis; can be identical to a natural compound found in the body, or may be synthesized to be chemically different and have different properties. Synthetic simply means "made by synthesis", it *does not* mean "artificial" (although common useage often implies "artificial" when the term synthetic is used to apply to a hormone).

TESTES: The male gonads; two reproductive glands located in the scrotum which produce the male reproductive cells or spermatozoa and the male hormone, testosterone.

TESTOSTERONE: The major male sex hormone produced in the testes and also in smaller amounts by the female ovary; plays major role in men and women for sexual arousal, maintaining bone and muscle mass, psychological wellbeing.

THYMUS: A gland located at the base of the neck that is important in development of immune response in newborns, with lesser activity as we get older. The cortex of the gland is composed of dense lymphoid tissue that produces the T-cells of the immune system.

THYROID GLAND: The endocrine gland situated in front of the larynx that produces the major hormones of metabolism; thyroxine (T4) and tri-iodothyronine (T3); also produces calcitonin that regulates calcium balance.

THYROID STIMULATING HORMONE (TSH): The hormone produced by the brain that regulates the production and release of thyroid hormones from the thyroid gland. TSH levels are low in *hyper*thyroidism, and high in *hypo*thyroidism.

TRANDERMAL: absorbed through the skin into the bloodstream from a cream or patch or injection; this form of delivery bypasses the liver's "first-pass" metabolism.

TRIGLYCERIDES (TG): One of the blood fats that the body can use to make cholesterol; elevated TG (from diet, alcohol intake, lack of exercise, and some drugs) are a significant and *independent* risk factor for heart disease in women and also increase the risk of diabetes. Consists of one glycerol and three fatty acids.

TRYPTOPHAN: An amino acid found in foods that is the major precursor ("building block") for the body and brain to make serotonin (5-hydroxytryptophan, 5-HT).

TUBAL LIGATION (BTL): The surgical procedure to cut or tie the fallopian tubes and prevent "eggs" released from the ovary from reaching the uterus. BTL is used as a method of contraception, considered permanent because it is difficult and expensive to reverse, with low probability of success. Some women notice "worsening PMS" and other symptoms of imbalance or decrease in ovarian hormones after tubal ligation, and this is thought to be due to changes in ovarian blood flow from the procedure.

TUMOR: An abnormal growth; may be cancerous or benign. An example is a uterine fibroid, a benign abnormal growth in the uterus. See also *fibroid*.

UP-REGULATION: The process of increasing the number or function of cellular receptors.

URETHRA: A muscular tube that carries urine from the bladder to the outside of the body. Inflammation of this tube is called urethritis, and causes painful, burning sensations on urination.

UTERUS: The womb or female reproductive organ that carries and nourishes a growing fetus; made up of an inner layer (see *endometrium*), and a thick muscular layer that undergoes rhythmic contractions during labor and delivery, during menstruation, and during orgasm (although not all women feel this).

ULTRASOUND SCAN: A method of using very high frequency sound waves to visualize internal organs, blood vessels, and the fetus in pregnancy. The sound waves used are more than 20,000 hertz, and above the level that humans can hear. Ultrasound images do not involve using radiation sources, so there is no exposure to radiation during the procedure.

VAGINA: The "birth canal" or genital passage leading from the uterus to the outside of the body at the vulva; it is muscular and elastic, expanding to accommodate the penis during intercourse, or to accommodate a baby during delivery.

VAGINAL DIAPHRAGM: A soft rubber cap that fits snugly over the cervix and is used for contraception.

VAGINAL RING: a small, soft plastic or silastic device containing hormones or other medication for direct topical delivery to the vagina and urinary system. An example is Estring, containing 17-beta estradiol, used to treat vaginal dryness.

VASOACTIVE HORMONE or DRUGS: Drugs or substances acting on the blood vessels to cause either dilation (e.g., estradiol, nitroglycerine) or constriction (e.g., nicotine) of the arteries.

VASOMOTOR: A term that refers to the way that nerve cells connect at the smooth muscle wall of arteries and govern the opening (vasodilation) and closing (vasoconstriction) of blood vessels to control blood flow.

VIRILIZATION: The development of masculine physical characteristics due to presence of male hormones. Virilization may occur in women if the androgen hormones are too high.

VULVA: Female external genitalia. Also known as the lips of the vaginal opening.

WILD (MEXICAN) YAM: A root vegetable that grows in many areas and contains precursor compounds that can be extracted and used in the laboratory as building blocks to make the hormones estradiol, testosterone and progesterone. Extracts of wild yam cannot be converted by the human body to the human forms of active hormones, since we do not have the enzymes to carry out these chemical reactions.

WAYS TO MEASURE BODY FAT

Body Calipers: Skinfolds are "pinched" in several areas of the body, the thickness measured, and then we use formulas to calculate total percent body fat. This measurement gives you helpful information, it is easy to do and readily available at health clubs and some doctor's offices. But keep in mind, if it is done by an inexperienced person, it can yield inaccurate results, especially if you are severely obese.

Electrical Impedance: This involves sending a harmless amount of electric current through your body to give a measure of the *bioelectric impedance* of the tissues. Since muscle, bone and fat conduct electricity differently, the computerized analysis tells how much of each type of tissue is present. This may be inaccurate if you are severely obese or if the machine has not been calibrated properly. The advantage is that it is easy, available, and inexpensive. It gives you a helpful baseline measure as well as a way to track your progress, and it is more reliable than trying to depend on scale weight in pounds to track loss of body fat.

DEXA (Dual Energy X-Ray): This is the same machine that tests your bone density; certain models of this equipment have the capability of also measuring your total body composition and giving a very reliable measure of percent body fat. It is one of the most precise methods available other than hydrostatic weighing, and if you are interested in having this done, you may be able to locate one of these state-of-the-art machines in hospitals, preventive medicine centers, and obesity research centers.

Hydrostatic Weighing: This involves having you sit in a special submersible scale in a large tank of water. You are then completely submersed and weighed underwater. This is the most accurate method of determining body fat but is limited in availability to laboratories with sophisticated equipment, and it is usually more expensive than the other methods.

Appendix II

RESOURCES AND REFERENCES

It is not possible to list the hundreds of medical and scientific peer-reviewed articles from reputable medical journals that I have read and studied for my clinical work and book writing. This is a list of *selected historical* and *current* articles that I think are key ones, and may be of interest for those of you who want a reference for your physician, or for your own reading of the medical literature. Many times I have included the older articles to illustrate how long this information has been available and how our current understandings have evolved from this historical foundation. Each article provides additional references if you wish to pursue a topic in more depth. I have focused on medical research articles published in the major, peer-reviewed national and international medical journals. In the consumer books section, I have primarily selected carefully researched, reputable books written by physicians or by formally trained health professionals in other fields who are recognized for their professional expertise. For the most part, I have not included books by laypersons who typically are not trained to evaluate conflicting medical information.

MEDICAL ARTICLES AND JOURNALS

Chapter 2

Fine J., Colditz G., Coakley, E., et al. "A Prospective Study of Weight Change and Health-Related Quality of Life in Women," *JAMA* 1999; Vol 282, No. 22: 2136-2142.

Greenberger, P. "SAM IX: More Information on Sex-Based Differences," *J Wos Hlth & Gender Based Med* 1999, Vol 8, No. 10 : 1223-1224.

Hu, F., Stampfer, M., Manson, J., et al. "Trends in the Incidence of Coronary Heart Disease and Changes in Diet and Lifestyle in Women," *N Eng J Med* 2000; 343: 530-537.

Kramer, R., Cook, T., Carlisle, C., et al. "Role of the Primary Care Physician in Recognizing Obstructive Sleep Apnea," *Arch Intern Med* 1999; 159: 965-968.

Kuskowaska-Wolk, A., Rossner, S. "Prevalence of Obesity in Sweden: Cross-Sectional Study of a Representative Adult Population," *J. Intern Med* 1990; 227: 241-6.

Lean, M., Han, T., Seidell, J. "Impairment of Health and Quality of Life Using New US Federal Guidelines for the Identification of Obesity," *Arch Intern Med* 1999; 159: 837-843.

Lee, Z, et al. "Obesity is the Key Determinant of Cardiovascular Risk Factors in the Hong Kong Chinese Population: Cross-sectional Clinic-Based Study," *Hong Kong Medical Journal* 2000; 6: 13-23.

Mokdad, A., Serdula, M., Dietz, W., et al. "The Spread of the Obesity Epidemic in the United States 1991–1998," *JAMA* 1999; 282: 1519–1522.

"National Task Force on the Prevention and Treatment of Obesity. "Overweight, Obesity, and Health Risk," *Arch Internal Med* 2000; 160: 898–904.

Phillips, G. "Hyperestrogenemia, Diet, and Disorders of Western Societies," *Am Jrnl Med* 1985; 78: 363–366.

Toda, Y., Segal, N., Toda, T., et al. "Lean Body Mass and Body Fat Distribution in Participants With Chronic Low Back Pain," *Arch Internal Med* 2000; 160: 3263–3269.

Wing, R., Matthews, K., Kuller, L. "Weight Gain at the Time of Menopause," *Arch Intern Med* 1990; 151: 97–103.

Chapter 3

Auwerx, J., Stales, B., Leptin. *Lancet* 1998; 351: 737–42.

Christiansen, C., Christiansen, M. "Climacteric Symptoms, Fat Mass and Plasma Concentrations of LH, FSH, PRL, Estradiol 17-beta, and Androstenedione in the Early Postmenopausal Period," *Acta Endo* 1982; 101: 87–92.

Crawford, S., Casey, V., Avis, N., et al. "A Longitudinal Study of Weight and the Menopause Transition: Results From the Massachusetts Women's Health Study," *Menopause: J N Am Meno Soc* 2000; 7 (2): 96–105.

Elbers, J., DeRoo, G., Popp-Snijders, C., et al. "Effects of Adminstration of 17-beta Oestradiol on Serum Leptin Levels in Health Post-Menopausal Women," *Clin Endo (Oxf)* 1999; 51:449–54.

Ferrara, A., et al. "Sex Differences In Insulin Levels In Older Adults and The Effect of Body Size, Estrogen Replacement Therapy, and Glucose Tolerance Status: The Rancho Bernardo Study, 1984–87," *Diabetes* 1995; 18(2): 220–225.

Folsom, A., Kushi, L., Anderson, K., et al. "Associations of General and Abdominal Obesity With Multiple Outcomes in Older Women," *Arch Intern Med* 2000; 2117–2128.

Gambacciani, M., Ciapponi, M., Cappagli, B. "Climacteric Modifications in Body Weight and Fat Tissue Distribution," *Climacteric* 1999; 2: 37–44.

Heymsfield, S., Gallagher, D., Poehlman, E., et al. "Menopausal Changes in Body Composition and Energy Expenditure," *Exp Ger* 1994; 29 (3/4): 377–389.

Kaye, S., Folsom, A., Soler J., Prineas R., et al. "Association of Body Mass and Fat Distribution with Sex Hormone Concentrations in Postmenopausal Women," *Int. J. Epidemiol.* 20, 151–6.

Ley, C., Lees, B., Stevenson, J. "Sex and Menopause-Associated Changes in Body-Fat Distribution," *Am J Clin Nutr* 1992; 55: 950–4.

Peiris, A., et al. "Relationship of Body Fat Distribution To The Metabolic Clearance of Insulin In Premenopausal Women," *Int J Obesity* 1985; 11: 581–589.

Reubinoff, B., Wurtman J., Adler D, et al. "Effect of Hormone Replacement Therapy on Body Composition Fat Distribution and Food Intake in Early Postmenopausal Women: a Prospective Study," *Fertil Steril* 1995; 64(5): 963–968.

Raison, J., et al. "Regional Differences In Adipose Tissue Lipoprotein Lipase Activity In Relation To Body Fat Distribution and Menopausal Status In Obese Women," *Int J Obesity* 1988; 12: 465–472.

Rosano, G. "Syndrome X in Women is Associated with Estrogen Deficiency," *Eur Heart J.* 1995; 16: 610–14.

Rodriguez, C., et al. "Effect of Body Mass on the Association Between Estrogen Replacement Therapy and Mortality Among Elderly US Women," *American Journal of Epidemiology.* 2001; 153: 145–152.

Rudman, D., et al. "Impaired Growth Hormone Secretion In The Adult Population: Relation To Age and Adiposity," *J Clin Invest* 1981; 67:1361–1369.

Schubring, C., Englaro P., Siebler T, et al. "Longitudinal Analysis of Maternal Serum Leptin Levels During Pregnancy, at Birth and Up to Six weeks After Birth; Relation to Body Mass Index, Skinfolds, Sex Steroids, and Umbilical Cord Blood Leptin Levels," *Horm Res* 1998; 50: 276–83.

Slopien, R., Warenik-Szymankiewica, A., Maciejewska, M., Wiza, M. "Serum Serotonin Level in Postmenopausal Women," Third International Symposium: Women's Health and Menopause. June, 1998.

Sorensen, T., Echwald, S., Holm J. "Leptin In Obesity," *BMJ* 1996; 313: 953–7.

Stock, S., Sande E., Bremme, K. "Leptin Levels Vary Significantly During the Menstrual Cycle, Pregnancy, and in Vitro Fertilization Treatments: Possible Relation to Estradiol," *Fertil Steril* 1999; 72:657–62.

Wing, R. "Obesity and Weight Gain During Adulthood: A Health Problem for United States Women," *WHI* 1992; 2 (2: 114–122.)

Chapter 4

Bray, G. "Pathophysiology of Obesity," *American Journal of Clinical Nutrition* 1992; 55 (2)(suppl): 488S–494S.

DeLeiva, A. "What are the Benefits of Moderate Weight Loss?" *Expl Clin Endocrinol Diabetes* 1998; 106(suppl 2): 10–13.

"Methods for Voluntary Weight Loss and Control," National Institutes of Health Technology Assessment Conference Statement, March 30–April 1, 1992. Available from the Office of Medical Applications Research, National Institutes of Health, Federal Building, Room 618, Bethesda, MD 20892.

Pirke, K., Schweiger, U., Laessle, R., et al. "Dieting Influences the Menstrual Cycle: Vegetarian Versus Nonvegetarian Diet," *Fertility and Sterility* 1968; 46(6): 1083–1088.

Serdula, M., Mokdad, A., Williamson, D. "Prevalence of Attempting Weight Loss and Strategies for Controlling Weight," *JAMA* 1999; 28(14): 1353–1358.

Yanovski, S.A. "Practical Approach to Treatment of the Obese Patient," *Archives of Family Medicine.* 1993; 2(3):309–316.

Chapter 5

Aloia, J.F., McGowan, D.M., Vaswani, A.N., Ross, P. and Cohn, S.H. "Relationship of Menopause to Skeletal and Muscle Mass," *Am. J. Clin. Nutr.,* (1991) 53, 1378–83.

Block, M., Schmidt, P., Danaceau, M., et al. "Effects of Gonadal Steroids in Women With a History of Postpartum Depression," *Am J.Psych* 2000; 157:924–930.

Cassidy, A. and Milligan, S. "How Significant are Environmental Estrogens to Women?" *Climacteric* 1998; 1:229–242.

Cauley, J.A., Pertini, A.M., LaPorte, R.E., Sandler, R.B., Baylers, C.M., Robertson, R.J. and Slemenda, C.W. "The Decline of Grip Strength in the Menopause Relationship to Physical Activity, Estrogen Use and Anthropometric Factors," *J. Chronic Dis,* (1982) 40, 115–20.

Christiansen, C., and Christiansen, M.S. (1982), "Climacteric Symptoms, Fat Mass and Plasma Concentrations of LH, FSH, PRL, Estradiol 17-beta, and Androstenedione in the Early Postmenopausal period." *Acta Endocrinol,* 101, 87–92.

Fink, G., et al. "Estrogen Control of Central Neurotransmission: Effect on Mood, Mental State, and Memory," *Cell Mol Neuroobiol* 1996 June.

Fotsis, T., Zhang, Y., Pepper M., et al. "The Endogenous Oestrogen Metabolite 2-Methoxytoestradiol Inhibits Angiogenesis and Suppresses Tumour Growth," *Nature* 1994; 368: 237–239.

Fonseca, E., Ochoa, R., Galvan, R. "Increased Serum Levels of Growth Hormone and Insulin-Like Growth Factor-1 Associated with Simultaneous Decrease of Circulating Insulin in Postmenopausal Women Receiving Hormone Replacement Therapy," *Menopause: J N Am Meno Soc* 1999; 6–1: 56–60.

Ganesan, R. "The Aversive and Hypophagic Effects of Estradiol," *Physiol Behav* 1994; 55: 279–85

Geary, N. "Estradiol and the Control of Eating," *Appetite* 1997; 29: 386.

Godsland, I., Walton, C., Stevenson, J. "Carbohydrate Metabolism, Cardiovascular Disease and Hormone Replacement Therapy," *The Modern Management of the Menopause*, The Proceedings of the VII International Congress on the Menopause, Stockholm, Sweden. 1994; The Parthenon Publishing Group, NY, NY: 231–249.

Genazzani, A.R., Bernardi, F., Spinetti, A., Stomati, M., Luisi, S., Tonetti, A., Petraglia, F. and Luisi, M. "The Brain as Target and Source for Sex Steroid Hormones," *Third International Symposium Women's Health and Menopause.* June, 1998.

Govoni, S., "Estrogens as Neuroprotectants: Hypotheses on the Mechanism of Action," *Third International Symposium Women's Health and Menopause*, June, 1998.

Jensen, J., Christensen, C., and Rodbro, P. "Estrogen-Progesterone Replacement Therapy Changes Body Composition in Early Postmenopausal Women," *Maturitas* (1986), 8, 209–16.

Jensen, M.D., Martin M.L., Cryer P.E., et al. "Effects of Estrogen on Free Fatty Acid Metabolism in Humans," *Am J Physiol.* 266, E914, 1994.

Kaye, S.A., Folsom, A.R., Soler, J.T., Prineas, R.J. and Potter, J.D. "Association of Body Mass and Fat Distribution with Sex Hormone Concentrations in Postmenopausal Women," *Int. J. Epidemiol.*, 20, 151–6.

Kenagy, R., Weinstein, I., Heimberg, M. "The Effects of 17-Beta Estradiol and Progesterone on the Metabolism of Fee Fatty Acid by Perfused Livers from Normal Female and Ovariectomized Rats," *Endo* 1981; 108–5: 1613–1621.

Knight, D.C. and Eden, J.A. "A Review of the Clinical Effects of Phytoestrogens," *Obstet Gynecol,* 1996: 87(5 Part 2): 897–904.

Kronenberg, F. and Hughes, C. "Exogenous and Endogenous Estrogens: an Appreciation of Biological Complexity," (editorial) *Menopause: The Journal of the North American Menopause Society*, 1999, Vol.6; no.1, 4–6.

Kyllonen, E.S., Vaananen, H.K., Heikkinen, J.E., et al. "Comparison of Muscle Strength and Bone Mineral Density in Healthy Postmenopausal Women: a Cross-Sectional Population Study," *Scand J Rehab Med* 23, 153–7, 1991.

Massafra, C., Buonocore, G., Gioia, D., et al. "Effects of Estradiol and Medroxyprogesterone-acetate Treatment on Erythrocyte Antioxidant Enzyme Activities and Malondialdehyde Plasma Levels in Amenorrhoic Women," *J Clin Endocrinol Metab* 1997; 82

Niki, E., Nakano, M. "Estrogens as Antioxidants," *Methods Enzymol* 186, 330, 1990.

Notelovitz, M. "Estrogen Therapy and Variable-Resistance Weight Training Increase Bone Mineral in Surgically Menopausal Women," *J Bone Mineral Research* 6(6); 583–590, 1991.

Ockner, R., Lysenko N, Manning J. "Sex Steroid Modulation of Fatty Acid Utilization and Fatty Acid Binding Protein Concentration in Rat Liver," 1980; 65: 1013–1023.

Petroianu, A. "Gallbladder Emptying in Perimenopausal Women," *Med Hypotheses* 1989; 30: 129–30

Phillips, S., Rook K., Siddle N., et al. "Muscle Weakness in Women Occurs at an Earlier Age than in Men, but Strength is Preserved by Hormone Replacement Therapy," *Clin Sci* 1993; 3: 84–95.

Phillips, S.K., Gopinathan J., Meehan, K. et al. "Muscle Strength Changes During the Menstrual Cycle in Human Adductor Pollicis," *J Physiol* 473, 125P, 1993.

Rosano, G., Collins, P., Kaski, J., et al. "Syndrome X in Women is Associated with Oestrogen Deficiency," *Eur Heart J* 1995; 16–5: 610–614.

Sarwar, R., Beltran-Niclos, B., Rutherford, O. "Changes in Muscle Strength, Relaxation Rate and Fatiguability During the Human Menstrual Cycle," *J Physiol* 493, 267, 1996.

Seumeren, I. "Weight Gain and Hormone Replacement Therapy: Are Women's Fears Justified?" *Maturitas.* 2000 34 Suppl 1: S3–S8.

Vliet, E.L., Davis, V.L.H. "New Perspectives on the Relationship of Hormone Changes to Affective Disorders in the Perimenopause," *Clinical Issues in Mid-Life Women's Health (NAACOG)*, vol. 2, no. 4, 1991, pp. 453–471.

Whitehead, Malcolm. "Oestrogens: Relative Potencies and Hepatic Effects After Different Routes of Administration," *Journal of Obstetrics and Gynecology* (1982) 3(suppl) S11–16.

Chapter 6
Barfield, R., Glaser, J., Rubin, B., et al. "Behavioral Effects of Progestin in the Brain," *Psychoneuroendocrinology.* 1984; 9–3: 217–231.

Bhatia, S.K., Moore D., Kalkhoff, R.K. "Progesterone Suppression of the Plasma Growth Hormone Response," *J. Clin Endocrinol Metab* 35: 364–369; 1972.

Crowley, W. "Progesterone Antagonism," *N Eng J Med* 1986; 315–23: 1607–1608. Editorial

De Lignieres B., Dennerstein L., Backstrom, T. "Influence of Route of Administration on Progesterone Metabolism," *Maturitas* 21, 251–257, 1995.

Gaspard, U.J., Wery O.J., Scheen, A.J., et al. "Long-Term Effects of Oral Estradiol and Dydrogesterone on Carbohydrate Metabolism in Postmenopausal Women," *Climacteric: The Journal of the International Menopause Society*, vol. 2, no. 2, June 1999, pp. 93–100.

Kalkoff, R. "Metabolic Effects of Progesterone." *J Obstet Gynecol* 1982; 142–6:735–738.

Wren, B.G., McFarland, K., Edwards, P., et al. "Effect of Sequential Transdermal Progesterone Cream on Endometrium, Bleeding Pattern, and Plasma Progesterone and Salivary Progesterone Levels in Postmenopausal Women," *Climacteric: Journal of the International Menopause Society*, September, 2000. Vol 3, pages 155–160.

Chapter 7
Arlt, W., Callies, F., van Vligmen, J.C., et al. "Dehydroepiandrosterone Replacement in Women with Adrenal Insufficiency," *N Engl Med.* September 30, 1999, 341 (14): 1013-20.

Nestler, J., et al. "Dehydroeplandrosterone: The 'Missing Link' between Hyperinsulinemia and Atherosclerosis?" *FASEB J* 1992; 6: 3073-3075.

McEwen, B., Biegon, A., Davis, P., et al. "Steroid Hormones: Humoral Signals Which Alter Brain Cell Properties and Functions," *Recent Progress in Hormone Research* 1982; 38: 41-83. Discussion: 83-92.

Nieschlag, E., Behre, H.M. (Editors) "Testosterone: Action, Deficiency, Substitution," *2nd Edition.* Springer-Verlag, Berlin, 1998.

Chapter 8

Bunevicius, R., Kazanavicius, G., Zalinkevicius, R., et al. "Effects of Thyroxine as Compared with Thyroxine Plus Triiodothyronine in Patients With Hypothyroidism," *N Eng J Med* 1999; 340-6: 424-429.

Divi, R.L., Chang, H.C., Doerge, D.R. "Anti-thyroid Isoflavones from Soybean: Isolation, Characterization, and Mechanisms of Action," National Center for Toxicological Research, Jefferson, AR, 72079. *Biochem Pharmacol,* 1997 54: 10, 1087-96.

Dong, B., Hauck, W., Gambertoglio, J. "Bioequivalence of Generic and Brand-name Levothyroxine Products in the Treatment of Hypothyroidism," *JAMA* 1997; 277-15: 1205-1213.

Fort, P., Moses, N., Fasano, M., et al. "Breast and Soy-Formula Feedings in Early Infancy and the Prevalence of Autoimmune Thyroid Disease in Children," (from Dept. of Pediatrics, North Shore University Hospital-Cornell University Medical College), in *J. Am. Coll Nutr,* 1990; 9: 2, 164-7.

Massoudi, M., Meilahn, E., Orchard, T., et al. "Thyroid Function and Perimenopausal Lipid and Weight Changes: The Thyroid Study in Healthy Women (TSH-W)," *J Women's Health* 1997; 6-5: 553-558.

Thyroid Disorders and Women's Health. *National Women's Health Report.* 2000; 22-56.

Reus, V.I. "Behavioral Aspects of Thyroid Disease in Women in The Psychiatric Clinics of North America," *Women's Disorders,* Vol. 12, No. 1, March, 1989; 153-166. W. B. Saunders Co., Philadelphia.

Cassidy, A., Bingham, S., Setchell, K.D. "Biological Effects of a Diet of Soy Protein Rich in Isoflavones on the Menstrual Cycle of Premenopausal Women," *Am J Clin Nutr,* 1994; 60 (3): 333-40.

Chapter 9

Birketvedt, G., Florholmen, J., Sundsfjord, J., et al. "Behavioral and Neuroendocrine Characteristics of the Night-Eating Syndrome," *JAMA* 1999; Vol 282 No. 7: 657-663.

Frank, C., Smith, S. "Stress and the Heart," *Psychosomatics* 1990; 31-3: 255-264.

Lipworth B. "Systemic Adverse Effects of Inhaled Corticosteroid Therapy," *Arch Internal Med* 1999; 159: 941-955.

Peeke, P., Chrousos, G. "Hypercortisolism and Obesity," *Ann NY Acad Sci* 1995; 771: 665-676

Post, R. "Transduction of Psychosocial Stress Into the Neurobiology of Recurrent Affective Disorder." *Am J Psychiatry* 1992; 149-8: 999-1010.

Rosenthal, N.E., Sack, D.A., Jacobsen, F.M., et al. "Melatonin in Seasonal Affective Disorder and Phototherapy," *J. Neural Transm Suppl* 1986; 21: 257.

Yager, J., "Nocturnal Eating Syndromes," *JAMA,* Editorial, 1999, Vol 282; No.7: 689-690.

Chapter 10

Bukowiecki, L., et al. "Insulin Resistance and Defective Thermogenesis in Obesity, in Obesity: Dietary Factors and Centrol," Japan Scientific Societies Press; Tokyo 1991, 107–117.

Campaigne, B.N. and Wishner, K.L. "Gender-Specific Health Care in Diabetes Mellitus," *Journal of Gender-specific Medicine* vol.3 Jan/Feb 2000, 51–58.

Deedwania, P. "Hypertension and Diabetes," *Arch Internal Med* 2000; 160: 1583–1594.

DeFronzo, R.A., Ferrannini, E. "Insulin Resistance: a Multifaceted Syndrome Responsible for NIDDM, Obesity, Hypertension, Dyslipidemia, and Atherosclerotic Cardiovascular Disease, *Diabetes Care* 14:3, 173, 1991.

Despres, J.P., Lamarche, B., Mauriege, P., et al. "Hyperinsulinemia as an Independent Risk Factor for Ischemic Heart Disease," *N Eng J Med* 334:952–957, 1996.

Escalante Pulido, J.M., et al. "Changes in Insulin Sensitivity, Secretion and Glucose Effectiveness During Menstrual Cycle," *Arch Med Res.* 1999 Jan–Feb;30(1):19–22. PMID: 10071420; UI: 99170814.

Gaspard, U.J., Wery, Scheen, et al. "Long-Term Effects of Oral Estradiol and Dydrogesterone on Carbohydrate Metabolism in Postmenopausal Women," *Climacteric: The Journal of the International Menopause Society*, vol. 2, no2, June 1999, pp. 93–100.

Kaplan, N.M. "The Deadly Quartet: Upper-Body Obesity, Glucose Intolerance, Hypertriglyceridemia and Hypertension," *Arch Int Med* 149: 1514–1520, 1989.

Ludwig, D., et al. "Relation Between Consumption of Sugar-Sweetened Drinks and Childhood Obesity: a Prospective, Observational Analysis," *Lancet* 2001, 1187:505–508.

Moller, D., ed. "Insulin Resistance," Chicester: John Wiley and Sons, 1993.

Pownall, H., Ballantyne, C., Kimball, K., et al. "Effect of Moderate Alcohol Consumption on Hypertriglyceridemia," *Arch Intern Med* 1999; 159: 981–987.

Rasmussen, J., et al. "Massive Weight Loss Restores 24-Hour Growth Hormone Release Profiles and Serum Insulin-like Growth Factor-1 Levels In Obese Subjects," *J Clin Endo and Metab* 1995; 80: 1407–1415.

Schmidt, M.I., Watson, R.L., Duncan, B.B., et al. "Clustering of Dyslipidemia, Hyperuricemia, Diabetes, and Hypertension and Its Association with Fasting Insulin and Central and Overall Obesity in a General Population," *Metabolism* 45 (6), 699–706, 1996.

Tarnopolsky, M.A., et al. "Carbohydrate Loading and Metabolism during Exercise in Men and Women," *J. Appl Physiol* 1995; 78: 1360–8.

Tchernof, A., et al. "Menopause, Central Body Fatness, and Insulin Resistance: Effects of Hormone-Replacement Therapy," *Coron Artery Dis.* 1998;9(8):503–11. Review. PMID: 9847982; UI: 99064448.

Visser, M., Bouter L, McQuillan, G. "Elevated C-Reactive Protein Levels in Overweight and Obese Adults," *JAMA,* 1999; Vol 282. No.22: 2131.

Yudkin, J. "Dietary Fat and Dietary Sugar In Relation To Ischaemic Heart-Disease and Diabetes," *Lancet* 1964; July: 4–5.

Yudkin, J. "Sucrose, Coronary Heart Disease, Diabetes, and Obesity: Do Hormones Provide a Link?" *Am Heart J* 1988; 115(2): 493–498.

Chapter 11

Ashwell, M., Chinn, S., Stalley, S., Garrow, J.S. "Female Fat Distribution: a Simple Classification Based on Two Circumference Measurements," *Int. J. Obes* 1982; 6:143–52.

Long, P. "The Great Weight Debate," *Health.* February/March, 1992, pp. 42–47.

Hakala, C. "Saliva Testing," Interview with Elizabeth Lee Vliet, M.D. in *Practical Reviews in Women's Health.* Oakstone Medical Publishing, July 1999.

Takunaga, K., et al. "A Novel Technique For The Determination of Body Fat By Computed Tomography," Int *J Obesity* 1983; 7:437–445.

Chapter 12

Bush, T.L., and Whiteman, M.K. "Hormone Replacement Therapy and Risk of Breast Cancer," (editorial) *JAMA* 1999, 281, pp.2140–2142.

Dickey, Richard P., M.D. "Managing Contraceptive Pill Patients," Seventh Edition, 1993. Available from: Essential Medical Information Systems, Inc., P.O. Box 1607, Durant, OK 74702–1607.

Halbreich, U. "Menopause and Psychopharmacology: Signs, Symptom and Treatment." Third International Symposium Women's Health and Menopause, June 1998.

Kritz-Silverstein, D., Barrett-Conner, E. "Long-Term Postmenopausal Hormone Use, Obesity, and Fat Distribution in Older Women," *Journal of American Medical Association, January 3, 1996, Vol 275, No.1, 46–49.*

"Low Biologic Aggressiveness in Breast Cancer in Women Using Hormone Replacement Therapy," *J Clin Oncol* 1998; 16(9):3115–3120.

Sellers, T.A., Mink, P.J., Cerhan, J.R., et al. "The Role of Hormone Replacement Therapy in the Risk for Breast Cancer and Total Mortality in Women with a Family History of Breast Cancer," *Ann Intern Med* 1997; 127:973–80.

Speroff, L. "Postmenopausal Estrogen-Progestin Therapy and Breast Cancer: a Clinical Response to Epidemiological Reports," *Climacteric: The Journal of the International Menopause Society,* 2000: 3: 3–12.

Chapters 13 and 14

"AACE Medical Guidelines for Clinical Practice for Management of Menopause," Endocrine Practice Vol. 5, No.6 November/December 1999, 355–366.

Chen, W.Y. and Colditz, G. "Hormone Replacement Therapy, Selective Estrogen Receptor Modulators and Breast Cancer Risk," *Menopause* 1999; 6: 279–281.

Duncan, A., Lyall, H., Roberts, R., et al. "The Effect of 17 Beta Estradiol and Norethisterone on Insulin Sensitivity in Postmenopausal Women," Third International Symposium Women's Health and Menopause, June 1998.

Fitzpatrick L., Pace, C., Wiita, B. "Comparison of Reigimens Containing Oral Micronized Progesterone or Medroxyprogesterone Acetate on Quality of Life in Postmenopausal Women: A Cross-Sectional Survey," *J Wos Hlth & Gender Based Med* 2000; Vol 9, No. 4: 381–387.

Godsland, I., Crook, D., Wynn, V. "Clinical and Metabolic Considerations of Long-Term Oral Contraceptive Use," *Am J Ob and Gyn* 1992; 166(6) Part 2:1955–1966.

Jensen, J., Christensen, C., and Rodbro, P. "Estrogen-Progesterone Replacement Therapy Changes Body Composition in Early Postmenopausal Women," *Maturitas* (1986), 8, 209–16.

Sulak, P. "Using OCs to Manage Perimenopause," *OBGyn Management* 2000; 41–50.

Sellers, T.A, Mink, P.J., Cerhan, J.R., et al. "The Role of Hormone Replacement Therapy in the Risk for Breast Cancer and Total Mortality in Women with a Family History of Breast Cancer," *Ann Intern Med* 1997; 127: 973–80.

Vassilopoulou-Sellin, R. et al. "Estrogen Replacement Therapy After Localized Breast Cancer: Clinical Outcome of 319 Women Followed Prospectively," *J. Clin Oncol* 1999; 117: 1482–1487.

Vihtamaki, T., Tuimala, R. "Can Climacteric Women Self-Adjust Therapeutic Estrogen Doses Using Symptoms as Markers?" *Maturitas: J Climacteric and Postmenopause* 1998; 28: 199–203.

Vliet, Elizabeth Lee, M.D. "An Approach to Perimenopausal Migraine," *Menopause Management* 1995; 4 –6: 25–33.

Vliet, Elizabeth Lee, M.D., and V. L. H. Davis. "New Perspectives on the Relationship of Hormonal Changes to Affective Disorders in the Perimenopause," NAACOG's Clinical Issues in Women's Health Nursing, Vol. 2, No. 4: *Midlife Women's Health*, October–December, 1991; 453–472. J. B. Lippincott Co., Philadelphia.

Vliet, Elizabeth Lee, M.D. "Screaming to be Heard: Hormonal Connections Women Suspect and Doctors Ignore, " M. Evans and Co., New York, 1995, revised edition 2000.

Vliet, Elizabeth Lee, M.D. Hormone Connections in Urinary Incontinence in Women." *Top Geriatr Rehabil* June 2000; 15(4):16–30.

Young, C.M., Blondin J., Tensuan, R., et al. "Body Composition Studies of "Older" Women, Thirty to Seventy Years of Age," *Ann NY Acad Sci* 1963, 110: 589–607.

Chapter 15

Ahrens, R. "Sucrose, Hypertension, and Heart Disease," *Am J Clin Nutr* 1975; 28: 195–202.

Allred, J. "Too Much of a Good Thing? An Overemphasis On Eating Low Fat Foods May Be Contributing To The Alarming Increase In Overweight Among U.S. Adults," *J Am Dietetic Assoc* 1995; 95 (4): 417–418.

Ames, B. "Paleolithic Diet, Evolution and Carcinogens," *Science* 1997; 258: 1633–34.

Berry, E., et al. "Effects of Diets Rich In Monounsaturated Fatty Acids On Plasma Lipoproteins– The Jerusalem Nutrition Study II monounsaturated Fatty Acids vs. Carbohydrates." *Am J Clin Nutr* 1992; 56: 394–403.

Borkman, M., Campbell LV, Chisholm DJ, et al. "Comparison of The Effects On Insulin-Sensitivity of High Carbohydrate and High fat Diets In Normal Subjects." *J Clin Endocrinol Metab* 72: 432–437, 1991.F.

Blum, M., Averbuch, M., Wolman, Y., et al. "Protein Intake and Kidney Function in Humans: its Effect on Normal Aging'. *Arch Intern Med* 149:211–212, 1989.

Brenner, R. "Nutritional and Hormonal Factors Influencing Desaturation of Essential Fatty Acids," *Prog Lipid Res*; 20: 41–47.

Campbell, L.V., Borkman, M., Marmot, P.E., et al. "The High-Monounsaturated Fat Diet as a Practical Alternative for NIDDM," *Diabetes Care.* 17(3), 177, 1994.

Carpenter, K. "Protein Requirements of Adults From An Evolutionary Perspective," *Am J Clin Nutr* 1992; 55:913–917.

Chen, Y., et al. "Why Do Low-Fat High-Carbohydrate Diets Accentuate Postprandial Lipemia In Patients With NIDDM?" *Diabetes Care* 1995; 18(1): 10–16.

Connor, W., et al. "N-3 Fatty Acids From Fish Oil: Effects On Plasma Lipoproteins and Hypertriglyceridemic Patients," *NY Acad of Sci* 1993; 683: 16–34.

Coulston, A., et al. "Persistence of Hypertriglyceridemic Effect of Low–fat High–Carbohydrate Diets in NIDDM Patients." *Diabetes Care* 1989; 12(2): 94–101.

Coulston, A., et al. Plasma Glucose, Insulin and Lipid Responses To High-Carbohydrate Low-Fat Diets In Normal Humans, *Metabolism* 1983; 32(1): 52–56.

Crapo, P., et al. "Comparison of Serum Glucose, Insulin and Glucagon Responses To Different Types of Complex Carbohydrate In Non-Insulin-Dependent Diabetic Patients," *Am J Clin Nutr* 1981; 34: 189–190.

Dulloo, A., et al. "Differential Effects of High Fat Diets Varying In Fatty Acid Composition On The Efficiency of Lean and Fat Tissue Deposition During Weight Recovery After Low Food Intake," *Metabolism* 1995; 44(2): 273–279.

Farquhar, J., et al. "Glucose, Insulin, and Triglyceride Responses To High and Low Carbohydrate Diets In Man," *J Clin Invest* 1966; 45(10): 1648–1656.

Flatt, J. "Use and Storage of Carbohydrate and Fat," *Am J Clin Nutr* 1995; 61(suppl): 925–928.

Garg, A., et al. "Effects of Varying Carbohydrate Content of Diet in Patients With Non-Insulin-Dependent Diabetes Melitus," *JAMA* 1994; 271(18): 1421–1428.

Horrobin, D. The Role of Essential Fatty Acids and Prostaglandins in the Premenstrual Syndrome. *J Reprod Med* 1983; 28: 465–469.

Hunt, J., et al. "High Versus Low Meat Diets: Effects On Zinc Absorption Iron Status, and Calcium, Copper, Iron, Magnesium, Nitrogen, Phosphorous, and Zinc Balance In Postmenopausal Women," *Am J Clin Nutr* 1995; 62: 621–632.

Hunter, B. "Some Food Additives As Neuroexcitors and Neurotoxins," *Clinical Ecology* 1984; II–2: 83–89.

Jenkins, D., et al. "Glycemic Index of Foods: A Physiological Basis For Carbohydrate Exchange," *Am J Clin Nutr* 1995; 34: 362–366.

Jenkins, D., et al. "Metabolic Effects of A Low-Glycemic Index Diet," *Am J Clin Nutr* 1997; 46: 968–975.

Lesourd, B. "Protein Undernutrition As The Major Cause of Decreased Immune Function In The Elderly: Clinical and Functional Implications," *Nutr Rev* 1995; 53: 86s–94s.

Muller, W., et al. "The Influence of the Anticedent Diet Upon Glucagon and Insulin Secretion," *N Eng J Med* 1971; 285: 1450–1454.

Parillo, M., et al. "A High-Monounsaturated Fat/Low-Carbohydrate Diet Improves Peripheral Insulin Sensitivity In Non-Insulin Dependent Diabetic Patients," *Metabolism* 1992; 41(12): 1373–1378.

Schubring, C., Prohaska, F., Prohaska, A., et al. "Liptin Concentrtions in Maternal Serum and Amniotic Fluid During the Second Trimenon: Differential Relation to Fetal Gender and Maternal Morphometry," *Eur J Obstet Gynecol Reprod Biol* 1999; 86–2: 151–157.

Slabber, M., et al. "Effect of a Low-Insulin-Response, Energy-Restricted Diet On Weight Loss and Plasma Insulin Concentration In Hyperinsulinemic Obese Females," *Am J Clin Nutr* 1994; 60: 48–53.

Smith, W., et al. "Dietary Fat and Fish Intake and Age-Related Maculopathy," *Arch Opth* 2000; 118: 401–404.

Thissen, J., et al. "Nutritional Regulation of the Insulin-Like Growth Factors," *Endo Rev* 1994; 15(1): 80-101.

Von Borstel, R. "Metabolic and Physiologic Effects of Sweeteners," *Clin Nutr* 1985; 4(6): 215-220.

Chapter 16

Abraham, G. "Nutritional Factors in the Etiology of the Premenstrual Tension Syndromes," *J Repro Med* 1983; 28(7): 446-464.

Blum, J., Averbuch, M., Wolman, Y., et al. Protein Intake and Kidney Function in Humans: Its Effect on 'Normal Aging'. *Arch Intern Med* 1989; 149: 211-212.

Cassidy, A., Bingham, S., Setchell, K. "Biological Effects of Isoflavones in Young Women: Importance of the Chemical Composition of Soyabean Products," *Br J Nutr* 1995; 74:587-601.

Iso, H., Rexrode, K., Stampfer, M. "Intake of Fish and Omega-3 Fatty Acids and Risk of Stroke in Women," *JAMA* 2001; 285(3): 304-312.

Ludwig, D., Pereira, M., Kroenke, C., et al. "Dietary Fiber, Weight Gain, and Cardiovascular Disease Risk Factors in Young Adults," *JAMA* 1999; 282(16): 1539-1546.

Mackey, R. and Eden, J. "Phytoestrogens and the Menopause," *Climacteric: J Int Meno Soc* 1998; 1:302-308.

Nagata, C., Kabuto, M., Kurisu, Y., Shimizu, H. "Decreased Serum Estradiol Concentration Associated with High Dietary Intake of Soy Products in Premenopausal Japanese Women," *Nutr and Ca* 1997; 29(3): 228-233.

Chapter 17

Pharmacist's Letter/Prescriber's Letter Natural Medicines Comprehensive Database. J. M. Jellin, F. Batz, and K. Hitchens, Therapeutic Research Faculty, Stockton, CA, 1999.

Boushey, C., et al. "A Quantitative Assessment of Plasma Homocysteine As A Risk Factor For Vascular Disease: Probably Benefits of Increasing Folic Acid Intakes," *JAMA* 1995; 274: 1049-1057.

Challen, J. "The Problem With Herbs," *Nat Hlth* 1999; Jan-Feb: 56-60.

Drapper, H., "Nutritional Modulation of Oxygen Radical Pathology," *Adv in Nutr Research* 1990; 8: 273-279.

Drinka, P., Langer, E., Voeks, S., et al. "Hypovitaminosis In a Control Subject," *So Med J* 1991; 85(11): 1368-1369.

Elam, M., Hunninghake, D., Davis, K., et al. "Effect of Niacin on Lipid and Lipoprotein Levels and Glycemic Control in Patients with Diabetes and Peripheral Arterial Disease," *JAMA* 2000; Vol 284, No. 10: 1263-1270.

Hansen, H. "New Biological and Clinical Roles For The n-6 and n-3 Fatty Acids," *Nutr Rev* 1994; 52 (5): 162-167.

Harris, et al. "Dietary Omega-3 Fatty Acids Prevent Carbohydrate-Induced Hypertriglyceridemia," *Metabolism* 1984; 33 (11): 1016-1019.

Hunter, B. "Some Food Additives As Neuroexcitors and Neurotoxins," *Clinical Ecology* 1984; II-2; 83-89.

Johnston, C. "Recommendations for Vitamin C Intake," *JAMA* 1999; Vol 282. No 22 : 2118 letters

Lardinois, C. "The Role of Omega-3 Fatty Acids on Insulin Secretion and Insulin Sensitivity," *Med Hypotheses* 1987; 24: 243-248.

McMahon, F., Fujioka, K., Singh, B., et al. "Efficacy and Safety of Sibutramine in Obese White and African American Patients with Hypertension," *Arch Intern Med* 2000; 160: 2185-2191.

Meagher, E., Barry, O., Lawson, J., et al. "Effects of Vitamin E on Lipid Peroxidation in Healthy Persons," *JAMA* 2001; Vol 285, No.9: 1178-1182.

Paolisso, G., et al. "Pharmacologic Doses of Vitamin E Improve Insulin Action in Healthy Subjects and Non-Insulin Dependent Diabetic Patients," *Am J Clin Nutr* 1993; 57: 650-656.

Stevinson, C., "Pittler M, Ernst E. Garlic For Treating Hypercholesterolemia is a Questionable Practice. *Ann Intern Med* 2000; 133: 420-429.

Wen, Y., Doyle, M., Harrison, R., et al. "The Effect of Hormone Replacement Therapy On Vitamin E Status in Post Menopausal Women." *Maturitas* 1997; 26: 121-124.

Chapter 18

Andersen, J., Schjerling, P., Saltin, B. "Muscles, Genes and Athletic Performance," *Scientific American* 2000; Sept; 49-55.

Baker, N. "The Fat Fixation," *New Woman* 1985; May: 60-62.

Berkman, S. "Body Image: Larger Than Life?" *Women's Health and Fitness News.* 1990; 4(8): 1-6.

Bullen, B., Skrinar, G., Beitins, I., et al. "Endurance Training Effects on Plasma Hormonal Responsiveness and Sex Hormone Excretion," *J. Appl Phys: Respirat.Environ. Exercise Physiol* 1984; 56-6: 1453-1463.

Duncan, J.J., Gordon, N.F., Scott, C.B. "Women Walking for Health and Fitness: How Much is Enough?" *JAMA* 266: 3295-3299, 1991.

"Exercise and Weight Control." The President's Council on Physical Fitness and Sports, Department of Health and Human Services, Dept. No. 176, 701 Pennsylvania Ave. NW, Washington, DC 20004.

Fine, J.T., Colditz, G.A., Coakley, E.H., et al. "A Prospective Study of Weight Change and Health-Related Quality of Life in Women," *JAMA* 1999; 282:2136-2142.

Fogelholm, M., Kukkonen-Harjula, K., Nenonen, A., et al. "Effects of Walking Training on Weight Maintenance after a Very-Low-Energy Diet in Premenopausal Obese Women," *Arch Intern Med* 2000; 160: 2177-2184.

Hardman, A., et al. "Brisk Walking and Plasma High Density Lipoprotein Cholesterol Concentration in Previously Sedentary Women," *BMJ* 1989; 299: 1204-1205.

Hersey, W., et al. "Endurance Exercise Training Improves Body Composition and Plasma Insulin Responses in Seventy to Seventy Nine Year Old Men and Women," *Metabolism* 1994; 43(7): 847-854.

Manson, J., Hu, F., Rich-Edwards, J., et al. "A Prospective Study of Walking as Compared with Vigorous Exercise in the Prevention of Coronary Heart Disease in Women," *N Eng Med* 1999; 341-9: 650-658.

Masand, P. Chr. Symposium. "Weight Gain Associated With Use of Psychotropic Drugs," *Therapeutic Advances in Psychoses* 1999; July 4.

Melissas, J., Christodoulakis, M., Spyridakis, M., et al. "Disorders Associated With Clinically Severe Obesity: Significant Improvement After Surgical Weight Reduction," *So Med J* 1998;

91(12); 1143–1148.

Norsigian, J. "Dieting Is Dangerous To Your Health," *The Network News* 1986; May–June: 4–6

O'Brien, S.J., Vertinsky, P.A. "Unfit Survivors: Exercise as a Resource for Aging Women. *The Gerontologist* 31, 347–357, 1991.

Prior, J., Vigna, Y., Alojada, N. "Conditioning Exercise Decreases Premenstrual Symptoms," *Eur J Appl Physiol* 1986; 55: 349–355.

Racette, S., et al. "Effects of Aerobic Exercise and Dietary Carbohydrate on Energy Expenditure and Body Composition During Weight Reduction in Obese Women," *Amer J Clin Nutr* 1995; 61: 486–494 .

Shangold, M. "Exercise and the Adult Female: Hormonal and Endocrine Effects," *Exer & Sport Sci Rev* 1984; 12: 53–79.

Sternhell, C. "We'll Always Be Fat But Fat Can Be Fit," *Ms* 1985; May: 66.

"The Facts About Weight Loss Products and Programs," (This brochure, produced by the Federal Trade Commission in conjunction with the Food and Drug Administration and the National Association of Attorneys General, has tips on evaluating diet claims and weight loss programs. Copies can be obtained from the FTC, Public Affairs Branch, Room 130, Sixth St. and Pennsylvania Ave. NW, Washington, DC 20580.)

Weber, M., et al. "Contrasting Clinical Properties and Exercise Responses in Obese and Lean Hypertensive Patients," *Journal of the American College of Cardiology,* 2001; 37: 169–174.

Wurtman, R. "The Ultimate Head Waiter: How the Brain Controls Diet," *Technology Review* 1984; 87–5: 42–51.

CONSUMER BOOKS, ORGANIZATIONS, AND WEBSITES

Screaming to Be Heard: Hormone Connections Women Suspect and Doctors Still Ignore. Elizabeth Lee Vliet, M.D., M. Evans and Company, New York, 1995; revised/expanded edition 2000. Comprehensive guide to the ovarian hormones and what they do, as well as current science regarding hormone connections in a variety of clinical syndromes such as fibromyalgia, migraines, PCOS, PMS, depression, bladder problems, heart disease, breast cancer, chronic fatigue, memory loss, osteoporosis. Also covers detailed description of getting hormones tested properly, what products contain natural hormones and when you may need to consider synthetic hormones in particular situations. Reviews available on Amazon.com.

The Thyroid Solution. Ridha Arem, M.D., The Ballantine Publishing Group, a division of Random House, Inc., New York, 1999. An excellent reference book on thyroid disorders, written by an endocrinologist with solid credentials and clinical experience. Dr. Arem validates what I have seen in my practice for my entire career: Many women in particular have subclinical forms of thyroid disorders that affect mood, fertility, weight and a host of other problems. In addition, Dr. Arem goes into more depth on the value of adding T3 to a thyroid medication regimen, as I have espoused and used for many years as well. I do not think Dr. Arem's information on estrogen therapy is either comprehensive or up to date, and I am very concerned about his emphasis on the use of Premarin and Provera based on the issues I have described in this book and in *Screaming to Be Heard.* I do, however, think his information on thyroid is outstanding.

Menopause and Midlife Health. Morris Notelovitz, M.D., and Diana Tonnessen, St. Martin's Press, New York, 1994. Written by a pioneer in osteoporosis and menopause, this book presents accurate and up to date information about managing your health, including the role of healthy lifestyle habits. Discusses hormone therapies, pros and cons of gynecological procedures, issues about breast cancer and other concerns of importance to women.

Menopause. Miriam Stoppard, M.D., Dorling Kindslerly Publishing, London and New York, 1994. A beautifully illustrated book that addresses the total woman during this important transition and the years beyond. Color charts and graphs make it easier to understand difficult medical concepts and help women manage their menopause in optimal ways.

The Female Heart: The Truth About Women and Coronary Artery Disease. Marianne Legato, M.D., and Carol Colman, Harper Collins Publishers, New York, 1996.

Nutrition, Hypertension & Cardiovascular Disease. Smith R., Lyncean Press, Beavertown, Oregon, 1989. Although this was published in 1989, it is clearly written, and provides understandable explanations of hypertension and cardiovascular disease, emphasizing risk factors you can control and ways to prevent development of disease. Dr. Legato does not address all the nuances of the differences in types of estrogens and progestins as I have discussed, but her heart disease information is quite good.

The Good News About Women's Hormones. Geoffrey Redmond, M.D., Warner Books, New York, 1995. There are many parallels in the work Dr. Redmond has done to identify and treat women's hormone problems and the hormone connections I have been addressing in my own work. This book is easily understandable, and has very good sections on androgenic disorders (excess hair growth, acne, and other problems) and alopecia (hair loss) as well as the many other hormone problems he discusses. He gives a balanced view of benefits and risks of hormone treatments, and a logical approach to helping women decide about hormone use and how to get reliable lab tests.

PCOS: The Hidden Epidemic. Samuel S. Thatcher, M.D., Ph.D. Perspectives Press, Indianapolis, IN., 2000. Dr. Thatcher is a renown expert in reproductive endocrinology and brings to this book many years of clinical experience as one of the early advocates for increased understanding of this complex and serious metabolic disorder. The book gives an overview of what PCOS is, our current understanding of causes, and information on helpful treatments based on research findings. This is an excellent resource, recommended by the Polycystic Ovarian Syndrome Association. Order from Perspective Press at 317-872-3055, or www.perspectivespress.com.

Why Zebras Don't Get Ulcers. Robert M. Sapolsky, W.H. Freeman & Co., New York, NY, 1998. Excellent and humorous review of the adverse effects over time due to high cortisol levels from stress. If you ever wondered just how "stress" affects your entire body, this is a terrific and well-written book.

Woman's Body: A Manual For Life. Dr. Miriam Stoppard, Dorling Kindersley, London and New York, 1994. Compiled by a team of health experts from many fields, this book covers physical and emotional concerns of women throughout the lifespan and is illustrated with hundreds of color charts, graphs, and photos. It is one of the most comprehensive and practical women's health books I have found.

Strong Women Stay Young. Miriam E. Nelson, Ph.D., Bantam-Doubleday-Dell, New York, NY, (paperback) 1998. An excellent book outlining the benefits of both aerobic and strength-training for women to preserve and build healthy bone and muscle. I highly recommend it.

Mind/Body Medicine: How To Use Your Mind For Better Health. Consumer Reports Books, Consumers Union of the U.S., Inc., New York, 1993. A well-researched book written by the leading authorities from the nation's top medical centers. Full of practical suggestions and descriptions of what works and how to find resources in your area.

The Bodywise Woman: Reliable Information About Physical Activity and Health. Written by the staff and researchers of the Melpomene Institute for Women's Health Research, Prentice Hall Press, New York, 1990. Well-researched and specific to the needs of women of all ages. Write to this organization for updates of their consumer materials.

40-30-30 Fat Burning Nutrition. Joyce and Gene Daoust, Wharton Publishing, Del Mar, CA, 1996. An excellent, easy-to-read, practical and easy-to-follow meal plan that helps you reduce the fat-storing insulin excesses caused by our current high-carbohydrate, low-fat diets. The Daosts have done a terrific job of providing healthy meal plans for both vegetarians and non-vegetarians, and they have also provided a list of prepared foods that fit well into the 40-30-30 balance. Our patients have found this book quite helpful. The authors have a new book that is more detailed in the exercise guidelines and receipes, called *The Formula: A Personalized 40-30-30 Weight Loss Program.* Their books are based on the concept of The Zone diet, popularized by Dr. Barry Sears, which has many sound concepts although the meal plans are more difficult to follow.

Note: Dr. Sears has recently published a new book, *The Soy Zone,* that I *do not recommend* because he does not take into account the latest science showing competitive inhibition of ovarian hormone production in premenopausal women by high dietary intake of soy protein or soy supplements. Nor does he address the potential for a high soy diet to markedly interfere with thyroid function, particularly a common problem in women. For these reasons, if you have any symptoms suggestive of either ovarian hormone imbalance or thyroid disorders, I suggest you do not use the "soy zone" meal plans.

Syndrome X: The Complete Nutritional Program to Prevent and Reverse Insulin Resistance. Jack Challen, Burton Berkson, MD and Melissa Diane Smith. John Wiley and Sons, New York, NY, 2000. An excellent resource for understanding the role that elevated insulin plays in causing heart disease, hypertension, elevated triglycerides, abnormal cholesterol patterns and diabetes. Gives helpful information on nutritional approaches to correct these problems and reduce later risk of diabetes and cardiovascular disorders.

Cooking Low Carb. Brenda Laughlin and Kelly Nason, Two N's Publishing, P.O. Box 35, Littleton, MA 01460, 1999. Order from *www.cest-bon.com.* A practical and easy-to-follow cookbook written especially for sufferers of PCOS, but useful for anyone with problems managing waistline weight gain.

Once-A-Month Cooking (Revised Edition): A Proven System for Spending Less time in the Kitchen and Enjoying Delicious, Homemade Meals Every Day. Mimi Wilson and Mary Beth Lagerborg. St. Martin's Griffin, New York. 1999. An excellent resource for making a month's worth of meals ahead and then having them quickly available when you are ravenous and too tired to make something healthy. Highly recommended by a close friend and mother of two active teenagers who said this book really works!

"Are You Eating Right?" Consumer Reports, October 1992. This article summarizes advice from 68 nutrition experts, including a discussion on weight control and health risks of obesity. Available in public libraries.

Women & Self-Esteem—Understanding and Improving the Way We Think and Feel About Ourselves. Linda Tschirhart Sanford and Mary Ellen Donovan, Penguin Books, New York, 1992. An excellent overview of issues affecting women, still relevant today. Helps women understand cultural sources of low self-esteem and provides practical approaches for building an enhanced self-esteem; a valuable resource.

Healing Words. The Power of Prayer and the Practice of Medicine, Larry Dossey, MD, Harper, San Francisco, 1993. A meaningful book about the ways that modern medicine has overlooked the crucial role of prayer in healing, and how to help you reconnect with your spiritual needs as you face life's challenges. I have read most of Dr. Dossey's books and have found they are inspiring and encouraging of the steps we need to take to make medicine and healing more focused on the whole person.

Sacred Journey. An inspirational journal of readings, prayers and reflections on life written by contributors of all faiths and published by the interfaith organization, A Fellowship in Prayer, Inc. 291 Witherspoon St., Princeton, NJ 08542. This little journal is a wealth of short, inspiring readings that will help facilitate your daily meditation and spiritual awareness.

Organizations and Websites

American Hemochromatosis Society, 777 E. Atlantic Avenue, Suite Z-363, Delray Beach, FL 33483, or read more about it on the Web (*www.americanhs.org*).

National Osteoporosis Foundation (NOF), 2100 M Street N.W., Suite 602, Washington, D.C. 20037, 1-800-223-2226, Web site: *www.nof.org.* An excellent source of cutting edge information about osteoporosis prevention and treatment. Join NOF and become an advocate in your community. I highly recommend their educational materials.

North American Menopause Society. Check their Web site at *www.nams.org* for information on hormone therapy, a list of health professionals specializing in menopause around the country, consumer educational materials and other helpful resources.

PolyCystic Ovarian Syndrome Association, Inc. An excellent resource for educational materials, support groups, web discussions of PCOS. The organization also hosts an outstanding annual conference on PCOS, with presentations from many of the leading experts in the field. Check out their Web site at *www.pcosupport.com*, or call 630-585-3690. Mail address is P.O. Box 7007, Rosemont, IL 60018

WIN: Weight-control Information Network E-mail: *win@info.niddk.nih.gov* Phone: (301) 984-7378 or 1-800-WIN-8098 Fax: (301) 984-7196. The Weight-control Information Network (WIN) is a service of the National Institute of Diabetes and Digestive and Kidney Diseases (NIDDK), part of the National Institutes of Health, under the U.S. Public Health Service. Authorized by Congress (Public Law 103-43), WIN assembles and disseminates to health professionals and the public information on weight control, obesity, and nutritional disorders. WIN responds to requests for information; develops, reviews, and distributes publications; and develops communications strategies to encourage individuals to achieve and maintain a healthy weight.

Newsletters

Alternative Therapies in Women's Health (published by American Health Consultants, a Medical Economics company) is a reliable resource for sound, balanced reviews of the literature and specific products. *Call 1-800-688-2421 for subscription information.* For those interested in *science-based information* on **alternative medicine therapies** in women's health, I recommend this newsletter because it does not appear to accept product advertising or to be sponsored by product manufacturers as far as I can tell. I have found it helpful for my own information in order to better answer patient questions about supplements and alternative therapies. I have no financial involvement with this publication.

The Harvard Women's Health Watch Newsletter. In my opinion, of all the many women's health newsletters that have been brought out since the first edition of my book, this is by far the best in terms of quality and depth of information. It is published monthly by Harvard Health Publications, 10 Shattuck Street, Suite 612, Boston, MA 02115. The authors provide timely, well-researched information on many topics of interest to women of all ages, and the content is provided in enough depth to make it useful to guide your discussions with your own health professionals.

Nutrition Action published by the Center for Science in the Public Interest, Washington, D.C. Web site: cspinet.org/nah. An excellent, progressive newsletter that is NOT supported by advertising. It is hard-hitting and unbiased by commercial influences. Contains practical advice on reading food labels, selecting healthy options, avoiding hidden sources of fat, salt and sugar and other pointers.

Pharmacists Letter/Prescriber's Letter Natural Medcines Comprehensive Database. This group publishes a newsletter and a comprehensive reference book of detailed information on vitamins, herbs, and natural medicine supplements. Their reference book has been prepared by pharmacists who have reviewed the medical studies from around the world and then compiled summaries of uses, side effects and symptoms of overdose for thousands of supplements. It is one of the most comprehensive, reliable, scientifically-based compilations of information on natural medicines that I have found anywhere. *It is not supported by advertising, is objective and medically sound.* For more information on how to subscribe to their newsletter or purchase a copy of the reference book, call 209-472-2244 or visit their Web site: *www.naturaldatabase.com.*

I subscribed to a number of other women's health newsletters for a year or so with each one so that I could evaluate their material over time. After this detailed review, I am not recommending any other women's health newsletters because in my professional opinion, they are either (1) pushing supplements and other products, (2) have unreliable medical information, (3) have too much "fluff" without enough depth to their content to be overly useful, or (4) they push a narrow point of view without sufficient balance to be objective.

To Locate Additional Resources on Obesity

The National Institute of Diabetes and Digestive and Kidney Diseases (NIDDK) is the part of the National Institutes of Health chiefly responsible for obesity research. NIDDK supports the study of obesity in its own labs and clinics and at universities, hospitals, and research centers across the United States. NIDDK-funded research has helped scientists learn more about the role of genes and metabolism in obesity. Other NIDDK-supported studies have examined the relationship between obesity and various medical conditions. Ongoing NIDDK research efforts include better ways to define and treat the various types of obesity and understanding how the body stores and uses fat.

NIDDK also oversees the *National Task Force on Prevention and Treatment of Obesity*. The task force comprises leading obesity and nutrition experts who gather and assess the latest information on obesity treatment and prevention. The task force also helps guide basic and clinical research on obesity. Scientific papers and general-interest brochures and pamphlets approved by the task force are available from the NIDDK's Obesity Resource Information Center. In addition to NIDDK, other sections of the NIH sponsor obesity research. They include:

> The National Heart, Lung, and Blood Institute (NHLBI)
> The National Center for Research Resources (NCRR)
> The National Institute of Child Health and Human Development (NICHD)
> The National Institute on Mental Health (NIMH)
> The National Cancer Institute (NCI)
> The National Institute on Aging (NIA)
> The National Institute of Nursing Research (NINR)
> The National Institute of Arthritis and Musculoskeletal and Skin Diseases (NIAMS)
> The National Institute of Neurological Diseases and Stroke (NINDS)
> The National Institute of Environmental and Health Sciences (NIEHS)

Other Materials

Polar Heart Monitor—a helpful device to monitor heart rate and keep you exercising in your target zone. They have various models at different prices, and some are waterproof, so they can be used with swimming as well as other exercises.

Aqua Jogger—a flotation belt with back support to keep you upright for "jogging" in the water. Particularly if you are overweight, this allows you to get a good aerobic workout without adding stress to the knees, hips, and ankles. Available at most pool supply stores.

SOURCES FOR NATURAL HORMONES

Belmar Pharmacy, Charles Hakala, R.Ph., Lakewood, CO (Denver area)
Phone 800-525-9473 Fax 303-763-9712

Charles Hakala has been a pioneer in compounding prescriptions for patients with challenging medical problems such as chemical sensitivities, multiple allergies to dyes/binders, in addition to his outstanding reputation in the field of compounding natural, bio-identical hormone preparations for thyroid, ovary, and adrenal hormones. For those with thyroid problems, Belmar

Pharmacy is the one I have used since about 1985 for individualized sustained release T3 preparations. Most commercial preparations containing T3 are fixed dose combinations that don't allow adequate flexibility in dose, and also may contain dyes, binders or animal proteins that adversely affect people with allergies and chemical sensitivities.

Charles is also knowledgeable about important differences between the more reliable *serum* methods of hormone testing versus methods such as saliva and urine that commonly give misleading results. He will discuss these issues with both consumers and physicians. He uses micronized natural forms of estradiol, testosterone, progesterone, and DHEA derived from soybeans and wild yams, and will make prescriptions in whatever form is needed for best results. Although I don't recommend estriol and estrone as desirable forms of hormone therapy, Charles does make these compounded prescriptions for those women who wish to use these types of estrogen. Belmar pharmacists will make up prescriptions using lactose-free hypoallergenic formulations with no dyes; they also make vaginal creams that are hypoallergenic and omit some of the common irritants found in most commercial products.

Spence Pharmacy, Daryl Spence, R.Ph., Ft. Worth, TX
Phone 800-209-7364 Fax 817-625-8103

Daryl Spence is another reliable compounding pharmacist who has created innovative topical pain relief medications, in addition to his work with bio-identical, natural micronized hormones such as estradiol, testosterone, progesterone, DHEA. Although I don't recommend estriol and estrone as desirable forms of hormone therapy, Daryl does make these compounded prescriptions for those women who wish to use these types of estrogen. In trying to find testosterone options for women, Daryl and I have collaborated on forms that will provide sustained effects over the day, and I am pleased with the success of his formulations for my patients. Daryl's sustained-release testosterone capsule formulation is one that many of my patients have found helpful. Spence Pharmacy will also make up prescriptions using lactose-free hypoallergenic formulations with no dyes, and no preservatives that are potentially irritating or may aggravate allergies.

Disclaimer: *I have no financial interest in any of these pharmacies or their products.* I provide this information as a service to you and your physician because reliable information on these topics has been difficult for the average consumer to obtain. Compounded and "natural" hormones are not new, in spite of all the recent marketing of such products. Many of these options have been around for forty years or more. I have been a longstanding advocate for the use of bio-identical, "natural" human forms of hormone preparations, and I have seen over many years of my practice the marked positive difference that occurs when women change from the animal-derived, conjugated estrogens and synthetic forms of progestins.

General Comments

Both Belmar and Spence Pharmacies are *full-service pharmacies* with ability to fill all of your prescription needs, not just compounded prescriptions. Both pharmacies also work with many major health insurance plans. In addition, I have found that both of these pharmacies often have better prices on common commercial prescriptions (such as estradiol patches) than my patients find at the big chain drugstores. I encourage you to do a little price-shopping to decide where you want your prescriptions filled before you automatically assume the big chain drugstores are cheaper.

There are many pharmacies around the country that are now providing compounding services. There are several important reasons I have continued to collaborate primarily with Belmar and

Spence pharmacies on prescriptions for my patients. First, both of these pharmacists have many years experience in the art and science of compounding and are not just starting these services in the wake of current interest. Second, each compounding pharmacist has his or her own formula for making the various forms of prescription hormones, and each formulation will vary in how it is metabolized in the body. Therefore, each formulation will act somewhat differently in a given person and adds yet another variable to the equation of trying to solve the problem when a person has side effects. It is difficult enough clinically to sort out individual differences in metabolism and response when I know the pharmacology of a given preparation. If the preparation also varies, it can become almost impossible to sort out the Gordian knot of factors that could alter a person's response. That's why I prefer to work with brand name products instead of generics, and to limit my prescriptions to just a few compounding pharmacists upon whose preparations I can rely for consistency.

Third, I am increasingly concerned at the degree to which some pharmacists are now practicing medicine by adjusting women's hormone doses based on questionable test methods, such as saliva and urine hormone levels, without having access to other laboratory measures that need to be included in decision making about appropriate hormone dose and route. Pharmacists who are advising patients on doses of various hormones are violating laws governing pharmacy practice. Pharmacists are not licensed to determine the *dose* that is correct for you; that function is by law the task of the physician. I have treated too many patients who have been significantly overdosed on hormones when getting their information from pharmacists making the dose changes, and I have chosen to put my prescriptions at pharmacies where the pharmacists do not engage in this practice.

The two pharmacies above are resources I have depended upon to provide individual prescriptions for my patients and family; we have been pleased with the results. These pharmacists are skilled, knowledgeable, and committed to providing quality service to you and your physician. I have found them to be ethical and responsible in working *with* the physician. Neither of these pharmacy owners allows their staff to go outside the bounds of pharmacy licensing and make dose changes on their own without consultation with your physician.

Comments about FDA-Approval

Women often ask, "Are these compounded hormones FDA-approved?" The answer is no, because the individual compounded prescriptions are not manufactured and distributed for sale in quantities that would require FDA-approval. At reputable compounding pharmacies, the ingredients used are *pharmaceutical-grade* (U.S.P.) bases that are then made up into tablets or creams or suppositories to your individual needs. Individual pharmacists operate within their training and state licenses when they prepare (compound) individual prescriptions based on your own physician's decision about dose and type of medication best for you.

Although many types of medications used to be compounded individually, it is no longer advantageous to do so with the current quality of manufactured products widely available. Much of the current use of individual compounding is for patients with allergies, marked sensitivities to dyes and binders in commercial preparations, patients who need smaller doses, and in particular, women who want to take natural, bio-identical human forms of hormones that aren't yet available in commercial products at regular drugstores.

Natural ovarian hormones have been in widespread use in Europe, Australia, Canada, Japan and other countries for many years, generally with better clinical response and fewer side effects than the synthetic progestins, conjugated equine estrogens, and synthetic methyltestosterone compounds used in the United States. When these natural, or bio-identical, forms of hormones are not available commercially at the chain drugstores, the compounding pharmacies can make up ones similar to those available in Europe and other countries.

For estrogen, however, there are several *brands* of the natural human form, *17-beta estradiol*, available in the United States that are FDA approved and made by commercial pharmaceutical companies (which means they are more likely to be covered by your health insurance plan as well as having the health benefits of being what your own body has always made): **Estrace and Gynodiol** tablets, **Estrace** vaginal cream, Vagifem vaginal tablets, Estring vaginal ring, **VivelleDOT, Climara, Alora, Esclim** and **Estraderm** transdermal (skin) patches. All of these products contain the same natural, bio-identical form of 17-beta estradiol that our ovaries made before menopause. These products are made with the precursor, or building block, molecules that come from soybeans. The primary difference in the various patches is the type of adhesive (which may affect frequency of skin rash and how well it stays on your body) and the duration of effect from the patch. We prescribe whatever brand a woman likes best.

There are also now available several generic versions of 17-beta estradiol tablets since **Estrace** has gone off patent. Unfortunately, I have found that the quality and potency varies widely from one generic manufacturer to another, and the dose you need may be more than what is required with Estrace to achieve the same effect. If you have been stabilized on one brand, it can lead to recurrence of your symptoms or to more side effects if you don't realize a pharmacist has switched your tablets to another manufacturer. For these reasons, I don't usually recommend the generic estradiol tablets. I have had many patients who had marked relapse of their symptoms when switched to a generic form of estradiol.

In addition to the commercial estradiol products, there are now two new FDA-approved commercial products for natural progesterone: **Prometrium** tablets and **Crinone** vaginal gel. You no longer have to turn to compounded natural progesterone products that are often not covered by insurance plans. Both Prometrium and Crinone are available through regular drugstores and are usually covered by most health plans that provide prescription plans. Both of these commercial products are made from yam and soybean precursors and are micronized for optimal absorption. They both work well for endometrial protection, so the choice of which product for your use depends on such aspects as personal preference and side effects, which will vary depending on whether progesterone is taken orally or is absorbed vaginally and therefore bypasses the liver "first-pass" metabolism.

If you are allergic to peanuts, you cannot use Prometrium, since the progesterone is dissolved in peanut oil. Compounding pharmacists can make tablets or capsules dissolved in other oils when needed. If Crinone vaginal progesterone is not available, or not covered by your health plan, a similar option can be compounded if you need a non-oral form to reduce side effects.

We do not have a major pharmaceutical company in the United States that has yet developed natural micronized testosterone preparation approved by the FDA for widespread consumer use. A *testosterone patch* for women is in development by several companies, and it is currently in clinical trials, but it is not yet available on the market in the United States. **Do not try to use the men's testosterone patch—the dose is far too high for women to use.**

It is my hope that as we understand more about the important differences between the native human forms for hormones and the synthetic or animal-derived ones, the women of this country will have better options widely available. Until that time, you may ask your physician to work with reputable pharmacists to compound the natural testosterone to suit your needs. It can be made up in creams, pills, capsules and suppositories.

Index

TO CONTACT DR. VLIET

For individual medical consultations:

1. We have a centralized appointment scheduling process for our consultations. This is managed from the Texas office, whether your consult occurs in Tucson or Texas. Please contact the patient services coordinator in Texas at *HER Place: Health, Enhancement and Renewal for Women, Inc.* To receive an information package, you may mail request to

HER Place
2700 Tibbets Drive, Suite #100
Bedford, TX 76022

or call

(817) 355-8008

or fax

(817) 355-8010

2. Visit our Web site at **www.herplace.com**. You may download and print the information forms and personal history forms that are used to schedule an appointment in either location. Then contact the Texas office as shown above.

To arrange speaking engagements, seminars, workshops, or a preceptorship for health professionals, please contact:

Kathryn A. Kresnik
Vice President, Director of Operations
HER Place
Phone: (972) 564-5089
E-mail: kkrez@aol.com, Web site: www.herplace.com
Mail: P.O. Box 64507, Tucson, AZ 85728

Arizona office (mailing address):

HER Place: Health, Enhancement and Renewal for Women, Inc.
P.O. Box 64507, Tucson, AZ 85728
Phone: (520) 797-9131, Fax: (520) 797-2948